W9-BOL-930

The Elements
of Bioethics

The Elements
of Bioethics

GREGORY E. PENCE

Professor of Philosophy
School of Medicine & Department of Philosophy
University of Alabama at Birmingham

Boston Burr Ridge, IL Dubuque, IA Madison, WI New York
San Francisco St. Louis Bangkok Bogotá Caracas Kuala Lumpur
Lisbon London Madrid Mexico City Milan Montreal New Delhi
Santiago Seoul Singapore Sydney Taipei Toronto

The McGraw·Hill Companies

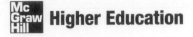

Higher Education

THE ELEMENTS OF BIOETHICS
Published by McGraw-Hill, a business unit of The McGraw-Hill Companies, Inc., 1221
Avenue of the Americas, New York, NY, 10020. Copyright © 2007 by The McGraw-Hill
Companies, Inc. All rights reserved. No part of this publication may be reproduced or
distributed in any form or by any means, or stored in a database or retrieval system,
without the prior written consent of The McGraw-Hill Companies, Inc., including,
but not limited to, in any network or other electronic storage or transmission, or
broadcast for distance learning.

Some ancillaries, including electronic and print components, may not be available
to customers outside the United States.

This book is printed on acid-free paper.

1 2 3 4 5 6 7 8 9 0 DOC/DOC 0 9 8 7 6

ISBN-13: 978-0-07-313277-8
ISBN-10: 0-07-313277-2
Vice President and Editor-in-Chief: *Emily Barrosse*
Publisher: *Lyn Uhl*
Senior Sponsoring Editor: *Jon-David Hague*
Editorial Assistant: *Liliana Almendarez*
Marketing Manager: *Suzanna Ellison*
Managing Editor: *Jean Dal Porto*
Project Manager: *Jean R. Starr*
Art Director: *Jeanne Schreiber*
Associate Designer: *Marianna Kinigakis*
Photo Research Coordinator: *Brian Pecko*
Cover Credit: *Francesco di Stefano Pesellino, (c. 1422–1457). St. Cosmas and St. Damian
treating a sick man. Panel from a Predella from Santa Croce in Florence, now in the Uffizi
Gallery in Florence. Oil on wood, 32 × 94 cm. © Erich Lessing / Art Resource, NY*
Production Supervisor: *Jason I. Huls*
Composition: *10/12 New Baskerville, by Interactive Composition Corporation, India*
Printing: *R.R. Donnelley & Sons*
Credits: The credits section for this book begins on page C-1 and is considered an
extension of the copyright page.

Library of Congress Cataloging-in-Publication Data

Pence, Gregory E.
    The elements of bioethics / Gregory E. Pence.
        p. cm.
    Includes bibliographical references and index.
    ISBN-13: 978-0-07-313277-8 (softcover : alk. paper)
    ISBN-10: 0-07-313277-2 (softcover : alk. paper)
        1. Medical ethics. 2. Bioethics. 3. Ethics.   I. Title.
    R724.P37 2007
    174'.957—dc22   2005043525

The Internet addresses listed in the text were accurate at the time of publication.
The inclusion of a Web site does not indicate an endorsement by the authors or
McGraw-Hill, and McGraw-Hill does not guarantee the accuracy of the information
presented at these sites.

www.mhhe.com

Contents

About the Author ix
Preface xi
Acknowledgments xiii

1. LYING TO PATIENTS AND ETHICAL RELATIVISM 1

1.1 Ethical Relativism and Ethical Subjectivism 3
1.2 Impartiality and Moral Reasoning 5
1.3 Kant on Lying 6
1.4 Utilitarian Ethics 9
1.5 Omitting the Truth vs. Lying 10
1.6 Apologizing for Mistakes and Taking Responsibility
for Mistakes 11
1.7 Virtue Ethics: Truthfulness, Complicity,
and Responsibility 14
1.8 Conceptual Issues: What Is a Mistake? 17
Further Readings and Resources 20

2. KANT ON WHETHER ALCOHOLISM
IS A DISEASE 21

2.1 The God Committee: Who Shall Live
When Not All Can? 22
2.2 Free Will 26
2.3 Kant on Human Dignity 31
2.4 Is Alcoholism a Disease? 34
2.5 Sociologists and Geneticists on Alcoholism 37
2.6 Kant's Critique of the Disease Model 40
2.7 Fingarette's Research 42
2.8 Harm Reduction vs. Moralism in Medicine 46
2.9 Liver Transplants for Alcoholics? 48
Further Reading and Resources 51

3.   KANT'S CRITIQUE OF ADULT ORGAN DONATION   52

3.1   Kant: Some Things Must Not Be Done   53
3.2   Background: Crossing the Ethical Bright Line
      in Organ Procurement   57
3.3   The Utilitarian Defense of Live Organ Donation   61
3.4   Act vs. Rule Utilitarianism   65
3.5   The Utilitarian Rebuttal   68
3.6   Autonomous Live Organ Donation for Kantians?   72
3.7   Utilitarians and Payment for Organs   73
3.8   Virtue Ethics and Live Organ Donors   76
3.9   Organ Transplantation and Race   78
      Further Reading and Resources   80

4.   UTILITARIANS VS. KANTIANS ON STOPPING AIDS   81

4.1   History of Utilitarian Ethics   83
4.2   Virtue Ethics, Medical Saints, and Paul Farmer   85
4.3   Utilitarianism and the Numbers: Applying Triage   87
4.4   Halting AIDS: The Challenge to Ethical Theories   90
4.5   Kantian and Utilitarian Ideals About Patient Care   91
4.6   Mill's Critique of Kantian Ethics   94
4.7   Farmer and Rawls on Just Medical Care   96
4.8   Placebos with AIDS Drugs on Vulnerable Africans   99
4.9   Cost of AIDS Drugs   104
      Further Reading and Resources   107

5.   EMOTIVISM AND BANNING SOME
     CONCEPTIONS   109

5.1   Background: Assisted Reproduction   110
5.2   Emotivism   112
5.3   Paradoxes About Conception   114
5.4   Multiple Embryo Implantation   119
5.5   Sex Selection   121
5.6   Age of Parents and the Good of the Child   124
5.7   Hume, Kant, and Aristotle on the Emotions   126
5.8   Surrogate Mothers and Compensating Gametic Donors   128
5.9   Reproductive Cloning   132
      Further Reading and Resources   136

6. TERRI SCHIAVO: WHEN DOES
   PERSONHOOD END?   137

   6.1   Cessation of Personhood   139
   6.2   Background: Brain Death and the Quinlan
         and Cruzan Cases   142
   6.3   Families, Criteria of Personhood, and Character Issues   150
   6.4   A New Category of Consciousness?   158
   6.5   Religious Issues   160
   6.6   Disability Issues   162
   6.7   Virtue Ethics: The Many Faces of Compassion   164
   6.8   The Politicization of the Schiavo Case   164
   6.9   What the Autopsy Showed   167
         Further Reading and Resources   171

7. ARE GENETIC ABORTIONS EUGENIC?   172

   7.1   Down Syndrome   173
   7.2   Roe vs. Wade and the Legalization of Abortion   175
   7.3   Choosing Against Pregnancy vs. Choosing Against
         Abnormality   177
   7.4   Abortion and Personhood   177
   7.5   New Genetic Tests, Disability Advocates, and Eugenics   181
   7.6   Eugenics   185
   7.7   Genetic Testing, Malpractice, and Insurance
         Companies   190
   7.8   Newborn Genetic Screening   197
   7.9   Sending the Wrong Message?   199
         Further Reading and Resources   202

8. CAN RESEARCH BE JUST ON PEOPLE
   WITH SCHIZOPHRENIA?   203

   8.1   Research to Cure Schizophrenia, Money, and Care
         for People with Mental Illness   204
   8.2   Nazi and American Research, and the Tuskegee Study   206
   8.3   Schizophrenia   211
   8.4   Informed Consent and Schizophrenia Studies   212
   8.5   Virtue Ethics, Integrity, and Conflicts of Interest   219
   8.6   Harm to Subjects and the Kantian Ideal of Patient Care   224

8.7   *Vulnerable Subjects and Social Justice*   225
8.8   *Structural Critiques of Modern Psychiatric Research*   226
8.9   *NBAC's Report on Psychiatric Research*   228
       Further Reading and Resources   231

9.   IS THERE A DUTY TO DIE?   233

9.1   *Gov. Lamm's Famous Remarks and His Historical*
       Predecessors   234
9.2   *John Hardwig: Defending a Duty to Die*   240
9.3   *Alzheimer's and Dementia*   245
9.4   *Rawls and Callahan on Justice and Natural Limits*   246
9.5   *Global Reallocation? Dying Simply So Others Can*
       Simply Live   251
9.6   *Mary Warnock vs. Felicia Ackerman on a Duty to Die*   255
9.7   *Within the Family: Our Parents' Keepers*   256
9.8   *Dworkin's Defense of Advance Directives and Autonomy*   257
9.9   *Medical Professionals and Medical Futility*   260
       Further Reading   262

10   TREATING JEHOVAH'S WITNESSES
     PROFESSIONALLY   263

10.1   *Jehovah's Witnesses and Medicine*   264
10.2   *Professionalism, Religious Minorities, and Tolerance*   267
10.3   *Parental Owners vs. Parental Stewards of Children*   270
10.4   *Virtue Ethics, Treatment Refusal, and Religious*
       Minorities   271
10.5   *Legal Issues*   272
10.6   *Medicine and Good of the Child/Adolescent*   273
10.7   *Bloodless Surgery and Jehovah's Witnesses*   275
10.8   *Consistency in Handling Cases of Minority Views*
       in Medicine   277
       Further Reading   278

Endnotes   N-1
Credits   C-1
Index   I-1

About the Author

Gregory Pence is professor of philosophy in the School of Medicine and Department of Philosophy at the University of Alabama at Birmingham (UAB), where he has taught for over thirty years. With McGraw-Hill, he has published *Classic Cases in Medical Ethics: Accounts of the Cases that Shaped Medical Ethics*, now in its fourth edition (2004), and *Classic Works in Medical Ethics* (1995).

At UAB, he served for twenty-two years on its Institutional Review Board for human experimentation and, for lesser terms, on its Hospital Ethics Committee and Animal Use and Care Committee. In 1994, he won UAB's highest award for best teaching in the classroom. He also directs UAB's BS/MD program.

In trade publishing, he has written (with G. Lynn Stephens), *Seven Dilemmas in World Religions* (Paragon, 1995). Rowman & Littlefield published his *Who's Afraid of Human Cloning?* (1998), *Re-creating Medicine: Ethical Issues at the Frontiers of Medicine* (2000), *Designer Food: Mutant Harvest or Breadbasket of the World?* (2002), *Cloning After Dolly: Who's Still Afraid?* (2005), and his anthologies: *Flesh of My Flesh: Ethical Issues in Human Cloning: A Reader* (1998) and *The Ethics of Food: A Reader for the 21st Century* (2000). A frequent writer of op-eds in national newspapers, *Brave New Bioethics* (2004) collects these.

He has given the Soundings Lecture at Castleton State College, the Thornton Lecture at Alma College, the Seidman Trust Lecture at Rhodes College, the Rutland Lecture at Clemson University, as well as invited talks in China, Israel, Switzerland, London, Portugal, and at over a hundred hospitals and universities in North America. He has discussed issues in bioethics on CNN, National Public Radio, and national morning television news shows, and has testified before committees of the U.S. Congress and California Senate.

Preface

For 30 years, I've been teaching, writing, and thinking about bioethics. Given how long I've been doing this, I should know more than I do. I do indeed know that I'm never satisfied with the available texts, so I keep trying to find new ways to reach students in bioethics.

This volume introduces bioethics by unfolding a paradigmatic case in each chapter amidst discussion of its key ethical issues. Curiosity about how the case develops pulls narrative learners through the philosophical analysis.

No great weight should be placed on "Elements." The word does correctly imply, however, that this book assumes no knowledge of either medicine or philosophy and is written for beginners. But bioethics is a big house, and this book does not cover each and every nook and cranny. This book is just one place and one way to begin.

The book weaves discussion of ethical theories into the cases and chapters in a new way. Rather than discussing Kant or utilitarianism in separate chapters or sections, several chapters force readers to think about how Kant, utilitarians, and virtue theorists approach lying, organ donation, stopping AIDS, and alcoholism. In Chapter 5, Leon Kass's emphasis on our emotional revulsion to new reproductive technology illustrates the ethical theory of emotivism. Other chapters center around personhood (Schiavo, genetic abortion) and justice (research on people with schizophrenia, a duty to die?).

Everyone will not agree about how I interpret and apply ethical theories to particular cases. However, at least we will have here a theory and a case developed for further discussion.

Although written at a beginner's level, almost all of the cases discussed in this book have never been discussed before in a text in bioethics: the Schiavo case, alcoholism and free will (the Crowfeather case), research on people with schizophrenia (Greg Friend's case), harm to live organ donors (Laura Giese's case), Paul Farmer's heroic efforts fighting for the world's poor, frequent abortions for a genetic condition in the first trimester, and a sympathetic discussion of Jehovah's Witnesses in medicine.

This short volume complements my other texts, *Classic Cases in Medical Ethics: Accounts of the Cases That Have Shaped Medical Ethics* (McGraw-Hill, 4th edition, 2004) and *Classic Works in Medical Ethics* (McGraw-Hill, 1995). Ninety percent of the material in this book is new and not in these texts. *The Elements of Bioethics* has both a simpler style than *Classic Cases* while paradoxically, it applies more theoretical analysis to its cases. The Contents reveals how this is done.

This book also complements an outstanding textbook for any course in introductory ethics, *The Elements of Moral Philosophy*, by the late James Rachels. *The Elements of Bioethics* both builds on, and is compatible with, this great book of my teacher, mentor, and friend. My book is not as good as Jim's, but his book inspired many ideas in mine.

Greg Pence, August 4, 2005
Email: pence@uab.edu

Acknowledgments

Physician faculty at the University of Alabama in Birmingham (UAB) improved virtually every chapter in the book. They included Ben Hippen (kidney surgery), Nathan Smith (psychiatry), Nat Robin (genetics), Charlotte William (geriatric medicine), and Keith Georgeson (pediatric surgery). Physician Kenneth Goodman of the University of Miami helped me understand issues about the Schiavo case.

I am indebted to Harold Kincaid and G. Lynn Stephens in the UAB philosophy department respectively for reading key chapters and making key suggestions and also Nathan Nobis.

Lawyer and bioethicist Connie Stockham helped improve the chapter on eugenic abortions. Reporter Deborah Shelton, whose groundbreaking series served as its main source, checked my chapter on live organ donation. Adil Shamoo, PhD, at the University of Maryland School of Medicine, made insightful contributions to the chapter on schizophrenia research, as did James Maddux, PhD, of the Psychology Department at George Mason University in Virginia.

Charles Cardwell of Pellissippi Community College in Tennessee did an extraordinary job as a reviewer of the final manuscript. I incorporated several of his points in Chapters 4 and 9.

I would also like to thank the following reviewers:

Kelly Armstrong, *University of Iowa*
Charles E. Cardwell, *Pellissippi State Technical Community College*
Phil Cox, *University of Massachusetts, Dartmouth*
David B. Fletcher, *Wheaton College*
Geoffrey Frasz, *Community College of Southern Nevada*
Ronnie Hawkins, *University of Central Florida*

Barbara Gail Joralemon, *Albuquerque Technical Vocational Institute*

Jason K. Swedene, *Lake Superior State University*

At McGraw-Hill, Jon-David Hague and Allison Rona have nurtured this project from the very beginning. I also especially want to thank Kathy Shackelford, the best senior sales representative any author could have, and a person who played an important role in getting this book done.

During the summer of 2004, Emily Taylor, Anand Iyer, Reema Hamid, Qin Zhang, and Roshan Patel served as my research assistants on this book. The following semester, Qin Zhang continued as my research assistant and did wonderful work. The next summer, Emily Taylor repeated her exceptional talents as proofreader and grammatical critic. She was aided by Nandini Raghuraman, Josna Haritha, and Felix Kishinevsky. First-year student Paula Province at the University of Alabama Medical School also carefully proofed the text, as did Benjamin Rogers.

Finally, 40 undergraduate students in my Intensive Bioethics Seminar for the spring of 2005, and 160 first-year medical students in the fall of 2005, all at UAB, beta-tested this book and made many useful suggestions.

CHAPTER 1

Lying to Patients and Ethical Relativism

All the chapters in this book use paradigmatic cases to focus attention on basic ethical issues in medicine. As the chapter unfolds, details of the cases progressively emerge and interweave with discussion of ethical issues. The book begins with a case that seems deceptively elemental and that serves to introduce discussion of relativism, subjectivism, Kantian ethics, utilitarianism, and virtue ethics.

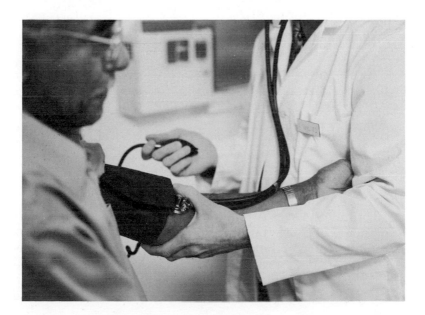

Mr. John Jones, a 48-year-old black male, has been in and out of the hospital since March for several minor problems.[1] He

1

now shows up at Christmas with complaints of chest pain. His chest X-ray reveals a large mass in the upper lobe of his left lung. Bronchoscopy and CAT scan confirm a stage III-A non-small cell cancer. At this stage, this cancer is inoperable and the patient's prognosis is for less than six months to live, probably much less.

Peter Thagard, a 27-year-old white male, is the consulting fellow in pulmonary (chest/lung) medicine. This is the first time he has ever seen Mr. Jones.

When Dr. Thagard tells Mr. Jones his diagnosis and prognosis, Mr. Jones comments, "This tumor must grow fast if they didn't see it last March." As a pulmonary consultant, Peter reviews Mr. Jones's chart and notes that the cancerous lung mass was indeed present (but much smaller) on a film from March.

Peter Thagard did not enter medicine to lie to his patients. Peter has completed four years of medical school and three years of residency in internal medicine.

Peter's classmate from medical school, Sam Peppard, was the resident who was responsible for Mr. Jones last March. Peter pages Sam, who calls him right back. Peter explains the situation and Sam responds, "Please don't tell him! You'll ruin my career. He'll sue my pants off!"

Peter replies that he thinks Mr. Jones should be told the truth.

Sam says, "I don't know how it happened, but it's too late now to do him any good. Medically speaking, he's a dead man. Please don't tell him. What good would it do?"

Should Dr. Thagard tell Mr. Smith that his cancer was evident on the old film and that another physician missed it?

The moral issues contained in this case occur frequently in medicine and illustrate the importance of medical ethics. Despite the case's technical aspects, this is a very human situation: one person in a room talking to another, thinking about whether to tell the truth, and in the same room, another person learning he is going to die and guessing that someone made a mistake.

Whatever your views about morality, you cannot deny that something profound is occurring between this young physician and this dying patient. Whatever that is, it seems to reveal something essential among humans.

Because a physician occupies a special place of trust at the beginning and end of our lives, as well as in between—in learning our secrets, in telling us of the unexpected problems, and in mediating all these with other physicians and our relatives—the physician–patient relationship constitutes one of the quintessentially moral relationships of our society, similar to the one between teacher and student. As such, violations of those relationships strike at the heart of our most basic moral practices.

1.1 Ethical Relativism and Ethical Subjectivism

Is it really true that lying is always wrong? How do you prove that? Isn't it just the way we feel about it? And don't people feel differently about lying?

What about the claim that the rightness or wrongness of lying is just how we feel about it? What is being claimed here? We could be saying that definitions of good and bad are relative to one's time in history and culture. This theory is called *ethical relativism*. For example, in 1927, physician Joseph Collins, in "Should Doctors Tell the Truth?" in *Harper's Monthly Magazine*, wrote that patients were better off not knowing the truth, especially about terminal cancer.[2] Several surveys of physicians during the early 1950s revealed that most physicians did not, in fact, tell patients the truth about their terminal condition.

During the 1970s in North America, some patients rebelled against such *medical paternalism*. Patients asserted the value of *autonomy* in making their own decisions. "Autonomy" comes from the Greek *auto* (self) and *nomos* (law) and refers to being self-governing. As Kant would put it, people are autonomous because they can be "law-givers unto themselves."

Autonomy became important in ethics as two strong currents merged into one. In ethics, the Enlightenment ethics of Kant celebrated the individual's reason, free will, and self as the seat of values, responsibility, and action. In politics, thinkers such as John Stuart Mill in *On Liberty* championed autonomy, especially in celebrating the individual's ability to know what is best over the paternalism of government, religion, or public opinion.

Since the mid-1970s, autonomy has become a crucial value in modern medical ethics. Since then, the culture of medicine has changed and has officially rejected medical paternalism. Routinely deceiving patients about a diagnosis of cancer has been abandoned.

Moreover, just because most physicians did not tell patients about cancer back in the 1950s does not mean that they were right to do so. It is possible for a whole culture to engage in a morally reprehensible practice, such as human slavery. Until recently, Japanese patients with terminal cancer were never told the truth so that anytime a grandfather visited physicians, he feared that they were withholding terrible news from him, making each visit to physicians an event filled with crippling anxiety.

It may also be thought that lying is not wrong because nothing is really right or wrong—it's all just a matter of how a particular person *feels* about such issues. This ethical theory is called *ethical subjectivism*. It holds that there is no objective truth in ethics. That is, there are no moral facts, no objective standards, and no way to settle disagreements in ethics. So where Peter wants to tell the truth, Sam feels differently, and that's the end of the matter.

To explore this theory, let us think about the difference between feelings and reasoning. This is a complicated issue because we have both good and bad feelings, and sometimes it is difficult to know which is which. Some people may have feelings making it difficult for them to accept male homosexuality, human cloning, or certain kinds of surgery, but these feelings themselves do not justify moral actions. Only when the feelings pass the test of rational reflection do they count as justified.

Consider Peter and Sam. Neither Peter nor Sam really wants to go back in the room and tell Mr. Jones the truth. It is likely that Mr. Jones will get angry. It is likely that a whole series of events will occur that may make both Peter and Sam agitated, worried, and tense. In particular, it is likely that Sam really does not *feel* like telling Mr. Jones the truth.

But what can we infer from Sam's feeling about truth telling? Very little. In this case, Sam's feeling is likely self-protective. He may believe it's right to tell the truth but may also have strong feelings against doing so. It is also possible, even normal, to have feelings that lead us to immoral actions.

Ethical subjectivism is a hard theory to defend in medical ethics, especially from the perspective of patients. A patient does not want physicians to serve her interests only when and if they feel like doing so. Instead, she wants physicians to do the right thing for her, whether that is telling the truth, ordering the extra test, or championing her case, regardless of what physicians feel about her on a particular day. (We will discuss the role of feelings more later in this chapter and also in Chapter 5 about reproductive issues.)

1.2 Impartiality and Moral Reasoning

Ethical subjectivism is also interpreted to claim not only that feelings ground ethics but also that no objective truth exists in ethics. Whether such truth exists in ethics must be separated from questions about appealing to feelings as justification. For now it can be observed that *good reasons* for a position can defeat bad ones in ordinary life, and therefore subjectivism can be defeated.

What would such good reasons look like? A central aspect of moral thinking is the requirement of *impartial reasoning*. For action based on feelings to be morally justified, we must give reasons that other people can accept. Moreover, those reasons must be of a special sort, impartial reasons. "Impartial" contrasts here with "partial" or biased. One familiar way that reasons may be biased is if they are self-interested.

To support a moral position, reasons cannot be partial but must have a wider scope than mere self-interest. The concept of morality normally stands in contrast with self-interest. When people talk about doing the right thing, or claim they acted because "it was the right thing to do," part of what they mean is that they did not simply act from self-interest.

The requirement of impartiality rules out a private morality internal to medicine, separate from public morality. A private morality would likely privilege the interests of physicians over those of patients. Inside medicine, one sometimes gets the feeling that medicine is for the sake of physicians, with internal skills that have their own excellences, and to this whole enterprise, patients are incidental. In reality, we know that medicine exists for the amelioration of human suffering and to help humanity, and as such, must be grounded in a morality common to both physicians and patients.

1.3 Kant on Lying

In our modern world, it is odd to hear people defending absolute rules in ethical theory. One person who did so was Immanuel Kant (1724–1804), the famous German philosopher of the Enlightenment, who argued that it was never right to lie to another person.

Kant was deeply impressed with Isaac Newton's discovery of universal laws of gravity. Thus, he searched for a similar discovery in ethics. In doing so, Kant asked a crucial question, one that has fascinated moral philosophers ever since: "What, if anything, makes an act morally right?"

In formulating possible answers, Kant laid down certain conditions. First, he thought that morality expressed the best and highest parts of humanity, and so must be a part of *reason*. It is in the act of thinking and reflecting, or of weighing the evidence for different ways of acting, that we are most distinctively human and different from the lower animals.

Second, he believed that morality was *universal*, the same across cultures. Even though he lived in an era when anthropologists were informing Europeans in great detail of the mores of different societies on the globe, Kant insisted that a core of rational morality existed that was the same for all humans.

Third, and more controversially, he thought that the commands of morality were *absolute* and unchanging. In this belief, Kant was a great enemy of moral relativism, which he thought attacked the foundations of civilization.

To the master question of, "What makes an act right?" Kant answered:

> Act only according to that maxim by which you can at the same time will that it should become a universal law.

By "maxim" Kant means a general rule covering an act. The quotation above expresses the requirement of *universalizability* in Kantian ethics. As Kant scholar Onora O'Neill writes, "the appeal of this principle to Kant was its combination of formality and fertility," meaning that this statement specified a certain form of a maxim that was ethical and that it ruled out many unethical maxims while allowing ethical ones.[3]

Universalizability at first glance seems like an abstract version of the Golden Rule. It is what your mother said when you made an unjustified exception for yourself in acting wrongly, "What if everyone did that?"

Kant's version is deeper than that, for it directs us to look at the "maxim" or rule under which we are acting and then asks if we can accept that all humans act on it. Kant expressed his views in language that sounds antiquated today; he wrote about morality as "imperatives" or commands that must be followed. In so writing, he distinguished between *hypothetical* and *categorical* imperatives.

A hypothetical imperative is one that is contingent upon some other good. For example, if you want to be successful in medicine, don't lie to your patients. The justification for not lying is achievement of success in medicine.

Kant thought people followed lots of hypothetical imperatives in pursuing their self-interest: I want a certain thing, so I act like X to get it. Hypothetical imperatives have the goal of fulfilling my desires.

In contrast, categorical imperatives are not about fulfilling my desires but about following the impartial dictates of duty. Even if I do not *want* to get up at 3 AM to care for an emergency, duty requires me to do so. Categorical imperatives are not contingent on any desire. They are right because our reason recognizes their universalizability, their "bindingness" on the conscience of all rational beings, and their intent of treating all humans as having infinite worth.

Consider now whether lying is universalizable. Although this is a complex subject for Kant, nonuniversalizable maxims were contradictory. What does this mean?

No human culture can exist, much less thrive, Kant argued, when most people routinely lie. If everyone routinely lied, communication and shared endeavors would be impossible. Moreover, Kant argued, it is irrational to think that practices such as promising and talking can continue when most people lie most of the time; it is *contradictory* to think that these practices are compatible with routine lying. So for Kant, rationality and morality go together.

This is also the problem with allowing physicians to lie to patients about a diagnosis of cancer. If the maxim is, "Lie to patients when the truth is unlikely to do them any good" or "Lie to patients when I may get sued for making a mistake," then such lying undermines all communication in medicine between doctor and patient. It also erodes all trust between physicians and patients.

To say such lying is contradictory for Kant is much more than saying that this practice makes a dent at the margins of the doctor–patient communication. As a harm, one lie to one patient probably does not do much damage. But for Kant, the deception goes much deeper because it strikes at the very heart of all communication.

Even if a murderer pursued a close friend and asked Kant where the friend was, Kant denied that it was right to lie to prevent the friend from being found by the murderer. In "On a Supposed Right to Lie from Altruistic Motives," Kant asserted that to be truthful is "a sacred and absolutely commanding decree of reason, limited by no expediency."[4] As philosopher Sissela Bok comments, "To breach that decree is to injure the system of communication among human beings and thus to endanger the very foundations of duty."[5]

In medicine, to deceive patients on the most crucial matters is to dissemble when it counts most: when patients most want to know the facts, and when the stakes are highest. In other words, it is like saying, "I enter this relationship committed to telling the facts" and "I do not enter this relationship committed to telling the facts."

Peter listens to Sam's pleadings, but he disagrees. Peter believes that as a physician, he owes Mr. Jones the truth. He also believes that as a person, he owes Mr. Jones the truth. That is, Peter believes he is morally obligated to tell the truth in this situation.

Peter asks himself how he knows it's right to tell Mr. Jones the truth and comes up with a time-honored answer. He asks himself, "What would I want to know if I were Mr. Jones?" Peter decides he would want to know the truth. Peter calls his own wife about the case and she agrees, "It's the right thing to do. I would want to know." Peter also calls his mother, who responds emphatically, "I can't even believe you're asking me this question! Of course you must tell him the truth!"

Basically, the Golden Rule is operating here, telling us to treat other people as we would like to be treated. Most people would want to know the truth about their condition and diagnosis so that they could make the best plans for the remainder of their lives. That is part of the reason why most people come to physicians about their health.

Unfortunately, the Golden Rule is not as clear-cut as it might seem; some people in this situation do *not* want to know because nothing can be done to help them. For such people, ignorance is bliss.

1.4 Utilitarian Ethics

In late 18th- and early 19th-century England, a reform movement started as a replacement for both Christian ethics and the class-focused, aristocratic ethics dominant at the time. Indirectly, it challenged Kantian ethics, which some utilitarians saw as an abstract form of Christian ethics. Jeremy Bentham (1748–1832) and James Mill (1773–1836), the father of John Stuart Mill (1806–1873), founded this movement, called *utilitarianism.* Its essence was that right acts should produce the greatest amount of good for the greatest number of beings, an idea that Bentham and Mill called "utility."

Utilitarianism analyzes what actions are right by focusing on the consequences to the people involved in a particular act, as well as on the consequences to general society in following a particular rule governing the act.

So how would utilitarians approach this case? For one thing, they would focus on consequences of telling versus not telling. The worst consequence in this case is that Mr. Jones is going to die, but nothing can change that. Indeed, the agony of his death may only be worse if he learns that he had a small chance last March of gaining a remission.

In this case, Mr. Jones would have needed radiation, chemotherapy, and perhaps surgery. Moreover, Mr. Jones had no medical insurance, and he is too young to qualify for coverage by Medicare (which does not cover people under age 65). Finally, even the best care for this kind of lung cancer gives patients only a 10 percent chance of another year of life, and the long-term prognosis five years out is almost 100 percent death. So Mr. Jones probably has not been robbed of any great stretch of life that he might otherwise have had. This is not like a drive-by shooting of a teenager that takes a whole life away.

Sam might also appeal to the good of himself, his family, the hospital staff, the reputation of the hospital, and even the reputation of medicine. "Everyone will be worse off if you tell," Sam implores Peter.

But that is not quite true, is it? If Mr. Jones learns the truth, he may tell his family, who may sue. They may gain a large amount of money from this malpractice suit and use this money to send Mr. Jones's grandchildren to college.

Sam could retort that any physician who has been through a malpractice case knows how psychologically traumatic it can be, with aggressive lawyers making ordinary physicians seem like Nazi doctors. "Surely," Sam says, "the *intensity* of our pain must also count for something?"

This shows that calculating the consequences for those affected is no easy matter. Even so, one could argue on utilitarian grounds for not saying anything to Mr. Jones.

1.5   Omitting the Truth vs. Lying

Pontius Pilate infamously asked, "What is truth?" In this arena, we also need to ask, "What is *un*truth?" In particular, is omitting the truth a lie? One could argue that a compromise could be found if Peter follows this line of inaction. Peter could never actively say anything that was false and just leave the room. Is that a lie?

It depends on how a lie is defined. Two important kinds of ethical theories evaluate actions by either results or intentions. Combining both theories, if lying has the *result* of leaving the patient with a false view, and if Peter *intends* to leave the patient with a false view, then Peter can certainly lie by saying nothing. It is also true that a convincing lie by omission would need to include the appropriate noncommittal, nonchalant body language, but assume that can be done.

What has arisen here is *the acts versus omissions doctrine,* a major theme in bioethics that includes the issue of whether omitting treatment for terminal patients is the same as actively assisting in their deaths. It is controversial to equate the two, but in the case of this chapter, the key moral issue concerns accurate communication of crucial information. In that regard, it seems clear that one can deliberately lie either by omitting crucial facts or by actively distorting the facts.

So Peter cannot easily get out of this situation by arguing that he is not really lying by ignoring Mr. Jones's questioning remark.

Peter tells Sam that there's no question that Mr. Jones will be told the truth. "The only question is whether you do it or I do it. I'm willing to let you have the chance to tell him. After all, he was your patient and it was your 'miss.' You'll come out better in the long run if you admit what you did and ask him to forgive you."

1.6 Apologizing for Mistakes and Taking Responsibility for Mistakes

Some professionals in Risk Management, the branch of a hospital that seeks to protect the hospital from lawsuits and legal damages, say that a physician's chances of being sued drop if he admits to a mistake and he honestly confesses the mistake to the patient and the patient's family. "Sorry Works," a policy in place at the University of Michigan hospitals since 2002, has dramatically lowered malpractice suits there.[6] Ordinary people do not expect perfection, but they do get angry when they cannot get a straight answer and when no one takes responsibility for an unexpected death.

A kind of theory called *virtue ethics* emphasizes that it takes strength of character to admit mistakes (more on this theory soon). For a teacher, it may involve loss of respect in front of a class. For a physician, it may involve that, too, but also acceptance of injury or death to another human being. Unlike plumbing or accounting, medicine is a special vocation in which mistakes can cause people to die.

In *Wrongful Death*, Sandra Gilbert writes about the unexpected death of her husband Eliot, the former chair of English at the University of California at Davis.[7] The 58-year-old man went in for a routine prostatectomy and bled to death in the recovery room. Because no one would explain to her how Eliot died, Sandra sued, and even though she won in court, she still didn't get a satisfying result. Ultimately, she had to write an exposé to get closure.

Sam refuses to talk face-to-face to Mr. Jones or to tell him the truth in writing or on the phone, so Peter is left to do it. Before Peter can go to Mr. Jones's room, the attending physician who supervises both of these young physicians asks to speak to Peter. He remarks that it is lamentable that this happened but that Peter should remember that it happened on June 30, the last day of Sam's residency. "Moreover, he had eight admissions that day, which is no excuse—he should have closed out his cases—but still, use the Golden Rule and put yourself in his shoes—it would be so easy to make the same mistake."

It turns out that radiology did in fact spot the cancer on Mr. Jones's X-ray and placed a note in Sam's box. But in this particular medical system, the responsibility of radiology ended with reading the X-ray and sending the note. It was then up to the physician who ordered the examination to read the result and to inform the patient.

The attending physician uses hospital parlance to say that what occurred was a "system error," not an error of a particular individual. As such, the system is to blame, not Sam. "In a sense, we're all responsible for that error," he tells Peter as he walks away.

Although the attending physician refrains from telling Peter not to tell the patient, Peter senses that he would rather Peter didn't. Peter realizes that his decision to tell Mr. Jones affects not only Mr. Jones and Sam, but also the attending physician and others on the hospital staff. It is beginning to seem complicated.

As noted, the attending physician implied that the mistake is a *system error,* and, as such, a problem of every physician and no physician. John Lantos, a pediatrician and medical ethicist at the University of Chicago, says he has made "quite a few mistakes in [his] time."[8] Both he and his colleagues have made similar mistakes, yet virtually none of them admit to them or discuss them with other pediatricians. While Lantos abstractly advocates truth telling, he also believes that truth telling about mistakes can destroy medical careers and even harm patients.

Traditionally, every patient in a hospital or clinic has a *physician of record* who is responsible for that patient's care and who, as a result, is blamed for any mistakes. Of course, things are more complicated in a teaching hospital when physicians rotate off a unit each month and where interns and residents leave at the end of June.

However, even if the system is to blame rather than Sam, does it logically follow that the attending physician is correct that Mr. Jones should not be told? Perhaps not.

The Institute of Medicine (IOM), a prestigious branch of the National Academy of Sciences, surveyed the problem in 1999 of mistakes in medicine and concluded that

> [A]s many as 98,000 people die in any given year from medical errors that occur in hospitals . . . more than [those who] die from motor vehicle accidents, breast cancer, or AIDS. . . . [M]ore people die annually from medication errors than from workplace injuries. Add the financial cost to the human tragedy, and medical error easily rises to the top ranks of urgent, widespread public problems.[9]

The committee of physicians who wrote the IOM report recommended "establishing a nationwide, mandatory public reporting system. Hospitals first, and eventually other places where patients get care, would be responsible for reporting such events to state governments. Currently, about a third of the states have their own mandatory reporting requirements." By 2004, a bill to create such a system was introduced in both houses of Congress, but even this voluntary system of reporting errors never became law.

Instead of the current culture of secrecy, which creates a climate that stifles study of how mistakes occur and how to avoid them, the IOM recommended creation of a "culture of safety" and a systematic attempt in medicine to lower the rate of mistakes.

A similar study in 2005 by the Urban Institute discovered that one-fourth of 1 percent of all physicians account for 13 percent of malpractice payments, suggesting that few physicians want to try to curb incompetent, rogue physicians (it takes tons of time, they can get countersued, they may be friends with the incompetent physician, etc.).[10] Another study by researchers at Harvard Medical School and the University of Ottawa found that many mistakes occur after release from a hospital, where 20 percent of 400 patients discharged had an "adverse event" that could have been prevented by adequate communication and planning.[11]

All of which is to say that the best way to deal with mistakes is not to sweep them under the rug or to deny that they occur but to open them up to peer inspection. So there are forces within medicine itself arguing against the attending physician's position.

1.7 Virtue Ethics: Truthfulness, Complicity, and Responsibility

Virtue ethics, a major theory of ethics, emphasizes that goodness consists of good character and its composite traits. One such trait of a good man is *truthfulness*, the willingness to tell the truth.

A large degree of truthfulness is essential for human communication. If most people lied most of the time, human communication would be difficult. For example, under such conditions, if a teacher told students, "Everyone passed the test," students would not know if they really had.

The ancient Greeks and their philosophers (Socrates, Plato, Aristotle) praised the nobleness of mind and spirit that disdained lying and deception. The person "whose soul squints" is always calculating about what to say and how, whereas the great-souled person is open and honest with everyone. For these Greeks, there is something fearful and small-minded about lying, especially as a trait of character. They would admire the modern saying, "His word is his bond" and the man who lives up to it.

Truthfulness or veracity also is essential to empowering the autonomy of patients. If patients do not possess accurate and complete information from physicians, they cannot make good decisions about their health and lives.

Another way to emphasize personal integrity or virtue is to mention the *can-you-look-him-in-the-eye? test*. Some people are uncomfortable directly lying to people in such an important situation. As such, when they lie, they avoid looking into people's eyes, lest their eyes give them away. Virtue theorists would emphasize that people with ideal integrity, even when giving bad news and dealing with awkward situations, manage to maintain eye contact. In a similar situation, people lacking in integrity do not personally deliver bad news but delegate this unpleasant task to someone else. Bellevue Hospital physician Danielle Ofri describes her anger when an old woman is referred to her because an oncologist did not want to tell the woman she had cancer.[12] In business, virtuous managers fire employees face-to-face, not by anonymous letter late on a Friday afternoon.

Another way to think about lying and ethical character is to act so that whatever you do could be printed on the front page of your local newspaper and you wouldn't be ashamed. This rule seems to apply to this case. How Peter and Sam should act may depend in part on whether each could feel comfortable at a later time—after Mr. Jones is dead—having everyone read about their actions.

Of course, it is likely that such public disclosure will never occur, but that is not the point. If one wants to determine what is right, thinking about transparency is a good way to start. If one is uncomfortable with the idea that one's private action suddenly comes under public scrutiny, it may be because one knows one is acting wrongly.

We have been discussing virtue ethics and thinking about one trait or virtue of a physician's character, truth telling or veracity. We can also discuss virtue ethics by looking at the physician's character in the patient relationship.

The typical way to think about the moral conflict in this chapter's case is one that involves tension, blame, and guilt, but there is also another way. Every case such as this is also an opportunity for moral learning. Existentialist philosophers such as Jean-Paul Sartre emphasize that in times of such moral crises, people shape their characters in profound ways (even in "choosing not to choose," they also shape their destiny, as choice is inevitable).

The physician–patient relationship is a paradigm of a moral relationship in all societies. To be a physician is in part to adopt a helping role toward patients, a moral role. In this role, communication is one of the most essential aspects of the physician–patient relationship. Falsehoods thwart that relationship, in both directions. If the patient does not reveal basic facts, the physician cannot make an accurate diagnosis. Nevertheless, revelation of such facts may be personally embarrassing to the patient (for example, revelation of risky behavior for sexually transmitted diseases) and, as such, can only be done if patients trust their physicians.

Deception by physicians deeply undermines trust by patients. Lying by one physician to one patient hurts all physicians and sabotages the trust at the heart of the physician–patient relationship. But most importantly, lying by a physician to his or her patients is a terrible flaw of character of the *physician as a physician*. If patients cannot go to a physician and get the truth about what is wrong with them, why should they go at all? Or pay physicians? What is the point?

Character is a big topic in ethics, and discussions of it play a big role in medicine. We shall discuss it later when we talk about physician Paul Farmer in Haiti, the integrity of researchers conducting medical experiments, and elderly people (as old as most grandparents) conceiving children.

Another aspect about character concerns complicity in a cover-up. As Peter thinks through his options, things begin to seem more complicated. He wonders about how complicit he can be in deceiving Mr. Jones. He realizes that if he participates in a conspiracy to keep Mr. Jones in the dark, and if the Jones family ever discovers the truth, then Peter, too, could be named in the suit. Peter then appreciates the famous line from Sir Walter Scott:

> Oh, what a tangled web we weave,
> When first we practice to deceive![13]

Peter realizes both on moral grounds and on grounds of self-interest that he can't be part of such deception. Better to tell the truth from the start, he decides, than go down the slippery slope of deception.

In the last decade, the mass media have celebrated whistle-blowers who courageously reveal corruption, incompetence, or fraud in public institutions. Generally speaking, the mass media present a rosy picture of what happens to such whistle-blowers, lauding them as heroes. In reality, being a whistle-blower requires tremendous courage and moral integrity, and frequently results in losing one's job and in being financially penalized. Congress recently created a special fund to compensate whistle-blowers in the federal government for money saved to the government (e.g., from Medicare fraud).

As a new issue, consider how personal responsibility for one's health enters this case. Sam confided in Peter at one point,

"Look, he was a smoker and smoked for decades. He brought it on himself. He took the risks and now he got burned. But why should I pay for his mistakes?"

The flip side of virtue ethics might be called examination of the vices, and when it comes to sickness, vices leading to ill-health are well known: smoking, drinking, abusing drugs, driving unsafely, and being overweight. A major question in bioethics concerns whether public policy should reward healthy behavior and punish unhealthy behavior. And when we drop down from the lofty level of public policy to the individual level of doctor and patient, to what extent should doctors punish patients for health vices?

At the level of public policy, one kind of question arises: Should alcoholics have the same eligibility for liver transplants as those who lost their livers through accidents or rare viruses? Should people who eat poorly and not exercise be forced to pay higher premiums for medical coverage?

At the individual level, another kind of question arises: Should physicians judge the behavior of their patients? Vent their anger at irresponsible behavior? In this case, is it Sam's job to judge Mr. Jones? To deny him information because of his past smoking?

Notice that it is possible to condemn something in public policy while tolerating it personally. One may think that punishments and rewards are appropriate *only* at the higher level of public policy (tax credits for adoption, higher premiums for smokers) and inappropriate for personal relations. One can compromise here and conclude that individual physicians should not judge behavior of patients, whereas national policy can still be crafted to discourage unhealthy behaviors.

Chapter 2 focuses on this question by asking if alcoholism is caused genetically, socially, or is chosen freely from a flawed character.

1.8 Conceptual Issues: What Is a Mistake?

Philosophical reflection often raises unexpected problems when it focuses on ordinary problems in life or in bioethics. In this case, such reflection raises the question of exactly what counts as a mistake.

This may seem nonsensical at first, but the deeper we delve into the question, the less that seems true. For example, suppose that Mr. Jones's cancer was an exotic one, which only a $10,000 test could have picked up. Because Mr. Jones had no medical insurance, he was a charity case for the hospital. As such, physicians would normally not order a $10,000 rule-out test for him. But if he turned out to have an exotic cancer, would it have been a mistake not to have given him the expensive test in the first place?

Defining mistakes can be controversial. Consider rare cancers. Suppose that if a hospital spends $10,000 on each indigent patient, it can rule out most rare cancers. But that $10,000 is not reimbursed and, as such, is a loss for the hospital. If the hospital continues to rule out rare cancers in all poor patients, it will go bankrupt. So which is the mistake: to practice to rule out rare cancers or to practice to go bankrupt?

Lately in developed countries, there is a tendency to view every death, every abnormal baby, as a mistake by some physician. But is every patient's death a mistake of some kind? That position is absurd, isn't it? No matter how perfect our medical treatment, each of us will eventually die.

In medicine, mistakes are legally defined as departures from the normal and customary *standard of care*. This practical standard is defined by how competent physicians act in the same specialty with the same kind of problem in a patient. Although at one time this standard applied only to a particular region or state, today it is a *de facto* national (and even international) standard.

Peter goes down the hallway to seek Mr. Jones to tell him the truth. Although he will not win praise from his attending physician for doing so, and although Sam may hate him, Peter has decided that he must tell Mr. Jones the truth. Ultimately, he decides, he can't look Mr. Jones in the eye and lie.

When Peter enters the room about 16 hours after he last saw Mr. Jones, no one is there, nor is any chart to be found. Peter walks down to the nursing station and asks the duty nurse. "Oh, that one. He left AMA (against medical advice) this morning."

"Can we call him at his home?" Peter asks. "That one was homeless with no known address," the nurse replies.

So far we have not discussed the fact that the major physicians in this case are white males and the patient is a black male. In the real world, race, gender, and class matter, and they matter in this case, too.

In a country where white Americans once owned blacks as slaves, slavery's historical legacy still influences both American life and American medicine. Black Americans still enter life with less wealth and opportunities than white Americans. Because whites kidnapped their ancestors and made them into slaves, blacks tend to regard white physicians with more suspicion in medicine than white people do.

In many states, if it could be proved that Sam missed a diagnosis that he should have made, this mistake could be the basis for a substantial malpractice suit against Sam, where Mr. Jones would sue for compensatory, and perhaps punitive, damages. As such, it is very likely that if either Sam or Peter tells Mr. Jones and his family about the missed diagnosis, then Sam will be sued.

Is that relevant to the ethics of the case? No, for the *ethics of lying must be separated from the legality of doing so,* and similarly, the ethics of truth telling must be separated from the legal consequences of doing so.

There is also a much bigger issue here: Would Sam act the same way if the patient were a white man? Would he act the same way if Mr. Jones were a rich businessman of his same social and economic class? There may be some evidence that he would not; thus, racism is an issue in the case. Again, this book will have more to say about racism in later chapters, for example, in describing the Tuskegee Syphilis Study by the federal government on black men in Alabama (see Chapter 8).

CONCLUSIONS

In real life, things don't always have neat endings the way they do on television shows or in movies. Indeed, messy endings may be the norm in real life. In this case, we don't know why the patient left, but we do know that, unlike in certain television shows, Peter did not then seek out Mr. Jones among the homeless people of the back alleys of his city. Realistically, hospital physicians just don't have the time to do such heroic actions.

Whether to tell the truth to a patient with a diagnosis of terminal cancer cuts to the heart of the physician–patient relationship. We have discussed the issue of whether omissions of truth amount to the same thing as deliberate lying, as well as discussed issues about race, complicity, relativism, responsibility for mistakes, system errors, and personal responsibility for health. Although the case did not end in a satisfying way because the patient checked himself out of the hospital and never returned, the use of the case was not designed to achieve a satisfying result; instead, it was to teach something about moral issues in medicine.

FURTHER READINGS

Bosk, Charles. *Forgive and Remember: Managing Medical Failure*, 2nd ed. Chicago: University of Chicago Press, 1979.

"The Emotional Impact of Mistakes on Family Physicians." *Archives of Family Medicine*, February 1996.

Gilbert, Sandra M. *Wrongful Death: A Memoir*. New York: W. W. Norton, 1997.

"The Internal Morality of Medicine," eds. Robert M. Veatch and Franklin G. Miller. *Journal of Medicine and Philosophy* 26 (Special Issue), no. 6 (December 2001).

Lantos, John. *Do We Still Need Doctors?* New York: Routledge, 1997.

Nuland, Sherwin B. "Mistakes in the Operating Room—Error and Responsibility." *New England Journal of Medicine* 351, no. 13 (September 23, 2004).

Ofri, Danielle. "They Sent Me Here." *New England Journal of Medicine* 352 (April 28, 2005), pp. 1746–48.

"Symposium: Patient Injury, Medical Errors, Liability, and Reform," symposium ed. Barry R. Furrow. *Journal of Law, Medicine, and Ethics*, 29, nos. 3 and 4 (Fall/Winter 2001).

Witman, G., et al. "How Do Patients Want Physicians to Handle Mistakes?" *Archives of Internal Medicine*, February 1996.

Wu, Albert, et al. "Do House Officers Learn from Their Mistakes?" *Journal of the American Medical Association* 265, no. 16 (April 24, 1991), pp. 2089–94.

Wu, Albert, et al. "To Tell the Truth: Ethical and Practical Issues in Disclosing Medical Mistakes to Patients." *Journal of General Internal Medicine* 12 (December 1997).

CHAPTER 2

Kant on Whether Alcoholism Is a Disease

This chapter has two goals. First, to bring together two topics normally discussed in separate fields of literature: free will and medical ethics. Many areas of medicine raise the issue of personal responsibility for illnesses such as cancer. The dominant moral issue of this chapter concerns whether patients are responsible for their own diseases, especially diseases caused by unhealthy lifestyles. This chapter uses the case of Ernie Crowfeather to focus attention on that question. A second goal of the chapter is to contrast views on alcoholism and free will by Kant, Alcoholics Anonymous, Herbert Fingarette, sociologists, and geneticists.[1]

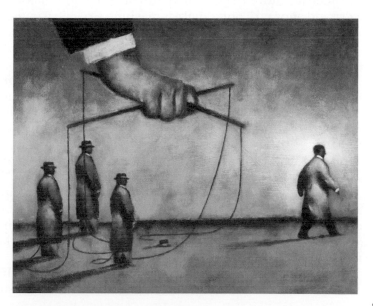

After a weekend of binge drinking, Ernie Crowfeather, a 26-year-old half-Sioux, half-white man, presented in the emergency room of Ellensburg, Washington, in October of 1968, coughing up yellow sputum and blood, with pain in his left kidney. "Binge drinking" describes two to seven days during which a person repeatedly drinks to the point of intoxication, during which he gives up his usual activities and obligations.[2]

Upon work-up, physicians diagnosed a urinary tract infection and anemia in Ernie Crowfeather. After being given antibiotics, they sent him home.

2.1 The God Committee: Who Shall Live When Not All Can?

In 1962 in Seattle, Washington, six years before Ernie came to the emergency room, physician Belding Scribner and other physicians had developed an artificial kidney machine.[3] The kidney cleans the blood of toxic by-products of metabolism and secretes them in urine. Without a functioning kidney, toxins accumulate in the blood and cause death.

Seattle physician Belding Scribner invented a spigot-like device called a "shunt" that permanently attached to a major vein or artery and allowed a hemodialysis machine to clean a patient's blood. Scribner's Teflon shunt, a U-shaped catheter stuck in an arm or a leg, allowed the machine's tubes to be attached and detached several times a week.

Unfortunately, during the early 1960s, few of these machines existed, and even in the state of Washington, renal failure caused hundreds of people to be sick. Ernie's seminal case in medical ethics centered around the question, *Who shall live when not all can?* By what criteria would physicians decide who received a machine and who did not? This question is one of *distributive justice* in the allocation of scarce medical resources.

After screening candidates for medical incompatibility, Dr. Scribner did not want to be in the position of turning down patients. So he famously turned over selection to a lay committee, dubbed "the God Committee." Dr. Scribner said he lacked the moral authority to decide who got a machine.

Neither Dr. Scribner nor anyone else at the time had any firm moral rule to use to make such decisions. As a result,

Dr. Scribner dropped from the level of *moral content* to that of *moral process,* giving a committee the right to decide who lived and who died. Subsequent decades saw similar moves when people disagreed about moral content in medicine and when solutions involved dropping a level to a process for resolving such disagreements.

In other words, we can visually imagine that solutions involving answers about right and wrong occupy one level, whereas solutions involving process occupy another level. For example, "Distribute machines by years on list" is an answer about content and an answer to the question, "How should such machines be distributed?" When too many people disagree about such answers of content, or such disagreement lasts so long that it seems irresolvable, one solution in ethics is to move to a meta-level beneath the level of content and to seek a process for arriving at a satisfactory content, where a fair process by definition creates the best answer (content) possible.

The most common process for resolving disagreements in bioethics is a committee, such as a Hospital Ethics Committee or Institutional Review Board (to oversee experiments). Advance directives are a common legal process to avoid disagreements about medical care at the end of life.

Publicity about this committee and its ethical issues began the new field of bioethics. Although medicine had always had ethical issues, bioethics would subject them to public debate and would create a new kind of professional to discuss these issues—the bioethicist.

The God Committee famously selected a criterion of content that came to be called *social worth.* Using criteria that determined social worth, the committee ruled that a divorced mother with three small, dependent children would receive a machine before a 60-year-old alcoholic, a cancer researcher before an unemployed day laborer. While they employed this method to select patients, physicians encountered Ernie Crowfeather in the dialysis program, who deeply affected everyone because he failed to get a machine by the social worth criteria. The God Committee twice denied Ernie a home hemodialysis machine because of his drinking and his unwillingness to learn home dialysis.

Decades later, the ethical issue that is central to this case appeared when surgeons with waiting lists had to decide whether lifelong alcoholics should be eligible for liver transplants. Did alcoholics have *any* responsibility for creating the cirrhosis that destroyed their livers over many decades of drinking? What about cigarette smokers, whom some surgeons consider for lung transplants? We shall return to these questions at this chapter's end.

> *Ernie Crowfeather was a heavy drinker. After his first visit to the emergency room, Ernie continued to drink heavily over the next several weeks. What is "heavily"? In his case, it was about two six-packs of beer on most nights. After a night of heavy drinking, he again presented to an emergency room on New Year's Day 1969. Still drinking the same amount, three weeks later he presented again to the same ER. There he complained of weakness, nausea, and fatigue.*
>
> *The liver filters out most of the toxic by-products of alcohol, but the alcohol certainly did not help his one remaining kidney (one had been previously removed because of an accident). He developed headaches, swollen hands and feet, and suddenly gained weight. When he developed intractable vomiting, physicians admitted him to the hospital.*
>
> *On admission, his blood urea nitrogen (BUN) levels were abnormally high, above 100, and his urine output was low, about 150 ml every 24 hours. Based on these symptoms, doctors suspected renal failure and transferred him to the University Hospital for dialysis.*
>
> *During the next three months in this hospital, Ernie had many problems: encephalopathy (brain swelling), clotting, infections, near cardiac failure, lots of pain, bloody urine, and possible renal cancer, necessitating biopsies. His physicians called him "a medical disaster."*

Hemodialysis is a form of dialysis that removes blood from the body by means of catheters (tubes). One catheter punctures an artery, usually in the arm, and the high blood pressure of the artery pushes blood into the catheter, which carries the blood into a dialyzer, a machine that uses a synthetic membrane and a high-dextrose solution to pull proteins and water from the blood.

Cleaned blood then returns through another catheter inserted into a vein in the body. Depending on a patient's needs, patients undergo hemodialysis three to five hours a day, three to four days a week. Because patients must be hooked up to machines during dialysis, they cannot go anywhere. Overall, and in comparison to peritoneal dialysis (see below), hemodialysis effectively removes most proteins and has fewer complications.[4]

Peritoneal dialysis, unlike hemodialysis, does not involve the removal of blood from the body. Instead, a catheter enters the peritoneal cavity of the abdomen, and dialysis solution drains into the cavity. Water and proteins diffuse from the blood through the peritoneal membrane of the body into the dialysis solution. After a while, the dialysis solution drains back out into another bag and fresh solution replaces it.

> Because peritoneal dialysis in 1968 carried fewer complications than hemodialysis, physicians preferred to use it on Ernie. In the hospital, they had to continually cut new openings for tubes into his peritoneal cavity. These openings frequently became infected, perhaps because of Ernie's poor compliance with medical routines. Had Ernie been more compliant, Belding Scribner could have stitched an in-dwelling shunt in Ernie, and he would have been eligible for a home-dialysis machine, but his drinking, his lack of personal responsibility for his health, and his insistence that others dialyze him precluded this possibility.[5]
>
> When physicians started Ernie on hemodialysis, he experienced clotting at both the cannula (tubing) site and in the artificial kidney. Then he developed a pericardial effusion, or fluid in the pericardium (a thick fibrous sac surrounding the heart). A pericardium filled with fluid competes with heart muscles for the same space and if swollen enough, compresses the heart's left ventricle and prevents it from refilling, causing (potentially fatal) cardiac tamponade (compression of the heart). So Ernie's physicians inserted an external chest tube to drain this fluid, and he went back on peritoneal dialysis. Through a renal biopsy, physicians discovered that his kidney had intravascular coagulation, a serious condition where blood clots inside veins.
>
> The pericardial effusion, and the general difficulty at this time of maintaining Ernie on dialysis, led physicians to decide that Ernie required a kidney transplant. At the time, even Scribner's shunt needed careful medical attention,

*damaged easily, and in a few weeks, destroyed the blood
vessels into which it connected. Had a kidney transplant
been possible, it would have solved many of Ernie's medical
problems.*

*Physicians who considered Ernie Crowfeather for a
transplant had to consider many nonmedical factors about
him, including alcoholism, being on parole for armed robbery,
and two common-law marriages, the first of which had resulted
in a child that he did not support financially. Though the rest
of his family seemed responsible and concerned about Ernie,
Ernie would likely not stop drinking and thus would not
be able to take care of himself on dialysis.*

2.2 Free Will

Humans have debated the existence of free will for a long time.
In Judaism, Islam, and Christianity, where God is seen as omniscient, humans struggle to understand how individuals are still
free to choose salvation or its opposite: If God knows in advance
what I am going to choose, am I really free to choose otherwise?
Wouldn't doing so violate God's nature?

Medicine need not take a stand on God's nature or existence, so the question of free will can be raised independently.
However, eliminating God from the picture does not eliminate
the problem of free will.

A key assumption of science is that every event has a cause.
In medicine, if a person's skin turns yellow, physicians would be
incompetent if they did not assume that some change in the patient's body caused this condition (most commonly, a problem
with the patient's liver).

Recently, medical science has delved ever deeper into the
causes of human behavior and increasingly looked for *genetic*
factors. Behavior previously thought to be voluntary, such as sexual attraction to a member of one's own gender, is now thought
to be partially determined by genetic inheritance. (Controversially, some people consider such sexual orientation not a discovery but a choice.)

A similar assumption can be made about the mind: In psychology, researchers assume that each mental event has a cause.
Whether investigating relations with parents in early childhood,
classical and operant conditioning, social roles and expectations,

or how the computer-like brain processes data to generate actions, psychologists seek the causes of human actions.

For both the body and mind, researchers do not assume a mysterious entity, free will, housed in some equally mysterious entity, the soul or mind. Instead, they assume that every action has a cause. Moreover, they assume that similar humans will act in similar ways from similar causes.

In an often-cited example, social psychologist Philip Zimbardo created a mock jail in the basement of a building at Stanford University in California and enrolled students in (what they were told was) an experiment about jails, prisoners, and guards.[6] In reality, the experiment was about social roles and authority.

Half the students became prisoners in cells, and the other half, guards. Within a short time, the powerful images of guards from movies such as *Cool Hand Luke* and *Escape from Alcatraz* provided a powerful model into which student-guards easily fell. Almost immediately, they began to abuse the student-prisoners. Thirty years later, the abuse of Iraqi prisoners by American military personnel in the Abu Ghraib jail in Baghdad showed the continuing relevance of Zimbardo's work.

But American citizens and military courts assumed that the abusive military personnel in Iraq *could have chosen otherwise.* They assumed the soldiers had free will to act decently toward Iraqi prisoners. Moreover, other military personnel overcame the power of the role of abusive guard and acted well toward prisoners. So how free are people to overcome genetics, early childhood, social conditioning, and social roles? More specifically, when it comes to their own health, how free are people to choose?

Historically, psychiatrist Thomas Szasz has accused psychiatry of undervaluing free will by making every wrong decision of lifestyle a mental illness.[7] Ivan Ilych in the 1970s also decried a similar "medicalization" of health that took away from patients control over their own lives and deaths.[8] More recently, physician Nortin Hadler in *The Last Well Person* accuses the medical system of undervaluing patients' ability to heal themselves without medical intervention.[9]

As we've said, the God Committee rejected Ernie Crowfeather for a home dialysis machine. It caught a lot of flak for doing

*so from critics, who thought it was biased against American
Indians and against lower-class drinkers. Critics accused it of
"playing God" in deciding who lived and who died (that may
have been the origin of this famous phrase).*

*By all accounts, Ernie was a charming person who was
liked by physicians, staff, and members of the God Committee.
Eventually, a group of physicians and leaders of local charities found Ernie a machine by fabricating a research protocol
particular to Ernie at another facility, University Hospital.*

*During the 30 months that Ernie was a dialysis patient
in hospitals around Seattle, physicians rescued him several
times in ways they never did for healthier, more compliant
patients. Why? In part because Ernie was half-Sioux; in part
because he was charming and what some people called "a con
man." Not only did physicians bypass the God Committee to
get Ernie a transplant, they jumped him ahead in the queue
to try to get him a kidney transplant.*

*When that failed and money ran out, two American Indian
medical professionals and a Jewish philanthropist spurred the
Seattle-area Native American community to rally around Ernie
and give funds for his dialysis, which they did. All in all,
Ernie received an extraordinary amount of time and money—
the equivalent of millions of dollars in today's money—for a
medical treatment that he was ambivalent about receiving.*

In bioethics, reaching out in this way to an identified person
that happens to be before you is called the *rule of rescue*.[10] It
involves ignoring other anonymous patients. It makes the physician the rescuer and the identified patient grateful. The rescue
of Ernie Crowfeather may be the primordial case of the rule of
rescue in American bioethics.

As Dr. Scribner wrote of Ernie's case, "You get locked into
these things and can't quit. At some point in time we become
committed to those patients. We don't know exactly when that is,
but once it happens, then we find it impossible to let them die."[11]

The rule of rescue may not be the best way to allocate
scarce medical resources such as dialysis machines. For one
thing, it does not give everyone an equal chance to get a machine and therefore does not treat everyone fairly.

Good reasoning in ethics offers *impartial reasons*. It is hard
to see why only giving a machine to people who first get on a

list, or who first walk through the hospital's door, and denying one to all others (for example, people who learned late of the machine's existence) is not an arbitrary, partial policy.

Kant would argue that a lottery is the right method to allocate such machines because that method treats everyone as an "end in himself" and with equal moral worth. In other words, that process has impartial reasons behind it. Utilitarians would also reject the rule of rescue, arguing that it would not result in the most lived years per organ. Utilitarians would complain that it was a waste to give Ernie Crowfeather a machine, because he was not going to stop drinking, and doing so condemned to death an unidentified nondrinker.

On the other hand, the rule of rescue grows naturally out of the traditional physician–patient relationship. After all, sick patients come to physicians to be rescued from illness and death. Physicians forced to adopt impartial criteria of selection, and hence forced to cease finding scarce resources for patients in their care, feel guilty of *abandoning their patients.*

In speaking of how physicians dreaded the point where they would simply have to turn Ernie away, Dr. Scribner said:

> Why can't we figure out a way to terminate a patient [from dialysis] when it seems reasonable to do so, when he's indicated that he wants it, too. It really isn't fair to a person to prejudge his ability to cope with dialysis. And yet we do this because we're afraid to get locked into a situation we won't know how to handle. We can't get out once we start. But for some reason, if you don't start a guy, if you don't get really involved with him, the fact you know he is going to die, and then does, doesn't seem to bother you so much. But once you've seen him on the machine, and walking around, then the thought of not dialyzing him and having him die just becomes overpowering.[12]

The existence of such feelings forces us to consider what role we want physicians to play. Do we want them to be patient advocates in a complex medical system, fighting for their sick patients against cold bureaucrats concerned with the bottom line? Or do we want them to be gatekeepers who not only ration expensive medical resources but who also judge the social worth of their patients?

Shana Alexander publicized the God Committee in a renowned *LIFE* magazine article, and Congress reacted shortly thereafter to avoid rationing of machines, and in 1972 guaranteed federal funding for dialysis machines for every American in the End Stage Renal Disease (ESRD) Act.[13] At the time, Congress incorrectly imagined the ESRD as an inexpensive program that would save the lives of young, mostly healthy people and enable them to go back to work and pay taxes. Rather than debate various theories of just allocation, Congress itself fell victim to the rule of rescue.

Belding Scribner described above how it seemed impossible for him and other physicians, once he accepted a patient, *not* to dialyze him or her. To do so felt like killing the patient. Yet he had no trouble with his God Committee or hospital admissions personnel screening would-be patients and denying them access to machines. That didn't seem to him like killing patients.

On the other hand, the rational part of him knew perfectly well that hundreds, even thousands, of patients in renal failure had died because they hadn't gotten a dialysis machine. The rational part knew that anytime he denied a person admission to his hospital for dialysis, that person would probably die.

So here we have both the rule of rescue and the actions versus omissions doctrine (discussed in the last chapter). Here, omitting a patient from a list of patients who get dialyzed doesn't seem as bad as actively cutting one from the list.

Behind both these issues lies the fact that once a person becomes identified in face-to-face encounters, his needs and death become real, whereas unknown patients exist to physicians as mere statistics.

One goal of bioethics is to reflect on these feelings and analyze their rationality. After such reflection, impartial reasons may enter ethical reasoning. The administrator of a Native American reservation who declined to help Ernie said he could do so only at the unjustifiable cost of not vaccinating all the reservation's children.[14] For utilitarians, he made the right decision.

So did the God Committee when it rejected Ernie twice for a home dialysis machine. Consistently noncompliant over his 30-month involvement, not only did Ernie keep on drinking, but during his last months, he also sought narcotics and barbiturates, and refused to learn home dialysis. Physicians spent a lot of money and time on this one person while other anonymous people died. Moreover, as Scribner said in another context, 95 percent of the others would have done well and learned home dialysis.[15]

Of relevance also to Chapter 4 on Paul Farmer's work in fighting AIDS, one member of the God Committee defended utilitarian selection criteria by contrasting its method with the usual approach of "throwing everything you've got at each patient who comes in the door until you're bankrupt. Then you stop." Isn't it more reasonable to husband resources and direct them to where they save lives, rather than go bankrupt saving one man at a time?

2.3 Kant on Human Dignity

Immanuel Kant articulated an ethical theory that gave a special moral standing to persons. As opposed to animals, humans had a unique moral value that for Kant was sacrosanct and inviolable. Kant's ethical theory has many implications, and in this chapter, we focus on what it means for human dignity, free will, and rationality.

Kant believed a number of things about morality: that it was *universal,* that it was *absolute* (or, as Kant put it, "categorical"), and that it was uniquely *rational.* In his *Foundations of the Metaphysics of Morals* (1785), he gave a crucial version of the one ultimate principle that he thought grounded all of morality. This version stated,

> Act so that you treat humanity, whether in your own person or in that of another, always as an end and never as a means only.[16]

By this statement, Kant meant to assert that humans have intrinsic value, not derivative or extrinsic value. For Kant, a human life is beyond all monetary price and, as such, cannot be the subject of a trade-off to secure other goods or even other lives.

In contrast, mere *things* have only indirect worth and are valuable only as a means to satisfying the desires of humans. Penicillin, a thing, only has value as a means to satisfy the human desire not to be sick from an infection, but it is not valuable in itself.

Kant recognized the duality of human nature, the fact that humans combine both a physical nature governed by laws of the natural sciences, and a mental nature, the seat of rationality, free will, spirituality, and morality. As a thing, a human body can be thought of as chemicals in motion, and thrown out a window; such a thing obeys the laws of physics in falling to the ground. But as a nonphysical *person,* a human is a much grander, more dignified kind of being.

Much more controversially, Kant thought that nonhuman animals lacked intrinsic value. For Kant, such animals only had value as objects of satisfying human desire and had no independent worth in themselves.

It is important not only to understand *what* Kant thought about the value of humans but *why.* Humans are special, as opposed to animals, because of several unique qualities. First, they are *rational,* meaning they are capable of weighing reasons, evaluating evidence, and reflecting on the best path to a goal. Second, they possess *free will,* meaning they can rise above their animal nature, their psychological conditioning, and social roles to make genuinely free decisions. Third, they are capable of rising above self-interest and doing the right thing simply because moral duty requires it. That is, they are capable of being *true moral agents.* Finally, they possess a deep self (some would call this a "soul") that is the subject of consciousness, conscience, reflection, and free will, making humans unique in the animal kingdom. For all these reasons, humans have moral value, unique in the universe.

All of these distinctively human qualities underlie the value of *autonomy* in Kantian ethics, a value that has become important in modern medical ethics. In the context of drinking, Kant believes humans can be "law-givers unto themselves" or give up on themselves, treating themselves as things. But in doing the latter, they voluntarily destroy something that is part of their essence.

It does not matter to Kant if most humans abuse their natures and do not act according to their highest parts. Even if most people voluntarily act irrationally, selfishly, and as if they had no free will, it does not mean to Kant that some humans cannot act correctly. Kant prefers to base his theory on what humans *can* achieve and how they *can* act, not on how they *actually act.*

Because each human is special, all humans are special. From this simple truth, enormous ethical obligations are generated. Each of us has a strict obligation to treat other humans as fully autonomous, equal moral agents, to not harm other humans, to go to the aid of injured humans, and in all ways, to respect humanity and persons therein.

Autonomy is a special word for Kant and in bioethics. It refers to the capacity of persons to be self-governing, independent, and self-contained. As Kant says, only persons are capable of voluntarily subjecting their desires to the moral law, and it is this capacity for voluntary self-regulation that makes persons different from animals and possessing intrinsic moral worth.

Kant's conception of human dignity flows from his view of human nature, and his view of morality is based on it. His view of dignity is fairly complex, and it will take awhile to understand it, but it has definite implications for some important topics in medical ethics.

Dialysis and Quality of Life

The stories of Seattle's God Committee in 1962 and the End Stage Renal Disease Act passed by Congress in 1972 are frequently told in terms of heroism and saving young lives in the face of rationing and tight finances. True, criticisms are made that, decades later, costs were hundreds of times greater than initial estimates, but that's usually the only criticism of the ESRD.

But another, darker side of kidney dialysis is more relevant to the case of Ernie Crowfeather and to today's typical patients, who are not young and white, but members of minorities, middle-aged, and often miserable. For example, African Americans make up 12 percent of the U.S. population but 33 percent of ESRD patients. Moreover, the fastest growing population on ESRD today is over 65 years old. As a result, nephrologists today treat patients who not only have failing kidneys, but also who have diabetes, hypertension, and the first stages of dementia.

The very success of dialysis over the last 30 years has given rise to these problems. People are being dialyzed today who would not have been considered candidates in a past generation. But it is this success, in maintaining older and sicker people for more decades, that engenders contemporary problems about quality of life.

One other fact helps us understand the Crowfeather case: Despite improvements over the last 40 years, many patients hate dialysis. It is especially unpleasant for people who, when they must face unpleasant things, turn to alcohol. Even today, life on dialysis has, to use the medical phrase, "a high symptom burden," meaning that quality of life is low. As one nephrologist reports about the unpleasant daily life of his patients on dialysis:

> Insomnia is extraordinarily common and many [patients] experience severe muscle cramping and pains of different sorts. Itching is an equally common phenomenon, along with nausea, vomiting, and poor spirits. Our data indicates that among the roughly 300,000 patients undergoing dialysis in any given year, about 65,000 (or 23 percent) will die.[17]

So many deaths of dialysis patients are quasi-suicides, where they cease taking their dialysis treatments and then die.

Consider another real case, that of a 49-year-old white woman who has suffered diabetes for the last 20 years, who has been on dialysis for the last 5 years, and who recently suffered both a stroke and a heart attack. These events left her partly blind and with loss of feeling in her hands and feet. Now, having trouble swallowing and in great pain, she decides to forgo further dialysis and die.[18]

Although not all dialysis patients suffer this badly, many do at the end of their lives, and the life expectancy for dialysis patients is between one-eighth and one-third of the rest of the population.[19] To avoid this low quality of life, patients seek kidney transplants, which offers them a return to normal life. But far more people want transplants than people who agree to donate, so many patients die waiting (Chapter 3 discusses this topic).

These facts about life on dialysis are stressed to emphasize that patients who do best are relatively healthy, young, resilient, with strong wills to live and supportive relatives. Noncompliant patients like Ernie Crowfeather, already ambivalent about living and dependent on alcohol, and who poorly tolerate a "high symptom burden," simply don't live long on dialysis.

2.4 Is Alcoholism a Disease?

Ancient peoples learned that fermented juice from grapes, potatoes, and other fruits and vegetables produced an intoxicating brew. Some ancient Greek worshippers of Dionysus thought that inebriation came as a gift from their god and celebrated accordingly. About the same time, people began to notice that some people liked this brew too much.

In Europe and colonial North America, people drank a lot of wine and beer because they did not have safe, clean water. Nevertheless, people came to understand the dangers of alcohol and preachers soon moralized against drinking. The traditional *Free Will View* held that anyone of good moral character could stop drinking. Today this is called the cold-turkey view, meaning that a person can simply and suddenly decide to stop drinking and hold out against temptation by sheer force of willpower.

Some psychiatrists reject free will about alcohol. They believe that predisposing genes, influences in early childhood, social stress, and physical addiction create a specific disease called alcoholism.

Alcoholics Anonymous, an organization dedicated to helping people stop drinking alcohol, completely agrees with this perspective. It holds that

> The explanation that seems to make sense to most Alcoholics Anonymous members is that alcoholism is an illness, a progressive illness, which can never be cured. But which, like some other diseases, can be arrested. Going one step further, many members of Alcoholics Anonymous feel that the illness represents the combination of a physical sensitivity to alcohol and a mental obsession with drinking, which, regardless of consequences, cannot be broken by willpower alone.
>
> Before they are exposed to Alcoholics Anonymous, many alcoholics who are unable to stop drinking think of themselves as morally weak or, possibly, mentally unbalanced. The concept of Alcoholics Anonymous is that alcoholics are sick people who can recover if they will follow a simple program that has proved successful for more than one and a half million men and women.
>
> Once alcoholism has set in, there is nothing morally wrong about being ill. At this stage, free will is not involved, because the sufferer has lost the power of choice over alcohol. The important thing is to face the facts of one's illness and to take advantage of the help that is available. There must also be a desire to get well. Experience shows that the Alcoholics Anonymous program will work

for all alcoholics who are sincere in their efforts to stop drinking; it usually will not work for those not absolutely certain that they want to stop.[20]

We shall call this the *disease model* of alcoholism. According to this view, Ernie Crowfeather did not really choose to drink heavily. Once he started drinking, he fell down a downward path to alcohol addiction, and he could not have done otherwise. Once he took his first drink, his fate was sealed.

The exact cause of Ernie's disease, whether genetic, physiological, social, or psychological, doesn't matter morally. The important fact is that Ernie had a disease and had no control over his actions. Sadly, he could not stop drinking, even to save his life.

The disease model logically implies several things. First, if alcoholism is a disease, then alcoholics cannot simply *decide* not to drink. Free will alone is powerless against alcohol, and alcoholics need help in conquering their disease, especially medical help such as drugs to ameliorate symptoms of withdrawal from alcohol.

Second, if alcoholism is a disease, then alcoholics should not be blamed for being sick. Leprosy strikes patients down, regardless of their virtue, and people should not be faulted for getting such diseases. To do so is to commit the classic moralistic sin of *blaming the victim* (for his disease).

Third, if alcoholism is a disease, then people with this disease should be called "patients" and should be treated like any other kind of patient. That is, they should be treated in a kind of institution called a "hospital" or "rehabilitation center," and the people treating them should be "physicians"—people specially trained to cure diseases.

Fourth, if alcoholism is a disease, medical insurance should cover its treatment. Group medical insurance both protects us against unexpected illness and subsidizes the sick by taxing healthy people. As such a moral enterprise, healthy nondrinkers should pay these premiums to help sick people recover from alcoholism.

This kind of model involves professions of helplessness in the face of the disease alone, requires both total honesty about one's behavior and confronting others with their deceptions, as well as calling upon others in a group for support.

The disease model of alcoholism has been powerful historically in developed countries, as well as in behavioral medicine. It has spawned various offshoots, such as seeing various eating disorders as diseases (bulimia, anorexia, morbid obesity) as well as certain kinds of compulsive behavior (sex addiction).

2.5 Sociologists and Geneticists on Alcoholism

In analyzing Ernie's case in their classic of medical sociology, *The Courage to Fail*, Professors Rene Fox and Judith Swazey devoted a chapter to Ernie's case. They extensively investigated the patient who so haunted physician Belding Scribner, his staff, and the God Committee. In their view:

> Ernie's response to his situation [his drinking, his non-compliance] was conditioned by his social background and his personality traits. These same factors [his Sioux background and personality] contributed to the ways physicians and the local community became involved in the case.[21]

During the time (1965–1975) when Fox and Swazey were writing, the environmental model of disease ruled in medicine. (Today explanatory fashion in medicine has swung to the other way and the genetic model reigns supreme.)

For Fox and Swazey, social factors explain a person's behavior more than anything else. In Ernie's case and in the staff's reaction to him, they think his "Indianness" mattered most.[22]

Many Americans feel guilty about the fact that white immigrants caused the deaths of 90 percent of Native Americans both directly through murder and forced marches to starvation and indirectly through introduction of diseases such as smallpox and yellow fever (against which Native Americans had no immunity) and theft of their lands by deception and broken treaties. Physicians in a state whose largest city is named for Chief Seattle understandably felt some guilt and made exceptions for this young charming half-Sioux male.

According to Fox and Swazey, as well as Ernie's own mother, this half-white half-Sioux rebelled against his Native American ancestry, disliked the name "Crowfeather," and tried to "look white." In addition to ambivalence about his Indianness, Fox and Swazey stress that his father was absent most of the time and died early, that he was one of six children, and that he was the only male in a female, Catholic household.

Ernie's sisters said that, as a smart, handsome but rebellious male child, Ernie often "got his own way" with his "great ability to manipulate people and situations for his own ends." Fox and Swazey believe that his mother's second marriage strongly influenced him. After a bicycle accident left him without a kidney, his stepfather became so angry at the care his mother lavished on Ernie that the marriage ended.

Ernie's social situation deteriorated after this accident. Because he lost a kidney, he could no longer compete in running events, football, or basketball, in which he previously excelled.

After his mother's divorce and his loss of his kidney, Ernie dropped out of high school and tried odd jobs. Then he robbed a bar, got 22 months in reform school, violated his parole, and got another 21 months for doing so. He spent most of ages 15 through 25 in jail, or when out, drinking and on the edges of criminality.

So these sociologists naturally believe that Ernie's social background caused him to drink, not his free choices. Any other half-Sioux, half-white, single-male child in such a female family, deprived of his athletic prowess and powerfully labeled as an "ex-con," would turn to alcohol.

Another scientific view of alcoholism comes from genetics. Some geneticists firmly believe that destructive drinking such as Ernie Crowfeather's stems not from free will but from inherited genes. They usually argue that alcoholism is *polygenic,* where more than one gene causes alcoholism.

As an overview, consider what happens physiologically when a person drinks alcohol. Basically, two important enzymes [proteins that catalyze reactions] begin to work. When ingested into the body, ethanol converts to acetaldehyde, which then converts to acetate.[23] An enzyme called *dehydrogenase* enables these conversions. Toxic to the body, acetaldehyde produces uncomfortable physiological responses: headaches, facial flushing, or profuse sweating.[24]

Some people react quickly and intensely to alcohol (this is sometimes called "alcohol sensitivity"). When they ingest alcohol, they produce too much actetaldehyde and not enough dehydrogenase. If they keep drinking, they build up a toxic level of acetaldehyde. For such people, their body's negative response makes them avoid alcohol.

Some people (often Asians) have a mutation in dehydrogenase that prevents acetaldehyde's conversion to acetate. This mutation increases the body's adverse reactions to alcohol, and lowers incidence of alcoholism. Asians have high alcohol sensitivity, which in them causes a low level of alcoholism.

Supposedly, Native Americans should behave the same. Evolutionary genetics says they originally migrated from Asia through Alaska. So they share most genes with Asians.

But Native Americans have both a high sensitivity to alcohol *and* a high incidence of alcoholism. Native Americans have a mutation and are not deficient in aldehyde dehydrogenase. Not being able to metabolize acetaldehyde, alcohol makes them flush and have headaches. But they still drink.

In a 2003 study in *Human Genetics* of 582 adult members of a southwest Native American tribe, 85 percent of males met "the DSM-III-R criteria for alcohol-dependence at some point in their lives."[25] Nearly 85 percent of adult males over age 35 also had met the same criteria, and nearly 65 percent of them had engaged in binge drinking. Nevertheless, all these Native American males also experienced the kind of flushing that makes many Asians sick from drinking alcohol. So why did these Native Americans keep drinking?

Geneticists don't really know. They speculate that American Indians may have a genetic variant that makes them susceptible to dependence on alcohol. They think that it's a downward spiral for many Native Americans. After the first drink, geneticists think a gene is activated that makes it almost impossible for them to stop drinking.

So geneticists believe Native Americans have an especially lethal combination of genes regarding alcohol: first, genes that make them alcoholics, and second, genes that make them unable to physiologically tolerate the effects of alcoholism.

What about this view? It is currently fashionable to think that every human trait, vice, or disease has a genetic basis. As mentioned, this is partly a fad. In the 1960s and 1970s, an opposite bias held sway, that environmental factors caused most diseases. Where funding agencies today encourage scientists to search for genetic causes of cancer, in the previous period they encouraged them to look for environmental carcinogens.

There is some reason to doubt the genetic explanation of alcoholism. What is that?

For some genetic diseases, if you have the gene for a lethal disease, you get the disease regardless of what happens in the environment. Huntington's disease, a lethal neurological condition, is like that. For other diseases, you crave something, and if it isn't around, you seek it out. If alcoholism were like that, a person who had never been exposed to alcohol would seek it out. Yet people raised in dry countries do not seek out alcohol.[26]

So, even if it's genetic, alcoholism is a peculiar disease. Even if heavy drinking is caused in part by genes, it is also true that alcohol must be introduced to the person and be part of his environment. So in a society of teetotalers, or a society where alcohol is forbidden, a person with a predisposition to alcoholism would never become an alcoholic.

More generally, we should ask what it means to say, "Alcoholism is gene-based." No pattern of familial inheritance, such as autosomal dominant or X-linked, has been established across generations of families. Moreover, alcoholism can skip generations, such that no children of alcoholic parents are alcoholics. How can a gene-based disease operate this way?

Finally, perhaps the most likely explanation is that researchers in genetics confuse the classic, AA-version of *alcoholism-as-a-disease* with the more moderate, controllable *heavy drinking*. Many people are heavy drinkers but not classic alcoholics. Perhaps this is part of the explanation.

In sum, heavy drinking might be caused in part by a gene-based predisposition to such behavior. Even so, such behavior leaves room for environmental and familial causes, as well as a window for some people of free will.

2.6 Kant's Critique of the Disease Model

Despite the growing popularity of the disease model, supporters of Kant think it philosophically flawed at its core. Why that is so will take some time to explain.

For Kant, the most important flaw of the disease model is in treating persons as mere things. That is, it treats Ernie as the cumulative result of the causal forces acting on his body and personality, such that his drinking inevitably flows from these causes. For Kant, this account loses the essence of persons—their rationality, their conscious reflection, and their real choices.

At its heart, the disease model treats people as if they have no free will. They are victims who are forced by bigger causes to drink, not responsible agents who made bad choices and who could make better choices in the future.

And that is precisely the second problem for Kant. People *do* have free will, and to treat them as if they do not is to treat them badly, like animals or things, and demeans their humanity. Sure, they chose to drink, and sure, they became dependent on alcohol, but that doesn't mean they forever lost their ability to choose otherwise. People make choices every day, including the choice to buy another bottle of whiskey.

Indeed, for Kant, Alcoholics Anonymous (AA) contradicts itself because its recovery program assumes that each alcoholic has the power to choose to be sober. Moreover, when AA agrees with Kant that alcoholics are responsible for their actions and should be treated as such, isn't it assuming a power to change?

And what about responsibility? You do not see members of Alcoholics Anonymous testifying at DUI (driving under the influence of alcohol) trials for manslaughter (where a drunk driver killed someone) that the alcoholic should go free because he was not responsible for his behavior.

Perhaps a kinder view of AA is to say that it assumes that free will is a necessary but not a sufficient condition of kicking alcohol. But if so, then this is a different kind of disease than, say, cystic fibrosis, where free will plays no role in contracting the disease or getting free of it.

Finally, Kant's theory emphasizes that the right actions are universalizable. That is, we should generalize the rule we are acting on so that all of humanity can and should act on the same rule. If we treat alcoholics as people who are not responsible for their actions because they have a disease, then we should absolve most of humanity because their actions also have prior causes.

But that method of treating humans is not only philosophically incorrect but also morally reprehensible: It treats people as if they had no human dignity, no rationality, no power of reflection, and yes, no free will. To treat people that way is not only false to real human nature but to human dignity and worth.

Put differently, the disease model's approach to alcoholism cannot be the real solution to curing alcoholism, *but, for Kant, is itself part of the real problem.* It is part of the problem because it ignores the key fact that must occur for an alcoholic to change: that he or she must consciously *decide* to change and to *decide* each day to stay sober.[27] So long as any model avoids this fact, it is doomed to failure.

That fact may explain why approaches to curing addictions that substitute one substance for another (methadone for heroin, marijuana for alcohol, a nicotine patch for cigarettes) fail most of the time. Ignoring the centrality of free will in human lives and morality explains the growing tendency to see everyone as a victim, whether it be persecuted atheists, Christians, Muslims, Jews, scientists, minorities, or liberals.

Kant would despise this cultural fixation on victims because it undermines human dignity and freedom. In a certain real sense, if you make a person think he is a victim, he will start to feel and act like one. On the other hand, if you make the same person think he is autonomous and responsible for himself, he will start to feel and act that way. Kant's insight is the moral truth behind all programs that try to teach youth personal responsibility and pride in exercising control over their lives and bodies.

2.7 Fingarette's Research

Philosopher Herbert Fingarette's *Heavy Drinking* analyzes alcoholism differently. Sympathetic to Kant, this modern philosopher empirically investigated whether most alcoholics follow the road predicted by the disease model. In doing so, Fingarette came upon some interesting findings.

Fingarette concluded that many beliefs about alcoholism are false: that alcoholics do not lose self-control, that alcoholism fails the criteria of a medical disease, and that alcoholics retain free will. Fingarette looked at many clinical studies and statistical comparisons between various methods of treating alcoholics and concluded that alcoholics *choose to be heavy drinkers* and are people who *choose* to make drinking a "central activity" of their lives.[28]

He specifically denies Alcoholics Anonymous's central claim that alcoholism involves *a specific progression of disease,* where the alcoholic cannot change until he hits rock bottom. Instead, he finds that most so-called alcoholics learn to moderate and control their drinking: They learn to eat before they drink, to drink only at home and not drive, or to drink alone to hide it from others.

In the above study in genetics about drinking by Native Americans, although the researchers implied that most of the Native American males they interviewed were alcoholics, the researchers did note that "many of these participants were in remission at the time of the examination."[29] Their alcoholism cannot be caused by several genes in the normal sense of "causation" and yet, at the same time, "many" are found to be in remission. Perhaps these Native American men have learned, like so many other heavy drinkers, to moderate their drinking. In any case, genes are not causing alcoholism here in the same way that a genetic disease such as Praeter-Willi Syndrome makes people crave food insatiably.

Fingarette argues that most heavy drinkers fail the AA criteria for alcoholism-as-a-disease. As an example, he says that one in five Americans at any given time drinks heavily enough to have alcohol-related problems, yet those people do not consider themselves alcoholics. Nor do they meet all the criteria for the disease model: They do not miss work due to intoxication, do not have blackouts, and have no obvious loss of memory.

Fingarette also denies that alcoholics lack free will over their drinking, citing studies that show that alcoholics moderate their drinking based on the rising cost of alcoholic beverages, an impending DUI court appearance, or the continuing embarrassment of passing out in front of their teenage children. According to one study done on hospitalized alcoholics who were given alcohol for performing a specific, monotonous task, alcoholics chose to moderate their drinking based on what they perceived as benefits and costs. In other words, the desire to drink first can be resisted, second, can be moderated, and third, the harmful effects of the desire can be reduced.

Fingarette also answers the argument that alcoholics can have self-control in a hospital environment that they could not have at home: If the alcoholic can gain self-control by being in a different environment, that implies that the loss of self-control is not due to an internal disease but due to external situations, for instance, job frustration or a poor home life.

Fingarette furthermore points out that if Alcoholics Anonymous works because alcoholics attend the meetings and abstain from alcohol, this implies that the alcoholic can exhibit self-control. In other words, the treatment plan of total abstention can only work properly if the alcoholic has sufficient self-control to abstain, which would be impossible if the alcoholic lacked that self-control due to an unstoppable disease. Finally, Alcoholics Anonymous's emphasis on abstention does not work better for its members in the long term than programs that emphasize moderate alcohol consumption.

Defending the Disease Model

This discussion mirrors a discussion between retributivists and utilitarians in the law about punishment. In this classic confrontation, Kantian retributivists believe that criminals *deserve* their punishment because they freely chose to commit crimes. To treat them as if they could not have chosen otherwise is to treat them as a mere thing, incompatible with their dignity. Similarly, when heavy drinkers harm others by driving drunk, they *deserve* censure because they could have done otherwise.

In contrast, utilitarians do not believe that punishment is good in itself, but merely a means to some greater goal, such as deterring future crime or protecting public safety. If we could achieve such goals without making criminals suffer (and that is a big "if"), utilitarians would favor that plan. Similarly for utilitarians, we should focus on reducing harms associated with heavy drinking, not moralistic condemnations of the character of drinkers.

Let us also discuss a different concept here: whether free will must be understood only as an all-or-nothing capacity. Although some people can resist temptation, life tempts some much more than others. For example, some may be genetically predisposed to love alcohol, whereas others cannot tolerate it.

More generally, how much free will should physicians assume in patients? Everything in medicine and psychology assumes that every human event has a cause, and this assumption has fueled great progress. Physicians once thought demonic possession caused schizophrenia, or bad parenting, but no longer. People with neurofibromatosis, phenylketonuria, and

Huntington's disease were stigmatized and punished until we learned the genetic causes of these diseases. Given this legacy, shouldn't we *presume* that alcoholism is polygenetically caused until we have overwhelming evidence otherwise?

From a structural or sociological perspective, some well-educated, healthy, intelligent, financially secure, mentally well-balanced people, blessed with good supportive families, may have some free will. People certainly seem more free, the more they have of these goods. On the other hand, ignorant, sick, stupid, poor, and mentally ill people all too easily become addicted to alcohol, nicotine, and other addictive substances.

So when it comes to a final decision, which way do we go? Do we say, yes, people have the free will to buy stocks or bonds, but no, they don't have the ability to just go cold turkey and kick the bottle?

In the chapter on Terri Schiavo, we will explore the idea that consciousness might not be an all-or-nothing quality but could exist on a gradient. In the same way, imagine free will on a gradient where genes, early childhood, social environments, and other influences can diminish or increase free will. From that perspective, the relevant question is not, "Are people free?" but rather, "To what degree was a particular person at a particular time and place free?" For example, "When, if ever, was Ernie free not to drink?" (Probably in high school before he lost his kidney.)

Kant's view seems too extreme in postulating that each person has maximal free will. He seems punitive, not only about rejecting alcoholism as a disease, but in rejecting degrees of free will. Kant seems to see alcoholics as wrongdoers in the same class as liars and thieves. In this sense, Kantian ethics is puritan.

For medicine, we must ask not whether an individual should see himself as free to stop drinking or whether public policy should see him that way, but *whether his physician should see him that way.* And that question may be easier to answer.

When an issue is so in doubt, do we want physicians to side with the puritans? Or do we want physicians to be non-judgmental and to help those who want to be helped? Do we want physicians or a God committee of laypersons deciding that people like Ernie are not worth a dialysis machine? Do we want physicians to be moral judges and deny liver transplants to alcoholics? Is that really what physicians are *for*?

2.8 Harm Reduction vs. Moralism in Medicine

Perhaps because of its puritan heritage, Americans generally pursue abstinence-only policies in fighting addiction. Canada, Britain, and Europe pursue less drastic strategies that try to reduce harms associated with various problems. The pragmatic, harm-reduction approach to medical problems sharply contrasts with a moralistic "preaching" approach. The former has come to be called in medical circles (especially in Europe) the *Harm Reduction Approach*, and the Harm Reduction Coalition (HRC) lobbies for this approach worldwide.[30]

Harm reduction parallels past moral debates in the history of medicine, for instance, combating syphilis, where physicians debated combating sin or combating merely spirochetes. So intertwined were syphilis and vice that some physicians in 1945 had difficulty understanding that good people could get syphilis and that spirochetes could be defeated without moral change simply by using condoms or penicillin.[31] Later in combating AIDS, debates erupted about the wisdom of giving drug-dependent patients clean needles for used ones. In high schools, similar debates emerged about whether giving teenagers birth control pills promoted extramarital sexuality or merely reduced harms associated with it.

So worldviews collide here. Harm reduction is pragmatic, nonmoralistic, and focused on reducing associated bad consequences of deviant behavior rather than eliminating the behavior itself or on moralizing about it. Its opponents see it as amoral, relativistic, and, as a result, as indirectly encouraging deviant behaviors.

Physician Alexander DeLuca was once chief of addiction medicine at St. Luke's Roosevelt Hospital in New York City, and there ran the Smithers Addiction Treatment and Research Center. Hired as an abstinence-only advocate, his medical experiences led him to embrace the moderation of HRC. At one point, he decided that most of the practice of medicine consists of harm reduction.

For example, one major approach to alcoholism offers brief intervention techniques and nonconfrontational therapy.

It provides emotional support and cognitive feedback from therapists. It rejects the disease theory of alcoholism.

Of great interest, Alcoholics Anonymous refuses to participate in scientific studies designed to prove its effectiveness. In contrast, HRC's methods have been extensively studied and proved somewhat successful.

The two approaches differ dramatically in how they think about control. AA emphasizes that the alcoholic has no control over his drinking and to cease drinking must acknowledge a higher power. HRC emphasizes that the drinker can control the consequences of his or her drinking, so it gives control to the person most affected. This can be important in dealing with alcoholic drinking by college students.

Like battles over AIDS, genetics, reproductive rights, and assisted dying, battles over the correct approach to alcoholism create ideological passions. Some AA defenders severely attacked Fingarette.[32] The television show *60 Minutes* later took this viewpoint in criticizing Mark and Linda Sobell, pioneering psychology professors in addiction research, and implied that their approach had killed some of their patients.[33] When Dr. DeLuca embraced the evidence-based HRC, St. Luke's fired him.[34]

As another example of these passions, any defense of Kant's view or harm reduction usually invokes strong responses by members of Alcoholics Anonymous, who see their way as the only way to stop drinking and who view these other approaches as enabling weak people to continue drinking. What may be closest to the truth is that AA's way works well for a minority of heavy drinkers and its cold-turkey, total-conversion approach may be the only way that can work for them. Having had such a method work, it is difficult for AA members to believe that Kant or HRC could have any part of the truth about drinking or that other methods might work for other drinkers.

Harm reduction also applies to other moral issues outside of medicine. In Europe, it lies behind the approach to marijuana and many addictive drugs, as well as to legalizing and regulating prostitution and gambling. The HRC approach is not to try to eliminate an age-old behavior, but to regulate it and reduce harms associated with it. Similar approaches might be used in America to control harms associated with handguns, teenage pregnancy, smoking, steroids in sports, and malpractice in medicine. For example, one researcher has advocated switching cigarette smokers who have repeatedly failed to quit to smokeless (chewing) tobacco, arguing that most of the harms associated with cigarettes come from the smoke and that the switch can prevent the onset of lung cancer or emphysema.[35] The American Lung Association and many pulmonary physicians opposed this HRC strategy, championing instead the cold-turkey approach.

> *Nephrologists in Seattle tried repeatedly to get Ernie Crowfeather to change his ways, to stop drinking, and to adopt healthy living habits so he could live on hemodialysis. But he wouldn't.*
>
> *Ernie's final day came on July 29, 1971. Eleven days before, after 30-months of being cut and re-cut painfully for dialysis, and after money raised for him had run out, in order to get money for more treatment, Ernie became very drunk and robbed a Hilton Hotel. Arrested immediately and released for dialysis, he never went to jail. A week later, he intercepted a check for $2,000 meant to pay his bills, cashed it, and paid off some debts to his second wife (by whom he had a second child) and to some friends.*
>
> *He then checked into a remote motel outside Seattle (as he told his sister later) "to drink myself into oblivion." Missing his scheduled dialysis appointments, his friends began searching for him to no avail. In his final phone call, he said, "I'm so alone. I can't go back to University Hospital, because they won't help me anymore."*
>
> *Ernie's sister figured out where he was and raced to find him. When she did, he was sick from having missed dialysis for several days and from his drinking. She got him alive to the local hospital, but at 11 PM that night, he died.*

2.9 Liver Transplants for Alcoholics?

Previously, we raised the question of whether alcoholic candidates for liver transplants should be excluded on the ground that they have voluntarily risked their health. In this case, blame can be hard to disentangle from medical criteria.

The liver is by far the most expensive organ to transplant. The surgery calls for a highly skilled team and takes a long time. A significant fact is that the most common cause of liver destruction, or end-stage liver disease (ESLD), is alcoholism. When alcohol causes liver failure, the condition is called *alcohol-related end-stage liver disease (ARESLD)*.

In the 1990s, controversy arose about whether patients with ARESLD and patients who were nondrinkers should be equally eligible for liver transplants. This is partly a medical issue, of course, since it can be analyzed in terms of which patients will live the longest from such a transplant, but there is also an element of social worth. Is a nondrinker more deserving of a donor liver? Can someone with ARESLD be held blameworthy for the loss of his or her liver and thus undeserving of a new one? Would a drinker keep on drinking, thereby destroying the new liver, or would drinkers be transformed by receiving the gift of life?

With ARESLD and liver transplants, the question of free will and personal responsibility gets practical. Even if alcoholism is a genetic predisposition, don't alcoholics have some free will to quit? And shouldn't we reward those who quit with a transplant?

In 1992, two teams of clinical medical ethicists battled over this point. In Chicago, physicians Alvin Moss and Mark Seigler argued that since ARESLD usually causes liver failure, since there is a dire shortage of livers for transplant, and since recidivism is likely among alcoholics, patients who develop liver failure through no fault of their own (that is, nondrinkers) should get livers before patients with ARESLD—whose condition "results from failure to obtain treatment for alcoholism."[36] In disagreement, two bioethicists at the University of Michigan with doctorates in philosophy, Carl Cohen and Martin Benjamin, maintained that alcoholics should not be blamed for drinking (because their alcoholism was a disease) and because alcoholics have satisfactory rates of survival after a liver transplant.[37]

Part of this disagreement is easy to dissolve: To do well during and after a liver transplant, patients must not have drunk alcohol for several months. Moreover, when patients get sick enough to need such a transplant, they usually do not feel like drinking or are in hospitals and cannot drink. So commonly, both former alcoholics and nondrinkers have been alcohol-free for six months before transplantation. (Some alcoholics who are too sick to drink will also die during the mandatory six-month period of abstinence.)

With a new liver, alcoholics may live out a normal life. They frequently die of nonliver problems, such as heart failure, accidents, strokes, or nonliver cancers. So surgeons may get the same years-per-liver from both types of patients.

With this in mind, the question of whether to give nondrinkers priority comes down to whether alcoholics should be blamed for destroying their livers and whether giving livers to alcoholics might, if it became generally known, discourage people from becoming organ donors.

The latter question is probably answered, first, by saying that the issue could be investigated, and second, by the fact that most such livers come from brain-dead patients. Since it won't benefit the dead patient, why not give the liver to the patient who matches best medically and then, by lottery?

Three months after Ernie's death, his story made the front page of the New York Times. An article by star physician-reporter Lawrence K. Altman began:

> SEATTLE, Oct. 23 [1971]—Ernie Crowfeather, a bright, charming part American Indian with a history of personal instability and brushes with the law, died recently at the age of 29 after he refused life-supporting therapy.
>
> By what was regarded as a suicide, Ernie averted the frightening possibility that his doctors would have had to purposefully turn off, for lack of funds and because of his irresponsibility, the artificial kidney that for two years had kept him alive on public money totaling $100,000.[38]

CONCLUSIONS

What, then, about moral blame? Should we penalize the alcoholic? Perhaps the best conclusion we should make is that, because it is an open question whether alcoholics can quit, we probably should err on the side of compassion and *not* blame them for drinking.

As for Native Americans, they likely have a genetic tendency to alcohol dependency which is toxic to them, yet they still have some free will over whether to take that first drink, whether to binge drink, whether to help or discourage other

Native Americans from taking a first drink, and whether to moderate the harmful effects of their drinking. The one thing that has not been emphasized in this chapter is how much this issue affects ordinary physicians in primary practice. "Not a day goes by," one physician says, "when I don't struggle with how much I can expect my patients to change their behavior. Sometimes I don't know whether to preach to them or to hug them."

FURTHER READINGS

Alcoholics Anonymous: http://www.alcoholics-anonymous.org/

American Society of Addiction Medicine: http://www.asam.org/

Cohen, C., and M. Benjamin. "Alcoholics and Liver Transplantation." *Journal of the American Medical Association* 265, no. 10 (March 13, 1992), pp. 1295–1301.

"Ending Dialysis: New Perspectives on End-of-Life Considerations." *Medical Ethics* (Lahey Clinic Medical Ethics Newsletter) 11, no. 2 (Spring 2004).

Fingarette, Herbert. *Heavy Drinking.* Berkeley: University of California Press, 1988.

Fox, Rene, and Judith Swazey. *The Courage to Fail: A Social History of Organ Transplants and Dialysis,* rev. ed. Chicago: University of Chicago Press, 1978.

Genetics and alcoholism
http://www.indiana.edu/~rcapub/v17n3/p18.html
http://alcoholism.about.com/od/genetics/

Moss, Alvin, and Mark Seigler. "Should Alcoholics Compete Equally for Liver Transplantation?" *Journal of the American Medical Association* 265, no. 10 (March 13, 1992), pp. 1294–95.

Pence, Gregory. *Classic Cases in Medical Ethics,* 4th ed., Chapter 14, "The God Committee." New York: McGraw-Hill, 2004.

Sobell, Linda, and Mark Sobell. *Problem Drinkers: Guided Self-Change Treatment.* New York: Guilford Press, 1996.

CHAPTER 3

*K*ant's Critique of Adult Organ Donation

This chapter's first goal is to discuss an issue in medical ethics that has been growing in importance over the last decade—use of adult organ donors (versus use of brain-dead patients) and the growing acceptance of this practice among surgeons who transplant organs. Its second goal is to explain how several ethical theories would view this change: how Kant might critique this growing practice, how a utilitarian would defend it, and how a champion of virtue ethics would celebrate it. As usual, to focus attention, the chapter uses a case (that of Laura Giese, an adult organ donor, and Willie Boyd, an organ recipient) and gradually reveals details about their experiences.

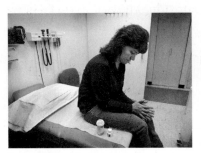
Laura Giese

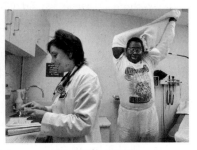
A nurse with Willie Boyd

Laura Giese was a 39-year-old Missouri woman who worked at an auto parts store and, on weekends, cleaned out foreclosed homes. One day near the start of 2002, she read a heart-warming story about a nurse who gave a piece of her liver to anybody who might need it, and the piece of liver saved the life of an 11-year-old girl. "I could do that," Laura told her husband, Bill.

Although Bill opposed it, Laura decided to give away one
of her (two) kidneys, even though she didn't know anybody who
needed one. She contacted various kidney centers, but at first
they all rejected her.

In her mind, she imagined the kind of person she would
help, how grateful he would be for her sacrifice, how the two of
them would bond together, and how she might even find a new
career as a spokesperson for organ donation.[1]

3.1 Kant: Some Things Must Not Be Done

As mentioned earlier, it is odd to hear people today defending
absolute moral rules. Recall that one person who did so was
Immanuel Kant, who argued that it was never right to harm one
person to benefit another.

In Chapter 2, we learned about Kant's view of personal responsibility. Recall also that Chapter 1 discussed Kant's view of
general moral rules. To review that discussion, Kant said that
these rules must be universal, absolute, unchanging, rational,
freely chosen, and in the form of categorical imperatives.

In a contemporary world that seems to champion ethical
relativism, someone might reasonably ask, "How can Kantians
think absolute moral rules are even *plausible* today?" To reply,
consider blackmail when terrorist groups take someone hostage.
As soon as kidnappers know that kidnapping can make countries
change their policies, they will start to kidnap, putting the lives
of innocent people at risk. So in international ethics, one ethical
bright line should be to resist giving in to hostage-takers.

This explains why, during the presidency of Ronald Reagan,
it was so damaging that Oliver North secretly conspired (by ship-
ping guns and arms to a trading partner of Iran) to satisfy the
demands of radical Iranians who had kidnapped Americans
(while publicly the Reagan administration denied that it would
ever negotiate with such kidnappers). Given the hundreds of
groups in the world who want something from America, and
given the visibility of Americans traveling around the world,
succumbing to the demands of such kidnappers would put
Americans around the world at risk.

As another example, the late James Rachels relates how
the great Catholic philosopher Elizabeth Anscombe protested
Britain's entry into World War II on the grounds that Britain

would end up acting immorally and unjustly.[2] In her view, that occurred when America's President Truman ordered atomic bombs dropped on Hiroshima and Nagasaki, killing thousands of innocent civilians in each city. So when Oxford University later gave Truman an honorary degree, Anscombe boycotted the ceremony and publicly denounced him as a "murderer." As she wrote, "For men to choose to kill the innocent as a means to their ends is always murder."

To use the hackneyed phrase, "the ends do not justify the means." Noble ends or goals do not justify employing horrible methods. Some means are always forbidden. For example, if we cloned a hundred identical children, gave them cancer, and tested various experimental cures for cancer on them, a great deal might be learned about cancer, but such means are absolutely forbidden.

In contrast, utilitarianism holds that nothing is wrong or right in itself, but instead, good or bad *consequences* make something wrong or right (more on utilitarianism below). Modern Kantians would retort that once you allow evil things to be done in the name of future good consequences, anything goes.

> *During the time when Laura Giese tried to donate an organ to a stranger, Willie Boyd spent most of his hours in one of two small places in Houston, Texas: an outpatient dialysis center in a strip mall or in a cramped studio apartment. One day in May 1998 while at work at a furniture warehouse, the 33-year-old man bent over in pain with severe stomach cramps and hot/cold sweats. At the emergency room, physicians said his skyrocketing blood pressure had ruined his kidneys. Within a year, his kidneys failed and he started dialysis, paid for by Medicare as part of its End Stage Renal Disease (ESRD) program.*
>
> *Being on that program qualified him as disabled, so he received special Social Security payments, as well as Texas Medicaid payments, that paid his rent and expenses.**

---

*Medicare is a federal program that pays for medical expenses for those over 65, plus monthly living and medical expenses for people who are disabled; states run *Medicaid*, with some matching money from the federal government, which pays for medicine and drugs for people who are poor or unemployed.

Few people enjoy life on dialysis, certainly not 30-something people whose independence had been yanked from them by life's random twists. Willie disliked life on dialysis—which meant not working and being tethered to a machine, and his whole life revolving around three appointments a week, lasting for four hours each. At age 33, he felt his life had stagnated.

When he learned that people with kidney transplants can live normal lives, like most patients on dialysis, he dreamed of getting a transplant. With their new kidney, many such patients live happily for decades.

Accordingly, after a few months on dialysis, he asked to be put on the list for a kidney transplant. He hoped that a transplant would return him to normal life.

As we saw in discussing Ernie Crowfeather, another way to put the central maxim of Kant's ethics is:

> Act so that you treat humanity, whether in your own person or that of another, always as an end and never as a means only.

This means not only that we do not exploit others to satisfy our own desires but also that we do not demean them as objects to do so. Importantly for Kant, this also means we cannot demean ourselves as things or objects. It is crucial to understand that, for Kant, respecting the humanity of oneself involves *preserving the integrity of one's own body.* As Kant says,

> To deprive oneself of an integral part or organ (to mutilate oneself), for example, to give away or sell a tooth so that it can be implanted in the jawbone of another person, or to submit oneself to castration in order to gain an easier living as a singer, and so on, belongs to partial self-murder.[3]

Respect for one's body, for Kant, is part of a more general respect for oneself as a member of the "Kingdom of Ends" and as a person having intrinsic worth:

> Man, however, is not a thing and thus not something to be used merely as a means; he must always be regarded in all of his actions as an end in himself. Therefore, I cannot dispose of man in my own person so as to mutilate, corrupt, or kill him.[4]

Regarding the practice of live organ donors, Kant would argue that it violates the absolute rule, "Never degrade your own body, even for a noble end."

What is wrong for Kant about the current obsession about enhancing oneself through plastic surgery is the identification of self with body. Take someone who justifies surgical enhancement this way, "I did it for myself. It made me feel so much better about myself." Kant would reply that the real person is not the body, the thing, and it is demeaning to humanity to identify one's self with one's body or to identify others with their bodies. If this trend generalizes, we become a society of bodies, not people.

But Kantian ethics also champions free will and autonomy, so wouldn't Kant allow free, autonomous donations of organs? Although modern Kantians might part ways with Kant on this point (see below), Kant himself would not allow such donation. He thought of persons as "members of the Kingdom of Ends," that is, people with absolute moral value. Constituent of that absolute value was mental and bodily integrity: one has a duty to oneself to preserve one's body and mind, as a member of the Kingdom of Ends.

We must also look at the practice of self-organ donation from the perspective of surgeons. Here Kant would argue, "Surgeons should never risk harming an innocent person, even with consent, to benefit another." Given the way the world is, there will always be many situations where surgeons could benefit greater numbers of people by harming an innocent person, for example, taking one person, killing him, and using his kidneys, liver, heart, skin, corneas, and tissue to save, say, a dozen other people. Such a practice might even speed up development of new, life-saving drugs and techniques, thus saving even more lives, but Kant thought it absolutely forbidden.

In 2001, Mid-America Transplant Services started Second Chance, a new program in St. Louis, Missouri, explicitly created to recruit live donors for people awaiting organ transplants. An active advertising campaign in print and visual media in St. Louis promoted the heroism and altruism of such donors.

As part of their desire for publicity, Mid-America and the two hospitals in St. Louis that perform transplants, Barnes and Jewish Hospitals, agreed to let St. Louis Dispatch *reporter Deborah L. Shelton follow the operation of their first adult donor and the donor's subsequent meeting with her organ's recipient. Neither Mid-America nor St. Louis transplant surgeons anticipated what happened with this case.*

Laura Giese was the first adult live donor that Mid-America matched to a recipient. Although over a hundred people requested information, few sent back the questionnaire, but Laura did.

Laura's AB blood type matched six people in the St. Louis area waiting for transplants. Willie Boyd topped the list. When she matched Willie, the system's wheels began to turn.

Some people wonder why someone would allow bodily harm to herself to benefit another human being. Because most kidney donors do not necessarily save lives, but merely improve the quality of recipients' lives (see below), skeptics question the sanity of such altruistic donors.

Thus a psychologist carefully screened Laura and put her through a battery of tests. She passed all of them. Ultimately, she impressed the psychologist with her unflinching commitment to helping somebody by giving up one of her kidneys.

Not only that, but a series of minor mishaps and setbacks tested her resolve. Each time she had psychological or physical workups, she had to drive from her home near Kansas City four and a half hours across Missouri to St. Louis. Laura also had many opportunities to back out: First scheduled for June, when her blood pressure skyrocketed, surgeons rescheduled her operation to July. When her surgeons had to be out of town, they rescheduled it to later in July, and then again, to August. Then Willie developed a gum infection, and $1,800 had to be found by Texas Social Services for his needed dental work, and ultimately the final date became September 25, 2002.

3.2 Background: Crossing the Ethical Bright Line in Organ Procurement

For many decades, an ethical bright line existed in transplant surgery of "First, do no harm," which in part meant "Do not harm one person to benefit another." In 1954, Dr. Joseph Murray successfully transplanted a kidney from Ronald Herrick, a 23-year-old man, into his identical twin Richard, who was dying of kidney disease. Since the transplantation involved identical twins, immunological rejection posed no problem, and Richard accepted the transplanted kidney. Since no compatibility barriers existed, and since a brother's life was saved, the benefits of this surgery appeared to outweigh possible harms to the donor, previous ethical concerns were overridden. This precedent demonstrated the viability of live organ transplantation and paved the way for alternatives to cadaveric transplantation.[5]

Half a century later, a remarkable change had occurred: By 2004, *the number of live donors had surpassed the number of cadaver donors* (brain-dead patients whose relatives consented to harvesting their organs).[6] In 50 years, transplant surgery has leapt from making one exception—an exception from a traditional rule (not to harm a life in order to save a life)—to a norm where the majority of organs today come from letting people volunteer to have surgeons risk harm to them to benefit another.

It is important to ask why medicine previously banned live organ donations. The answer is one that resonates in Kantian ethics: A surgeon who cuts part of a liver from a healthy person unequivocally risks real harm to the donor.

Donors tend to be altruistic, idealistic, and optimistic. No matter how much the surgeon explains the risks, most donors don't expect anything bad to happen to them.

Fundamentally, the wrongness of live organ donation for Kantians does not center on medical risks to the donor but on the impermissibility of her using her body as a thing for another. But from another perspective in Kantian ethics, the surgeon's, risk is relevant because the surgeon is using one person as a means to helping another, subjecting one person to risk for the sake of another.

Consider the first transplant from a healthy parent (a mother) to a daughter—from Teri Smith to Alyssa Smith in 1989. While he was removing the lobe of Teri's liver, surgeon Christopher Broelsch of the University of Chicago nicked Teri's spleen and had to excise it. Broelsch called the loss of Teri's spleen a "major complication," saying it gave him "the sickest feeling to have trouble with the first patient."[7]

Also in 1989, Marissa Ayala was conceived to provide stem cells for her sister Anissa, who had leukemia.[8] Preimplantation genetic diagnosis (PGD), the practice of analyzing artificially fertilized embryos, allowed Anissa's parents to choose an embryo that could serve as a compatible bone marrow donor for Anissa. Should Marissa have been conceived as a resource for Anissa? Marissa's bone marrow was taken and given to Anissa, which saved Anissa's life, but does one happy result justify creating a thousand more children to serve as resources for dying siblings?

In 1993, transplant centers accepted and recruited adult relatives of children for organ transplants, and Nilda Rodriquez gave one-quarter of her liver to her sick granddaughter. In the same year, James and Barbara Sewell each donated part of a lung to their 22-year-old daughter, whose own lungs had been damaged by cystic fibrosis, a genetic disease that is typically fatal by age 30 (the patient usually dies from infection and collapse of the lungs). By 1997, as the practice became more accepted, California surgeon Vaughn Starnes had taken lobes from 76 donors for 37 recipients. One commentator in the same year noted that the practice was "ethically problematic," implying that a norm had not yet been established.

From 1990 to 2002, surgeons in St. Louis performed 207 lung transplants on 190 children.[9] All 190 children were under age 18, 121 were ages 10 to 18, and the most common reason for transplantation was cystic fibrosis. This means that surgeons took lung lobes from 207 healthy adults for these children. Italian surgeons reported similar results for 1996 to 2002, giving 55 people of mean age 25 years a lung transplant.[10]

Similar things happened with liver transplantation among relatives. From a few isolated cases in 1993–1994, such requests eventually became the norm: "There now exists an ethical imperative to develop this [live-donor donation of livers]," said Jean Edmond, MD, director of liver transplantation at New York Presbyterian Hospital in 1999.[11] Between 1996 and 1999, surgeons performed over 70 transplants among adult relatives, with 45 in the first half of 1999.

In 1999, officials confirmed the first death from adult-to-adult liver donation and they estimated that two to three other adults had died from donating parts of organs to their children.[12] By 2003, at least five people had died.[13] Exact figures are unknown.

The surgical journal *Transplantation* reported in late 2002 that 56 people who had previously been living organ donors later required a kidney transplant.[14] (This does not mean that the donation itself caused the failure of their remaining kidney, only that they were unlucky enough to damage it and had no second one to fall back on.) Of the 56 people, only 43 received transplants, and of these, 36 worked (the other 7 are presumably on dialysis or died). Of these 56 candidates, two died while waiting for an organ and one died after the operation.

Consider the sad case of Walter Wood, 45, who donated to his brother under the impression that kidney transplants were first, relatively safe, and second, done only to save a life. Walter Wood sadly experienced an unexpected outcome during surgery: His abdominal muscles ruptured. He has since been in constant pain and has been unable to perform the simplest of tasks. As a result of his severe disability, Walter lost his job, had to sell his house, and approached bankruptcy. "I'm in constant pain from the surgeries I've had. I can't even move around in bed," Walter says.

Protecting patients such as Walter Wood is a problem in the system because the transplant team understandably focuses on the sick recipient of the organ, not the donor. Not only that, transplants occur only on people who have medical coverage, so the transplant team and its hospital get paid for medical services to the recipient. In contrast, it receives nothing for caring for donors and gives such care at a financial loss. In sum, transplant teams have asymmetrical relationships to donors and to recipients.

After he donated part of his liver to this brother in 2002, newspaper reporter Mike Hurewitz of Albany, New York, died a gruesome death at Mount Sinai Hospital in New York City. Also, 69-year-old Barbara Tarrant from North Carolina disastrously donated a kidney to her son with mental retardation and wound up paralyzed on her left side and without coherent speech.[15]

Widely regarded as heroic in the popular media, living donor transplantation carries real dangers. Surprisingly, no one knows how many donors have ended up like Mike Hurewitz, Barbara Tarrant, or Walter Wood. Why? Because living-donor transplant centers have no obligation to report deaths or injuries to the United Network for Organ Sharing (UNOS), nor does

UNOS have any legal obligation to monitor such deaths and injuries.

Amazingly, no hospital, transplant center, or medical department tracks deaths and injuries from live donors such as Walter Wood. Once donors leave the hospital, they are on their own—for medical care, for insurance, and for follow-up, and no one has done a long-term study on their problems.

Given the lack of such studies, an obvious question arises: Without such data, how can donors really give *informed* consent about the risks of donation? If there is no long-term follow-up of the medical problems of past adult donors, how can new donors be accurately informed of the real risks of organ donation?

The day finally came when Laura was able to give someone one of her kidneys. She still had no idea whom the recipient would be.

Willie Boyd flew to St. Louis, where his mother and brother from North Carolina had driven all night to join him. Willie also had a grown sister, Yolanda. At 54, his mother had already survived a heart attack and a stroke. Unlike Willie, his brother and sister had children.

Willie did not ask any of these relatives to donate a kidney to him, nor did they urge him to take one of theirs.

All his life, Willie had problems controlling anger. Perhaps this was caused by, or caused, his high blood pressure. In any case, his anger had gotten him into problems in the past.

Now he hoped to get Laura's kidney for a second chance in life. He wanted to prove to himself, to his family, and to the world that he could control his anger and that he was now a better man than he had been in the past.

3.3 The Utilitarian Defense of Live Organ Donation

The ethical theory of *utilitarianism* (discussed initially in Chapter 1) sees these matters differently. To the master question of "What, if anything, makes an act right?" utilitarians answer: the greatest amount of good consequences for the greatest number of beings. This means that consequences, not motives or intentions, make an act right and that the numbers matter morally.

With these adult organ donations, utilitarians argue that Kantians lose sight of the fact that adult organ donations save many lives. Although some problems arise for donors, the gain in lives and happiness to recipients so vastly outweighs the harm to donors as to be a no-brainer. Utilitarians wonder why the same autonomous free will that Kant champions to blame drinkers for alcoholism can't justify free, autonomous choices to donate organs. And no one is coercing anyone to donate— everyone makes a *free* decision. All in all, the new medical practice is justified because it saves lives and makes existing lives happier.

The numbers tell the whole story here, especially when we remember that each number has a face with a real human being behind it. Nearly three thousand Americans die each year waiting for an organ transplant. The great good that can be achieved by live organ donors is to allow some of these three thousand people to live for decades more. Even if surgeons injure a small number of donors, the compensating good to the people saved makes the practice worthwhile.

And as said, these are *voluntary* organ donations. No one is coercing or bribing anyone to donate his or her kidney to someone else. Surgeons explain the risks to potential donors and rule out unstable people by hiring psychologists to test candidates.

Finally, just focusing on the few cases of injury or death from donation doesn't accurately tell the whole picture. The risk of serious disability or death from, say, kidney donation is only 3 in 10,000. In contrast, and for example, the risk of death from complications from elective liposuction in Florida is almost the same, 2 in 10,000.

Organ Donation Among Nonrelated Adult Donors

By the late 1990s, surgeons crossed yet another line by transplanting organs between *nonrelated* adults. In 2000, a North Carolina high school science teacher gave a student in her class one of her kidneys, supposedly to save his life but probably to make his life free of dialysis.[16] In 2001, a Connecticut schoolteacher donated one of his kidneys to the mother of one of his students in an act described as "saving her life."[17]

Also in 2001, a 51-year-old Arizona woman gave one of her kidneys to a fellow member of her church whose polycystic kidney disease left her with a transplant as her only option to live.[18] In 2003, a man nearly 70 years old gave one of his kidneys to a former student, age 35, so that she would no longer have to endure dialysis three times a week.[19] In 2003, and to spare his son from donating, a St. Louis man gave part of his liver to his ex-wife, who had primary biliary cirrhosis, a genetic liver disease.

Back in 1999, surgeons crossed a new ethical line when a healthy female nurse volunteered to allow surgeons at Johns Hopkins Hospital to remove one of her kidneys *for an unknown recipient.*[20] After the first such *altruistic donor* was accepted as a donor by transplant surgeons, the floodgates opened. In 2001, Mittzi Nichols, a Virginia woman, became an anonymous kidney donor—donating her kidney to whomever needed it.[21] A Web site for live organ donors in 2004 listed 90 programs where nonrelated healthy adults could donate a kidney or part of a liver or pancreas to a stranger. In St. Louis in 2004, Mid-America Transplant Services launched its campaign for people in St. Louis to become live donors.

Six of Laura's relatives surround her at 8 AM as she's about to be wheeled into surgery. Both her mother and her husband oppose her decision, but Laura is adamant.

Around 10 AM, the surgeon opens her side to prepare to remove her left kidney. He removes her twelfth rib, which blocks access to the organ, and then spends 30 minutes slicing through skin, fat, and muscles while cauterizing small vessels and tying off larger ones.

Then he discovers that Laura's pancreas drapes atypically in front of her kidney, compelling him to use a circular steel retractor to pull it aside. (Just as surgeon Chris Broelsch accidentally nicked Teri Smith's spleen back in 1989 and had to excise it, the atypical location of Laura's pancreas will create problems for her.) The rest of the operation is uneventful.

Around 11 AM and down the hall, other surgeons open Willie Boyd. Around 1 PM, they begin the two-hour operation to suture veins into his new kidney.

Surgeons transfer Laura's kidney, which is in perfect condition. In less than two days, Willie is up walking around, feeling like a new man. By the third day, he eats solid food. Ten days later, he is full of pep and his spirits soar.

Things go less well for Laura. After the operation, physicians told Laura's relatives that everything went fine, so they went home. Allergic to morphine and most pain relievers, Laura cannot take these drugs and becomes increasingly uncomfortable as her pancreas becomes increasingly inflamed.

As a result of her family's departure and her refusal to take pain killers, while Willie took his first solid food, surrounded by a happy family, Laura lay alone, in great pain, vomiting, itching, and miserable.

During this time after the transplant, the medical team seemed to lose interest in her. Nor did Mid-America Transplant Services call or come around to see how she was doing. During this time, Laura felt abandoned.

Kant's Critique, Continued

As explained previously, for Kant it is always wrong for surgeons to risk harm to one person to benefit another. It makes no difference that the people are children in the same family or relatives. People are being treated as means to benefit others.

For Kant, it is also wrong for a parent to use one child to save another. Once one child's health can be sacrificed to save another, one has embarked on a kind of justification that leads to dark corners. In the same way, injuring an innocent child to benefit another is totally wrong. These acts cannot be universalized as a maxim for all parents to act on. Thus as we have seen, once the ethical bright line was crossed in 1954, allowing one twin to donate a kidney to save another, the door opened to intrafamily kidney, lung, and liver transplants.

If one follows the path of this reasoning, one arrives at a place that may be a reductio ad absurdum conclusion of getting on the path in the first place. Consider the tragic situation where a single mother is dying of liver disease and the only compatible possible "donor" is her 8-year-old son. Is it justified to take part of the son's liver to try to save the mother? Acting like this unquestionably uses the child as a means or tool to benefit the mother. It also may harm the son, although it probably won't kill him or leave him with a lifelong disability. But the operation *could do so*, and that is the ethical problem. Once we cross this line, will all children be seen as solid organ, bone marrow, and skin resources for their dying parents? If we could do so, would it be right to transplant an eye from a two-eyed child to his blind mother?

Consider also the tragic situation where parents have two children dying, both of whom need organ transplants, as well as a healthy third child who is a compatible organ donor. In this situation, does not utilitarian or cost-benefit reasoning justify killing the third, healthy child to save the dying two? And what if the tragedy is even greater? Suppose some kind of explosion has occurred and a family of seven will die unless one healthy child is sacrificed.

Even though utilitarians argue that saving seven lives is good, and that the good of two outweighs the good of one, Kant believes that it is absolutely wrong to act in this way. Killing innocent children is intrinsically wrong, even to save other innocent children. It treats children not as ends-in-themselves but as means to benefit the health of parents. As Elizabeth Anscombe said of such matters, *some things may not be done, no matter what.*

The real, deep problem here is that such cost-benefit reasoning leads one further and further down a slippery slope with dubious goals at the end. Consider a more subtle point, not the actual practices or the actual results, but the *kind of justification* behind utilitarianism. For Kant, once one accepts the justification that one child can be harmed to save another, justification easily gets corrupted, such that other wrong actions can be justified.

3.4 Act vs. Rule Utilitarianism

Consider again the case where parents have two children dying, both of whom need organ transplants, as well as a healthy third child who is a compatible organ donor. Utilitarianism seeks both to *guide* moral reasoning and to *explain* the best part of it. We know it is wrong to chop up a healthy child to save two others, but can utilitarianism explain this?

Because of this case and others, some defenders champion *rule utilitarianism* over *act utilitarianism*. The former holds that what makes an act right is following the general moral rule that produces the greatest good for the greatest number. In our case, the rule that a surgeon can sacrifice an innocent, healthy person to save two others would lead to massive fear of surgeons and hospitals, and hence, be a bad rule.

In contrast, an act utilitarian wants to reserve the right to judge each unique case and figure out which action creates the greatest good. Although he or she may agree that general rules commonly should be followed ("don't lie," "Treat people with respect," etc.), he reserves the right to break them, should extraordinary circumstances arise where a great good for a great number of people would be created by doing so.

Some critics have said that any true utilitarian must always be willing to make exceptions in extraordinary circumstances and therefore no moral rule can be exceptionless and sacrosanct, at least, if one is a real utilitarian.[22] For that reason, such critics believe that rule utilitarianism ultimately may collapse into act utilitarianism.

Transplant Surgeons Cross Other Ethical Lines

During the last decades, transplant surgeons have crossed even more ethical bright lines. At first, kidney transplants were done to save lives, but then, they began to be done to get people off dialysis and give them a better quality of life. As we saw in the previous chapter, although dialysis is uncomfortable and disruptive, people can live on it for decades and live normal lives. While it is one thing for a brother to donate to a sister, with the understanding that his sister's life is not saved but merely improved, it is quite another for strangers to do the same and, moreover, do so under the false impression that they are saving lives.

Sometime in the past decades, another line was crossed when adult children were allowed to donate to save the lives of their parents. A similar corruption in reasoning occurred, and another ethical bright line was crossed when physicians and society slid from harming one child to *save the life* of another to harming a child merely to benefit the adult parent. In 2001, *New York Times* reporter Denise Grady reported that

> Children donating livers to parents are surprisingly common, and the process brings up difficult issues for some families. This is particularly true if the cause of the failure has been hepatitis C, the leading reason for liver transplants in the United States. Many people with the disease contracted it long ago through drug abuse, which they never revealed to their children.[23]

Admittedly, we are talking about adult children donating their organs to their parents, not children below the age of consent. Even so, as with the ethical issue of asking parents of teenagers dying of cystic fibrosis to donate a lobe of their lungs, the ethical correctness of even asking some questions would trouble Kant. How can an adult child *not* agree to donate an organ to save his mother or father? Similarly, how can a parent *not* agree to donate a lung lobe to save a son or daughter? Should some questions not be asked? Given the power of the parental role and its expectations, as well as the bond between parent and child, isn't the answer predictable, if the question is allowed to be asked in the first place?

What about an adult man with mental retardation dependent on his competent mother, who is slowly dying from polycystic kidney disease? Utilitarians would say that the man would be better off minus one kidney and with his mother alive and taking care of him than with two kidneys and her dead. But there is no doubt that this man is being used as an organ resource for his mother and that he cannot truly give normal, informed consent. Kant would oppose this transplant, not in the specific case, but because the maxim "Take organs from the cognitively vulnerable to ensure that their guardians live" cannot be universalized.

On October 5, 10 days after the two operations and surrounded by members of both families, Laura and Willie meet for the first time in the hospital. According to Deborah Shelton, the reporter who witnessed the event:

The two awkwardly shake hands, then embrace.

"Thank you so much," Willie says. "I really appreciate it."

"No problem. It's yours," Laura says in his ear. "Just take care of it."

Willie slowly rocks Laura in a bear hug, right to left, left to right. Laura pats his back.

Laura is disappointed to learn that Willie is neither married nor has children. "He don't want none," Willie's mother said, also disappointed.

Fortunately for everyone, Laura actually hears the words from Willie that she's been waiting for, that she fantasized

about hearing. He says, "I feel like I'm on cloud nine. You really saved my life. The second or third day, it hit me. I can walk, I feel like I can fly. I really understand the gift of life."
Laura is happy to hear this. She feels wonderful about what she has done. She's really helped another person have a second chance at life.

3.5 The Utilitarian Rebuttal

Let us consider a similar case of using one person as a means for another, the Ayala case. In 1989, Marissa Ayala was created in part to be a bone marrow donor for Anissa, who would likely have died without Marissa's bone marrow. The Ayalas claim they love little Marissa just as much as Anissa, and both children now seem fine. Although less than ideal, Marissa's conception stemmed from as good a reason as conception from unprotected sex, which creates far too many unwanted babies around the world.

The rule in Kantian ethics that was broken in the Ayala case is that every child should be wanted for herself, not as a means to something else. Because Marissa was wanted as a means to save Anissa, in Kantian ethics, her conception was wrong. A noble motive and a happy result do not justify breaking the rule.

Why not? Because the rule cannot be universalized that children should be created as resources for other children in a family. Imagine a family with a baby slowly dying of a defective heart. If this rule were not important, the same family could create another baby and transplant its heart to save the first. Or to take a more extreme example, every family that uses in vitro fertilization could create an embryo twin of each child, keeping the embryo twin frozen until a time of need arose, then gestating the twin to be used as a resource for the adult, for example, as a liver donor.

For utilitarians, rules are not sacrosanct and must be reevaluated as facts and interests change. Yes, they say, the original "First, do no harm" rule served its purposes, but surgeons justifiably first broke it in 1954 to save the twin Richard Herrick. Thirty years later, both twins still lived, and isn't the alternative, one twin dead, the other grieving because he could have saved his twin, just awful?

Slightly harming one adult twin, who consents to this harm and who understands the risks, is justified to save his identical twin, with whom he is emotionally bonded.

Nor do utilitarians care about the change over the last half century to where the number of organs donated from adult donors surpasses the number of organs harvested from brain-dead patients. Utilitarians care about maximizing life in a tragic world—a world where insufficient resources do not allow medicine to maximize life for many people. Each hospital, each unit, each country is a lifeboat in which decisions must be made about giving medical resources and about who lives and who dies.

So, yes, thousands of adults have donated lobes of their lungs to children with lung diseases. Hundreds of people have undergone the somewhat traumatic surgery involved in donating a kidney or bit of a liver (which usually can regenerate) to save the life of another person. So what?

As a result, thousands upon thousands of people now live, taking care of families, working and paying taxes, and contributing to the general happiness. If we had listened to Kantians years ago, these people would all have died long ago. Even if surgeons unexpectedly injured some donors, or even killed some, the vast number of lives saved outweighs the small harm to the few.

In the month after the transplant, Willie's spirits have soared and he feels great. Meanwhile, Laura's life has gotten worse.

While she was calm and self-confident before the transplant, she is now riddled with anxiety, nightmares, and depression. Since leaving the hospital, she has had to inject herself in the abdomen 73 times with a drug to help her pancreas heal.

Because her own medical insurance won't cover this self-inflicted injury, she has to drive four and a half hours across Missouri back to St. Louis, every two weeks, in order for doctors to test her and try to heal her pancreas with drugs.

Reglan, the drug Laura has been taking for her pancreatitis, causes anxiety, and Laura showed unusual sensitivity to it. A co-worker called the transplant coordinator in St. Louis, worried about Laura's health: "You don't understand," she tells the coordinator. "It looks like all the life has been sucked out of her."

Over the next few months, Laura unexpectedly meets Willie at two clinic appointments and learns how happy he is.

Laura's husband, Bill, is saddened by the comparison: "It seems like we've traded places with the recipient," he says.

Worst of all, Laura eventually realizes that she feels no bond with Willie. A year later, he never calls to tell her how he's doing or to say how grateful he is.

Perhaps Laura naïvely hoped for a long-term relationship with Willie, a person who before was a complete stranger. Other than the transplanted kidney, they come from two different backgrounds. And what would they talk about? After all, Willie can only say he's grateful so many times and they have little in common other than Laura's kidney.

Kantians Respond

If we accept utilitarian reasoning as legitimate in ethics, where does it end? Such reasoning cannot explain why it is intrinsically wrong to cut up one innocent child and transplant his kidneys, liver, heart, eyes, and skin to save a half-dozen dying children with whom he is a compatible match. In Kantian ethics, we know that it is absolutely forbidden. Is it forbidden in utilitarianism? It seems utilitarians must either admit it is not or be hard-pressed to show how their theory can explain its wrongness.

All these cases and the utilitarian reasoning behind them inevitably lead to crossing yet another ethical line with organ procurement: paid organ sales. Already, rich people are paying poor people in India to sell a kidney, and in America, proposals abound for allowing rewarded cadaveric donation (paying families of brain-dead people to encourage them to agree to donate organs).

If the world can save a hundred, or a thousand, or a million lives by allowing paid organ donation, and if donors are not harmed too much and gain some financial capital, shouldn't utilitarianism—with its emphasis on numbers and consequences—condone and even advocate that? Kant would say, "I told you so!" and be aghast at the picture of thousands of organs from poor, brown and black people being exported for rich, light-skinned people in developed countries.

Consider again liver donation, which poses categorically different problems than kidney transplantation. When surgeon Broelsch first removed part of a mother's liver to transplant in her daughter in 1989, surgeons treaded carefully in this new terrain. In the 1990s, the practice took off like a rocket. The good news for utilitarians is that no child now dies on a waiting list for a liver, whereas before, about 25 percent did.[24] By 2001, at least 1,500 children had received liver transplants, mainly from parent to child (providing a good match).

That change in turn led to another, liver transplants to adults from adults. Now surgeons were giving liver transplants not only to 12-year-old children but also to 60-year-old adults. Because this kind of operation requires a larger piece of liver from the donor, "in the immediate post-op period, the donor is suffering from borderline liver failure."[25] Some children, some as young as 10 years old, have donated to their parents.[26]

The risks of liver donation differ dramatically from those of donating kidneys. In one St. Louis study, nearly two in three liver donors had complications, some of them major and including nerve damage, cardiac arrhythmia, pericardial infections, and pneumonia.[27] Only about 12 percent of cadaveric donors possess livers suitable for transplantation, which has increased the demand for livers.

In another crossing of ethical bright lines, surgeons expanded the class of acceptable donors, long ago leaving perfectly healthy donors and now venturing into donors with medical problems such as high blood pressure. "If we say, we'll [only] do the best cases—people at lowest risk, donors with no disease at all—we won't do very many transplants," says a kidney physician at the Mayo Clinic.[28]

> *If Laura had lost her job as a result of donating, she would have lost her medical insurance. Nothing in any organ recipient's medical policy covers the costs of injuries to organ donors. As a result of organ donation, donors (such as Walter Wood, who did lose his job and his employment-based medical insurance) must deal with such difficult consequences themselves.*
>
> *Even if the donor did not lose her job, the organ procurement system is not set up to help her. After the organ is transferred, the procurement system is finished. Mid-America promised to be Laura's advocate, but failed to do so. Afterward, it changed its literature to say it only "facilitated" donations among adults and omitted saying (as it had said previously) that it would act as "advocates" for donors.*

*When complications occur, donors are thrown back on
their own physicians, who may only then learn that their
patient has donated an organ. Some insurance companies
may not pay for complications, considering them "self-
inflicted injuries."*

*In Laura's case, the hospital absorbed the $3,000 cost of
her drugs (perhaps because of the newspaper article following
her case on the front page).*

3.6 Autonomous Live Organ Donation for Kantians?

Modern Kantians do not necessarily agree with Kant's actual
conclusions. Kant lived for 80 years during the 18th century
(1724–1804). Medicine has changed a lot since his death over
two hundred years ago, and some modern Kantians believe that
Kant could not have foreseen the altruistic possibilities of modern organ donation.

Such Kantians argue that the highest form of autonomy is
to give up one of one's kidneys, or to risk one's liver by donating
a part of it, for the good of another. Wouldn't we want someone
else to do this for us, if we needed an organ to live?

Kant himself does not reason in this way. Not everything
can be done in the name of autonomy. People are not allowed
to sell themselves into slavery because it makes a person into a
mere thing. Kant also believes that suicide is forbidden because
it is self-interested (escaping life's pains), because it disrespects
life, and because it destroys the seat of all values. And as the previous quotations from Kant have shown about the body, Kant
forbids selling or destroying parts of one's body for another's
good.

A modern Kantian might still allow live organ donation
because the good created, saving a life, is so good and would
argue that saving lives treats everyone as an end-in-himself.
More important, in another formulation of his ethics, Kant
stressed that right acts not only were those that treated everyone as an end-in-himself but also were governed by maxims or
rules that could be universalized. As some donors such as Zell
Kravinsky (see below) argue, we can universalize the maxim,
"Don't keep two kidneys when others have none and need one
to live." Another formulation of this maxim might be, "If one

can save innocent human life at little cost to oneself, one should."

Of course, kidney donation often doesn't save life but instead allows people to get free of dialysis machines. And with liver and bone marrow donations, the risks to donors start to become significant. Some modern Kantians think Kant's original prohibition was correct, especially when they contemplate surgeons risking harm to an innocent person to help others.

The disagreement we are discussing here actually stems from a deeper ambiguity in Kant's ethics. Kant thought that the essence of morality could be expressed in one supreme principle, which he called the Categorical Imperative. One of his characterizations of this Imperative was

> Act only according to that maxim by which you can at the same time will that it should become a universal law.

However, in the same book (*Foundations of the Metaphysics of Morals*), Kant expressed this same Categorical Imperative as

> Act so that you treat humanity, whether in your own person or in that of another, always as an end and never as a means.[29]

As James Rachels noted, "Scholars have wondered ever since why Kant thought these two rules were equivalent. They seem to express different moral conceptions."[30]

All in all, most modern Kantians are likely to go against Kant's original position and side with modern virtue ethicists, all of whom hold that people who donate organs are exemplars of compassion and altruism. The idea of freely offering one's organ for another rests squarely within the emphasis in modern medical ethics on personal autonomy, even if such individualistic decisions might alienate some families (as it did with Zell Kravinsky's family, see below). Thus, we will distinguish between Kant's original position and those of many Kantians today.

3.7 Utilitarians and Payment for Organs

For Kantians, payment for organs is just as bad or worse than allowing adults to donate their own organs, but utilitarians are at least willing to look at the consequences of such a new practice. In particular, utilitarians willingly consider rewarded cadaveric donation, where families of brain-dead patients receive money, say enough to cover funeral expenses, to encourage them to donate.

What is the strongest utilitarian argument for rewarded organ donation? The answer is a direct one, appealing to life itself and not simply to indirect benefits. It's quite simple: Doing so would save many lives. Well over 3,000 Americans die each year while waiting for an organ transplant that never occurs.[31]

At this moment, over 11,000 Americans become jaundiced while waiting for a donated liver. Every year since 1998, 1,000 of them have died while another 4,000 Americans are turning ash-gray from failing circulation as they wait for a heart. During the 1990s, 750 or more of them died each year.[32] From 1988 to 2000, over 40,000 Americans died waiting for organ transplants.[33]

So year after year, thousands of people die unnecessarily. Medicine has the scientific capacity, the facilities, and the personnel to save them, and for utilitarians, this taboo against rewarded donation is irrational and antilife.

In reviewing past discussion of paid organ transfer, few people emphasize the huge numbers of lives lost by not having financial incentives. Indeed, this loss is sometimes treated by opponents almost as mundane, as if it is obvious that thousands of lives must be sacrificed on some altar of abstract value.

It is impossible to overemphasize the immediate, tangible, and direct good that is being lost here. It is the good of life itself, something that both secularists and sanctity-of-life theorists should think worth saving. Not only is saving lives an intrinsically good thing, but it is a morally commendable goal, against which few other such goals count for much.

Life is precious. Utilitarians think that to allow it to be wasted, when simple changes in our medical-legal system could save it, is a tragedy of human-making, not divine fact. True, we didn't cause the diseases that destroyed the organs, but we continue to allow the system to operate that prevents lives from being saved. If we changed the system just to allow rewarded cadaveric donation, many lives would be saved. (Perhaps this is all the change we need to make for a few years, while we acquire data on how the change works and study unanticipated consequences.)

TABLE 1   **Patients Who Died Waiting for an Organ**[34]

Organ	1988	1989	1990	1991	1992	1993	1994	1995	1996	1997	1998
Heart/lung	61	74	66	41	43	51	47	28	49	56	41
Heart	493	517	613	778	779	761	724	769	745	772	767
Intestine	0	0	0	0	0	3	15	19	21	41	45
Kidney	721	—	749	—	915	—	975	—	1,045	—	1,275
Kidney/ pancreas	0	0	0	0	14	59	70	84	01	121	93
Liver	196	282	317	435	495	560	655	797	956	1,130	1,319
Lung	16	38	50	137	218	251	286	340	386	409	486
Pancreas	5	21	19	35	32	2	8	3	3	11	9
Overall	494	1,659	1,958	2,351	2,573	2,883	3,053	3,414	3,896	4,313	4,855

One of the great problems of ethics is to make judgments between incommensurable values, that is, values of different kinds. On the negative side, financial incentives may coarsen society by forsaking the wonderful ideal of altruistic donation. On the other side lies the richness, creativity, beauty, and wonder of human lives saved. The number of such lives lost each year—whether 3,000 American or 50,000 worldwide—counts powerfully in utilitarian calculations of correct moral action.

Indeed, in any moral framework emphasizing consequences to humans, for any competing value to be strong enough to trump this value, *it would have to involve an equal number of human lives saved or lost.*[35] But we are not in the situation here of philosopher Judith Thomson's famous Trolley example, where the driver of a runaway trolley can divert the trolley to the left and hit two people or to the right and hit a dozen.[36] Our situation resembles one where a hundred people wait on the right and on the left lies a magnificent morgue.

The great good of saving the lives of thousands would be accompanied by indirect goods. Thousands of members of families would value the people saved. Some patients could continue working, paying premiums for medical plans and taxes, contributing to the economy and the costs of their transplant.

Families who received payment for cadaveric donation would get something out of the death, helping pay for education of their children, perhaps.

Not only would monetary incentives increase the quantity of lives saved, they would also increase the quality of life of those living. Currently 80,000 people live on dialysis in America, but less than 10 percent of those are listed as "clinically suitable" for kidney transplants. Were donations to grow tenfold, many more could be listed, and life with a new kidney would be far better for all of them than dialysis. (Moreover, one study suggests that it costs less in the long run to transplant people than to dialyze them.[37])

From a utilitarian point of view, where the number of people affected and the consequences matter, offering payment to families for rewarded cadaveric donation increases both the number of lives saved and the quality of life lived for those getting transplants. Many of the consequences of offering payment are positive. Using this theory, utilitarians argue that we should begin experiments in a few states to see if rewarded cadaveric donation works to save lives.

3.8 Virtue Ethics and Live Organ Donors

A new kind of hero and a new kind of altruism has been born of altruistic organ donations, encouraging people to be heroes, not only in their own extended families but also at work and in religious groups. Laura Giese is not a victim, but a hero and saint. Virtue ethicists say people should emulate her.

Consider Zell Kravinsky, a man worth $15 million, who gave away all his money and who gave away one of his kidneys to a complete stranger (even though his wife, a psychiatrist, threatened to divorce him for doing so).[38] Indeed, Zell had to deceive his family and sneak out of the house to donate the organ (after which, his psychiatrist-wife objected that the transplant team should work more with families who object to the relative's donation). Zell stood firm about his decision and the reasoning behind it: "No one should have a vacation home until everyone has a place to live. No one should have a second car until everyone has a first car. And no one should have two kidneys until everyone has one."

His attitude benefits society and shows ideal character. Of course, such donors should be informed about risks, long-term studies should be done about risks to donors, and donors should be protected if, as a result of donating, they lose their jobs and medical coverage. Children should also not be donors to adult parents because they are put in impossible situations. But these are fine-tunings of the new practice, not refutations of it.

Rather than dwell on the small number of people who have been harmed or killed by donating an organ, we should celebrate the growing number of heroes who save lives and who live out their own lives happily knowing that their action immensely benefited another human. So virtue ethicists say.

Fourteen months after her donation, Laura still had persistent, sometimes intense, pain on her left side, which may be from excessive scarring that developed after the operation. Her pancreas still had problems. She also suffered from diverticulitis, an intestinal infection that may or may not have been related to the transplant.

Three years after the transplant, not much about her life has changed. Once honored at one local chapter meeting of the National Kidney Foundations, she resumed work at the auto parts store and cleaning foreclosed houses on weekends.

She has had little contact with Willie Boyd. She wishes him well, and would like to know how he's doing and if he's taking care of himself.

Nor did everything go as well as Willie Boyd hoped. When he left dialysis, he left Medicare and Social Security's special disability benefits for dialysis patients. In the eyes of the United States government and the state of Texas, he became a healthy, able-bodied man who should be working. So he received no more disability or welfare checks.

Unfortunately, Willie Boyd could not go back to work. For one thing, the immunosuppressive drugs he had to take caused him to gain 25 pounds, and he soon weighed 285 pounds. These drugs also prevented a bad open sore on his ankle from healing.

In general, he worried that standing on his feet for eight hours would put too much stress on his new kidney and cause his blood pressure to soar again (which caused him to lose his original kidneys). "I haven't put this kidney, this health, to

*the test," he said, and he felt reluctant to do so. After all, he
would be unlikely to get another.*

*For her part, Laura Giese claims, "I would do it again
in a heartbeat." She is not bitter about her outcome: "What
happened to me was just my bad luck. The chances of it
happening to someone else are slim."*

3.9 Organ Transplantation and Race

Laura Giese was white and Willie Boyd was black. If Laura had
known she was donating to a black male, would she have still
donated? Almost certainly. Would other whites do the same?
Should altruistic donors be allowed to know the race of the
recipient? To specify the race of the recipient?

Publicly discussing issues of race in organ donation, especially kidney donation, has bordered on taboo among bioethicists and transplant surgeons, yet once the issue is probed a bit,
issues of consistency arise. For decades, it has been widely
known that black Americans consent less often to cadaveric donation than white Americans.[39] Moreover, black Americans pro-
portionally receive more kidneys than white Americans.[40]

So should the system allow people to donate only to members of their own race? UNOS forbids doing so. Currently, a
white supremacist cannot specify a white recipient. However, a
member of someone's extended family (a son-in-law, a second
cousin) or church may indeed specify a particular recipient.
The big question for UNOS concerns why some personal bonds
are allowed to justify a designated person to receive a donation
and not others. What about LifeSharers, whose members are
committed to donating their organs at death to other members
of this group but not to anyone else?

Obviously, the transplant system does not want to reify or
encourage racism in citizens and that is why race-specific donation is not allowed. On the other hand, if transparency is a
virtue in moral systems, the present system is not transparent
and frequently masks underlying problems, such as injuries to
live donors and racial tensions within the system.

*All of the above story about Laura and Willie came from
Deborah Shelton's multipart story in the* St. Louis Dispatch.

Contacted about the story, in the summer of 2005, Laura confidently says "it was worth it" and that she has no regrets.[41]

Contacted about the same story, Willie feels it made him look bad and left out his perspective.[42] *The most important part omitted, Willie believes, is that many people around him assumed that when he got a new kidney, everything would be perfect. His girlfriend and family seemed to regard it as a miracle, not only for replacing dialysis but for solving all other problems in life. "It was like, now that you've got a new kidney, what do you have to complain about? You don't have any real problems now," he says.*

But it wasn't that way. All the problems with family members, job skills, and his girlfriend did not go away by getting a new kidney. What did go away was disability checks and welfare subsidies. The political system treated him as if, overnight, he had become the perfect, self-sufficient man, when in reality, he had been financially dependent on this system for nearly five years. And now that it was suddenly gone, everyone around him expected him to be happy and self-sufficient.

At last contact in the summer of 2005, Willie was trying to pull his life together. His kidney was doing fine, but the rest of his life was a constant struggle for healing and fulfillment. His main message to readers is that, like Laura, his life didn't end up perfect, either. And even though he doesn't call Laura, he says he really is grateful for her gift to him.

CONCLUSIONS

Medicine is rife with ethical controversies, and this chapter has revealed only the tip of one ethical iceberg. What Kant saw as bad, virtue ethicists champion. One constant source of controversy is when the Kantian imperative never to harm the innocent for the benefit of others clashes with the utilitarian charge to maximize the greatest good for the greatest number. In the next chapter we will see another version of this clash, where we discuss contrasting strategies for stopping the spread of AIDS.

FURTHER READINGS

Fox, Rene, and Judith Swazey. *Spare Parts: Organ Replacement in American Society.* Oxford, England: Oxford University Press, 1992.

Ingelfinger, Julie. "Risks and Benefits to the Living Donor." *New England Journal of Medicine* 353, no. 5, pp. 447–49.

Kantian ethics
http://plato.stanford.edu/entries/kant-moral
http://www.kuleuven.ac.be/ep/page.php?LAN=E&FILE=
ep_detail&ID=28&TID=107

Living Donors Online
http://www.livingdonorsonline.org/liver/liver.htm
http://www.livingorgandonor.org/default.htm

Living Organ Donor Advocate Program
http://home.earthlink.net/~thedonornetwork/

Mid-America Transplant Services
http://www.mts-stl.org/

Picoult, Jodi. *My Sister's Keeper.* New York: Washington Square Press.

Shelton, Deborah. "Trying to Give a Kidney Tests Woman's Resolve." *St. Louis Dispatch* (3-part series), December 1, 2, and 3, 2003; "Man's Second Chance Hasn't Turned Out Like He Expected." *St. Louis Post-Dispatch,* December 21, 2003. See also her series, "Lives on the Line: Living Organ Donors," *St. Louis Post-Dispatch,* May 6, 2005, May 11, 2005.

Troug, R.D. "The Ethics of Organ Donation by Living Donors." *New England Journal of Medicine* 353, no. 5, pp. 444–46.

CHAPTER 4

Utilitarians vs. Kantians on Stopping AIDS

This chapter discusses the ethical problem of stopping the spread of acquired immuno deficiency syndrome (AIDS) and emphasizes clashes between utilitarian and Kantian ethics. It uses the work of Paul Farmer to illustrate Kantian and virtue ethics, and discusses how these ethical theories differ from utilitarianism in trying to arrest the global spread of AIDS.

Ceasing the spread of this deadly virus challenges medicine more than ever before. If an effective strategy could be found and implemented, more lives could be saved by curing AIDS than by all other surgery, drugs, and public health efforts combined. Ending AIDS is also one of the greatest challenges to medical ethics, for, as we shall see, part of the problems of ending AIDS are also moral ones.

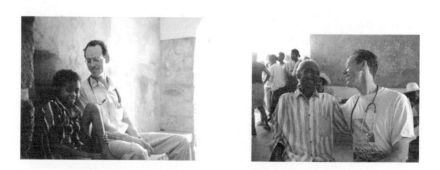

In 1959, a young boy named Paul Farmer was born in the western Massachusetts town of North Adams. He was one of six children whose mother was the daughter of a farmer. His

*father, an itinerant salesman, dominated the children, who
affectionately called him "The Warden."*

*When Paul was seven, his family moved to Birming-
ham, Alabama, to escape the unemployment from the
closed mills in North Adams. They then rented a house
and used a large bus that had once been a mobile TB
clinic for family vacations. In the fourth grade, Paul
entered a class for gifted children and became fascinated
with herpetology.*

*When Paul was 11, the Warden took a job in a public
school in the Florida panhandle. For the next decade, the
family lived inside the bus, which sat in a rural campground
surrounded by southern pines near the Gulf of Mexico.
His mother worked nearby as a cashier at a Winn Dixie
grocery store.*

*Awarded a full scholarship to Duke University, for his
first two years Paul joined a fraternity and became its social
director. He next spent one summer and fall in Paris, where
he learned to speak French fluently.*

*Friends said he had a photographic memory. He
majored in biology and anthropology. In his junior year,
the premed student came to admire the public health
philosophy of Rudolf Virchow (1821–1905), a German
medical reformer who focused on eliminating social
conditions of disease. That year he also met a nun who
introduced him to poor Haitian laborers, who worked in
fields not far from Duke.*

*He soon became interested in Haiti, read everything about
it, and joined those at the Krome Detention Center in Florida
in 1981 who protested the policy that welcomed Cuban refugees
as heroes but sent Haitian refugees home. Graduating
magna cum laude from Duke, in 1984 he entered Harvard
University's MD/PhD program. Despite spending many
months during the ensuing years in Haiti, six years later
in June of 1990, he received both his MD and his PhD in
anthropology.*

*In 1983, while in medical school, he first visited Haiti
and met Ophelia, his first great love. In Haiti, he found his
life's goal of bringing the best modern medicine to the world's
poor.*

While citizens of the developed world increasingly live longer and better, people in the developing world fare differently. Because of AIDS, life expectancy of Botswanans has declined from 61 years in 1993 to 39 years in 2001.[1] While a newborn Japanese baby can expect to live 81.5 years, a Zambian baby can expect to live only 32.5 years.[2]

In these two worlds, different diseases kill people. In developed countries, the main killers are heart disease, strokes, and pulmonary diseases such as emphysema and lung cancer. In developing countries, the three killers are AIDS, respiratory infections, and heart disease.[3] In developed countries, non-communicable diseases cause the majority of deaths (77 percent), while in developing countries, communicable diseases such as AIDS and tuberculosis cause most deaths. ("Communicable diseases" are contagious and can be transmitted from one source to another by infectious bacteria or viruses.)

In general, the world's poor die from diseases such as influenza and tuberculosis that are typical of past Western societies.[4] Such disparities show that many diseases in the developing world cannot be treated only by drugs and surgery, but require improving social conditions and encouraging behavioral changes.

The same year that Paul Farmer was born, 1959, in Kinshasa in the Democratic Republic of Congo, a man died of a strange disease that gave him fever, rapid loss of weight, and strange sores. Rumors abound that others in the 1940s and 1950s died the same way. Scientists stored a sample of this African's blood and later discovered that it contained the virus HIV-1, which causes AIDS.

4.1 History of Utilitarian Ethics

As we said in Chapter 1, utilitarianism began in early 19th-century England as a reform movement that defined right acts as producing the greatest amount of good for the greatest number of beings, what Bentham and Mill called "utility."

The Puritans in England and America wanted to organize society so that everyone obeyed their rules, which they held to be from God, but utilitarians thought that many of the inherited ideas were outdated. For example, Puritans forbade dancing.

For Christians, Jews, or Muslims, morality cannot be conceived without God's existence. In contrast, utilitarians saw morality as a human construct that should minimize harm and maximize group welfare.

Nevertheless, utilitarianism is compatible with many aspects of theistic ethics. If a believer thinks that God meant for humans to make the world better by eliminating starvation, torture, dictatorship, and unnecessary pain, then he and utilitarians will agree on many ideas.

Likened to the counterculture movement of the 1960s and 1970s, utilitarianism humanized outmoded institutions of its time. It scorned virtues cherished by England's aristocracy: stylish dress and manners, fetishes about personal honor, and unthinking patriotism.

Its greatest reforms came in 1832 in eliminating pocket boroughs under the control of one great landlord and in extending the vote to 20 percent of the adult male population who had some property (propertyless males and women still had no vote). Utilitarian reformers campaigned against slavery in the British empire and the intolerable factory conditions described by Charles Dickens in novels such as *Hard Times*. Their Factory Act forbade employment of children under age 9 in cotton mills and declared that 13-year-olds could work no more than 12 hours a day. Similar bills were passed to make mining and industrial machinery less lethal to workers.

They also attacked the penal system, passed the Corn Laws, ended debtor's prison, opposed capital punishment for petty thefts, and advocated the vote for women. They urged creation of public hospitals for the poor, proper sewage disposal, the penny post so that everyone could send and get mail, and created a central board of health, so that municipalities could create facilities for clean water, waste disposal, and sewers.

Utilitarians today still see many of our basic ethical feelings as out-of-date. For example, they oppose capital punishment, our treatment of animals, and bans on physician-assisted dying for terminal patients. Insofar as it critiques these practices in ethics and politics, utilitarianism still functions today as a reform movement.

Finally, then and now, utilitarianism inspires its followers to work to relieve world suffering. As Mill wrote in 1861 in *Utilitarianism:*

> Yet no one whose opinion deserves a moment's considera-tion can doubt that most of the great positive evils of the world are in themselves removable, and will, if human affairs continue to improve, be in the end reduced within narrow limits. Poverty, in any sense implying suffering, may be completely extinguished by the wisdom of society com-bined with the good sense and providence of individuals. Even that most intractable of enemies, disease, may be indefinitely reduced in dimensions by good physical and moral education and proper control of noxious influences, while the progress of science holds out a promise for the future of still more direct conquests of this detestable foe.[5]

In June of 1981, the Centers for Disease Control and Prevention (CDC) identified the first three cases of—what it called—GRID (Gay-Related Infectious Disease).

At the time, CDC scientists did not understand how the disease spread or what caused it. Hypotheses included sharing blood, sexual contact without condoms, use of stimulants, and even mosquito bites.

The first three men with GRID (later to be called AIDS) soon died. Within a month, 46 more men were dead and 108 were known to be infected. Because at the time CDC did not know the incubation period, it did not know how many people were infected.

Because most of those infected were gay, drug users, or pros-titutes, public figures such as the Reverend Jerry Falwell and Patrick Buchanan blamed these victims for the disease. These lead-ers claimed that because the deviant behavior of these victims had caused the disease to spread, the victims deserved what they got.

4.2 Virtue Ethics, Medical Saints, and Paul Farmer

Virtue ethicists and Kantians regard a person's motives as a sign of his character. In contrast, John Stuart Mill, who inherited the mantle of utilitarianism from his father and Bentham, says that the drowning man doesn't care why the lifeguard is swimming

out to sea to rescue him, just that the lifeguard really is coming.[6] Utilitarians think motives only count insofar as they tend
to produce the greatest good. For utilitarians, good character is
good because people who have it usually act in ways that produce good for other people. But it's not good in itself.

In medicine, the official view is that it makes a difference
whether a physician listens because she really cares about patients or because she's found that satisfying patients is an effective way to maximize income. A utilitarian might argue that if
the physician's techniques are good enough, whether she really
cares about her patients matters little; in either case, patients get
served. However, many utilitarians would also agree that a good
person determined to do good has high utility in the world and
should be emulated.

Virtue ethicists retort that it is not enough for the physician
to just go through the motions of caring for patients. Eventually,
her patients will see the difference between just going through
the motions and really caring. You can't fake real virtue.

Paul Farmer's life illustrates virtue ethics. Against almost
an entire world of nay-sayers, Farmer single-handedly started a
medical clinic deep in the countryside of Haiti and helped
thousands of people to live better lives. His example inspired
dozens of physicians to join him. Some, such as Jim (Yong)
Kim, went on to become equally lauded and had great careers
of their own (in Kim's case, as director, HIV Department, WHO,
the World Health Organization).

Farmer inspired many medical students and physicians
who thought, "There must be more to medicine than making
money and filling out forms." They left comfortable practices
in pediatrics and nephrology and traveled to dangerous places,
such as Haiti, to make a difference—all because Paul Farmer
wouldn't take "no" when critics said it couldn't be done.

*By 1987, Paul Farmer had become a well-recognized Harvard
professor of infectious diseases, as well as an anthropologist
specializing in Haiti. For his humanitarian work in Haiti, he
received a MacArthur "genius" grant, with which he founded
Partners In Health (PIH), a nonprofit organization dedicated to improving health care in developing countries.[7]*

*During subsequent decades, Dr. Farmer traveled from
Harvard around the world preaching that "the only real*

*nation is humanity" and the obligation of those in privileged
nations is to save the lives of sick people in developing
countries. Undeterred by most people's indifference, Farmer
succeeded well beyond the predictions of his critics.*

4.3 Utilitarianism and the Numbers: Applying Triage

A controversial tenet of utilitarianism is its maximization principle. For utilitarians, numbers matter: It's better to save more
people than fewer. Obviously, that attitude has important implications in public health today when the world faces AIDS, an
out-of-control, lethal communicable disease.

The maximization tenet can get utilitarians into trouble.
Wouldn't utilitarianism be willing to violate the traditional
sanctity-of-life principle to save many people? Here, utilitarians
bite the bullet. They think that the Nazi generals who tried to kill
Hitler in 1944 at Wolf's Lair were justified. They think that on the
expedition to the South Pole in 1913, Commander Robert Scott
should have allowed his crew member with the gangrenous leg to
die, rather than slowing down the whole party by taking turns
carrying him, which resulted in the death of all. They think that
if an FBI sniper saw a terrorist about to detonate a bomb in a bus
full of innocent people, the sniper should shoot the terrorist.

The maximization principle seems to imply that one
should always maximize lives saved, even by doing controversial
things. If we can take the organs from one man and save two
people rather than one, shouldn't we save two? What about a
Jewish mother hiding a family of six from the Nazis outside?
Should she smother her crying baby to save the whole family?
Or is Kant right, that such things should never be done?

What is a defect in some situations can be a virtue in another. When one thinks about the worldwide crisis of halting
the spread of HIV infection, an ethical theory that gives importance to the number of beings affected seems right on target.
With tens of millions of people infected, and equal numbers at
risk, talk about treating each person as "an end in himself," and
giving him or her the highest standard of medical care seems an
outdated luxury, especially if the opportunity cost of this high
care for an individual is *no* care for many others. Perhaps utilitarianism has finally found its time.

*In 1983, Luc Montagnier of the Institut Pasteur in France
discovered that a virus, named the human immunodeficiency
virus (HIV), caused AIDS. In 1984, a test was created to test
for antibodies to HIV.*

*By 1989, more Americans had died of AIDS than had
died in the Vietnam War, over 60,000. The CDC estimated
then that 10 million people might be infected on the
planet.*

*By 2001, AIDS had killed 500,000 Americans and
20 million humans on the planet. Another 40 million had
been infected.*

*According to data released at the 15th World AIDS
Conference in the summer of 2004, 70 million individuals
were infected by HIV, 30 million of whom were already
dead.*

*In the five countries with the greatest concentration
of HIV infection—China, India, Russia, Ethiopia, and
Nigeria—if no strong measures are taken, 75 million people
could be infected by 2010.*

Triage Medicine

In medicine, utilitarianism applies powerfully in public health
and triage situations. Both of these apply to AIDS.

As for the first, improvements in public health almost
certainly have helped more people live longer (created more
"utility") than all the drugs and surgeries ever invented. As
an example, consider the work of English physician John Snow.
In 1849, he advocated clean water to prevent cholera epidemics,
which spread by contaminated water. Although it took 40 years
and several more cholera epidemics for Snow's ideas to prevail, eventually they did, and as a result, millions of people
have been saved from cholera, and contemporary people in
developed countries now take clean water (and longer life) for
granted.

A second application involves *triage*. Triage involves the
apportionment of scarce resources during emergencies when
circumstances preordain that not all victims will live. Because
consequences count, utilitarianism says a physician should *not*
treat each patient equally, but should focus only on those whom
he can actually benefit. Rigorous application of this principle

gives utilitarianism its controversial hard edge: A physician should abandon those who will die anyway, even if he could soothe their pain, and just as ruthlessly, abandon those who will live anyway without his help. He should help only those who waver between life and death and for whom he can make a difference. The goal is to save the most lives.

So in the classic scenario of a lifeboat in the middle of the Pacific Ocean after a shipwreck, with an officer at the helm with a gun and too many people outside the lifeboat trying to get in, utilitarians say that the officer should only choose those who will be the strongest rowers. Before that, he must deny others entry into the boat to prevent it from sinking. Although harsh, this thinking is designed to maximize the number of lives saved rather than to let all die by having chaos reign. The officer may even have to do something wrong according to Kantian ethics: Kill innocent people attempting to enter the overloaded boat.

If you were in the water, you would want a utilitarian lifeboat captain rather than a Kantian one, as the former would try to save the most people. The latter might just keep letting each identified person into the lifeboat, such that it would soon sink and everyone would drown.

A compromise would be for the Kantian lifeboat captain to draw straws about who was allowed in the lifeboat. Even then, he could not throw people overboard who got short straws because that would be a direct killing of the innocent, a violation of Kantian principles.

This point illustrates an ambiguity in sanctity-of-life ethics. Traditionally, sanctity-of-life ethics such as Kant's emphasize the absolute value of each individual, implying that the physician should at least comfort those who are beyond his help. But utilitarian-triage ethics maximizes the value of life in saving the maximal number of people who can actually live. In some contexts, utilitarianism can be more pro-life than Kantian or Christian ethics.

Finally, triage ethics in medicine has seen a resurgence after the bombing of the World Trade Center in 2001.[8] A new subspecialty in emergency medicine, disaster medicine, trains physicians and nurses to assess situations where tens of thousands of people have been injured from explosions or exposed to lethal biological agents. In some situations, physicians must first protect themselves (e.g., from SARS), lest they themselves rapidly succumb and die. After that, triage ethics must prevail.

> *Even though Partners In Health began as a one-person mission, Paul Farmer always sought international support. He persisted and obtained financial aid from the Gates Foundation, the Soros Foundation, and the World Health Organization. Farmer traveled to the countryside of Haiti, the slums of Peru and Cuba, and the prisons of Russia to promote equity of health care.*
>
> *He also addressed the alarming spread of multidrug resistant (MDR) tuberculosis (TB) in poor countries. Farmer emphasized to international health-care providers that partial treatment of TB patients with the standard four TB medications was producing resistant strains of TB. He focused on the poorest areas of the world and advocated community-based approaches to fighting MDR-TB and AIDS, with full treatment for all TB patients.*

4.4 Halting AIDS: The Challenge to Ethical Theories

As we have said, modern medicine faces its greatest challenge in delaying and eradicating the spread of AIDS. Physicians could save more lives by keeping AIDS in check than by all other efforts combined.

Bioethics is also challenged by the problem of how to halt the spread of AIDS. Consider some ethical dilemmas caused by AIDS: Does giving out condoms and clean needles solve the problem or inflame it? Do we attack behavior or the virus in trying to stop the spread? Do we use nonmoralistic education or moralistic condemnation? Does giving infected people medicine encourage them not to take precautions against infection? Is giving expensive antiretroviral medicine to each HIV-infected person futile with such large numbers of the infected?

Arresting the spread of AIDS is also a moral issue of global distributive justice. In developed countries, HIV infection has become a treatable disease. But for most people in the developing world, because they have no access to AIDS medications, infection from HIV is a death sentence. So the world's medical leaders and heads of state face this challenge: Do they cast a blind eye to the rest of the world, watching a billion or two billion people succumb to AIDS? Or do they finally wake up and start a massive, realistic effort to break the back of this disease?

As Paul Farmer says, the HIV-infected are seen as "Other," not like us. Most have brown or black skins and do not speak English. Does our moral concern extend to those infected with HIV in sub-Saharan Africa? How much are we willing to change to help them?

On some level, preventing HIV infection is also an issue of virtue ethics. Many North Americans and Europeans drive vehicles worth $30,000 or more. How many lives could be saved in Africa from the money diverted to AIDS medications from one such vehicle? Or is this just a ridiculous example, since the money diverted might never get there, or help, or if it did at first, the people might still later make the wrong decisions and die? Virtue ethicists say that good people should "live simply so that other people can simply live."

4.5 Kantian and Utilitarian Ideals about Patient Care

Dr. Farmer's approach to patients in rural Haiti is to treat them as if they were patients in his clinic at Harvard. That is, he endeavors to deliver to his patients the best of medical care, no matter what the cost and no matter where they are.

Paul Farmer does not assume, for example, that a procedure that requires strict compliance and help would be unfeasible in Haiti. So patients in renal failure, who might be left to die in most poor countries, get put on dialysis machines at his clinic. He might even try to get a promising young patient a kidney transplant, even though such a transplant costs a quarter of a million dollars.

Although he does not call it this name, Farmer's approach is essentially Kantian. Each HIV-infected patient is treated as an end-in-himself and each is given the best possible treatment. That is, we must have no double standard with HIV-infected Haitians or Africans. Each must be given the gold standard for HIV treatment: A cocktail of antiretroviral drugs several times each day with close monitoring by physicians.

Utilitarians see things in a different way. The biologist Garrett Hardin has argued that the planet is like a lifeboat with so many people wanting to get in that if we adopt Christian or Kantian ethics, which value each individual as an end-in-himself, we will let everyone in the boat and the boat will sink.[9] Developed countries are the lifeboat, with limited amounts of resources, and the developing countries of the world are survivors of the wreck at sea, all wanting to get in.

In this situation, Hardin advocated that we should not give money to save victims of famine because they will only have more children later who will fall victim to another famine in their lifetime. Instead, we should triage large parts of the world, letting them save themselves if they can, but generally not wasting our resources on them. Like good triage officers, we should only expend our limited charity on countries where the people are willing to change and become self-sufficient.

Controversies about the environment illuminate Hardin's ideas. Some environmentalists think we should not aid Catholic countries that ban birth control. For them, giving aid to such countries is pouring money down the drain.

Other environmentalists, for example Colorado governor Richard Lamm, think we should close our borders and not let millions of unskilled, illegal immigrants enter America, not for racial or ethnic reasons, but because added millions of people use up our limited water, clean air, and natural resources. To save the American environment, we must reduce human consumption. How to do that? One answer: reduce the number of Americans.

What are the implications, then, for treating HIV infection on Lifeboat Earth? First, for utilitarians, we cannot afford the Kantian approach to patient care with the 40 million HIV-infected people worldwide. Using this approach is like giving one lucky patient in your hospital 6 quadruple organ transplants, desperately trying to save him over and over, while ignoring 25 anonymous people who never received one organ.

Second, and truth to tell, the Kantian approach makes the individual physician feel like a hero riding to the rescue of the victim: He is the dispenser of the magical medicines, not the cold bureaucrat. But perhaps this psychological satisfaction is too costly in the face of this huge, expanding tragedy of AIDS.

In Boris Pasternak's *Dr. Zhivago*, and the great movie of the same title by director David Lean, the good Dr. Zhivago follows the Kantian approach with each patient he meets. But he lives in the terrible time of the overthrow of the czar and the beginning of communist Russia. To free the people from the iron grip of the White Russians and their army, the new Russia needs hard-headed, unsentimental men, as symbolized by Pasha, who changes his name and becomes the tough communist general Strelnikov, the kind of man whom Russia needs at its critical transition. To prevent a world with a billion HIV-infected people, utilitarians suggest, we need some medical Strelnikovs.

Instead of the Kantian approach, we should pick out strong rowers for the long row across the ocean, and try to save their lives, so that some live rather than all die. In this way, we pick pragmatic countries with educable citizens willing to learn and to change their behaviors, such that the whole country is spared. Or we choose strange bedfellows, such as Fidel Castro, whose quarantine program gave Cuba, despite a large sex tourism business over the last decade, a miniscule incidence of HIV infection.

Kantians can defend themselves against utilitarians in various ways.

First, does the world really need more hard-headed Strelnikovs to fight AIDS against sentimental Kantian physicians? Well, every arrogant researcher who has ever abused research subjects under his medical care has used the same utilitarian appeal to the distant, general good. (Stalin is reported to have said, "*Everything* is justified in the long run, if you take a long enough view.")

In the 1996 movie *Extreme Measures*, the arrogant medical researcher played by Gene Hackett justifies his violation of traditional medical ethics and the Kantian ideal of the doctor–patient relationship by retorting, "If you could cure cancer by torturing and killing one person, wouldn't you have to do it?"

Kant answers, "No." Even if the sky will fall and the world will perish, people should always do what is right. No amount of good consequences justifies torturing and killing an innocent person, especially by a physician charged with his care.

Despite his general interest in international health care, Farmer has placed much of his focus specifically in the Central Plateau of Haiti. In the poorest countryside of

Haiti, his clinic, "Zanmi Lasante" (Creole for "Partners In Health"), prospers. Once a small clinic, it has now expanded beyond the village of Cange and into a multifaceted health complex that includes a school, surgery wing, infirmary, and pediatric care facility. Zanmi Lasante treats approximately 1000 patients daily free of charge, and is focused on the prevention and treatment of TB, malaria, and HIV/AIDS.

Realizing early in his experience in destitute situations that health care involves more than clinical treatment, Farmer and his staff have established housing, water, food, and even education programs. As a result of Zanmi Lasante's success, Haiti received financial award from the Global Fund to Fight AIDS, Tuberculosis, and Malaria. Since then, the clinic has spread into neighboring communities, where it serves as the only hospital for patients miles away. In his original medical clinic in Cange, his small medical staff often sees close to 220,000 patients each year.[10]

4.6 Mill's Critique of Kantian Ethics

John Stuart Mill was aware of Kantian ethics and referred to it in his great essay, *Utilitarianism*. Mill denies that any logical contradictions occur from adopting evil maxims:

> He (Kant) fails, almost grotesquely, to show that there would be any contradiction, any logical (not to say physical) impossibility, on the adoption by all rational beings of the most outrageously immoral rules of conduct. All he shows is that the consequences of their universal adoption would be such as no one would choose to incur.[11]

This is a powerful point. One can logically will that everyone be selfish and not contradict oneself: Of course, in doing so, when one's car breaks down on a deserted stretch of highway, one cannot expect any help. Similarly, one can will without contradiction that everyone should steal when they think they can do so without detection. One will then take precautions and act as if everyone is trying to steal his property. But there is no contradiction in so acting and believing.

From a utilitarian point of view, Kantian ethics has another big problem. Conflicts among maxims cannot be solved by logic, but must either be irresolvable or appeal to consequences. Kant does not say much about this problem, but he denies that appeal to consequences is proper in determining morality.

Utilitarians think Paul Farmer's approach is noble but misguided. For them, the road to hell is paved with good intentions. Instead of focusing on providing the best care for the particular patient before him, Dr. Farmer should attempt to save the maximal number of lives with the resources he has.

That is to say, physicians should not approach AIDS using the traditional rule of rescue and doctor–patient relationship. Recall from Chapter 2 about Ernie Crowfeather that the Rule of Rescue is where physicians give arbitrarily identified patients maximal resources, but ignore anonymous patients outside the system, who die.

One way of seeing Farmer's and the Kantian approach to patient care is simply as an instantiation of the Rule of Rescue. The patients Farmer happens to see at this clinic get the best care, while those on the other side of the island get nothing and die.

Idealistic, nonutilitarian approaches aren't helping the world's poor or delaying the spread of HIV infection. We can keep screaming and pleading for more resources, but the fact is, the number of people infected by HIV keeps dramatically growing while the world gives only a small amount of resources to fight AIDS. Given those facts, those resources should be used in utilitarian-triage fashion to save the most lives possible and, sadly, to ignore the rest. In reality, what that means is allocating all the existing money to preventing the spread of HIV in countries with cooperating leaders and attitudes, while triaging countries with bad attitudes and uncooperative leaders.

Nothing else can work. The World AIDS Conference in 2004 in Thailand reported one failure after another. Most impressively, in the preceding year, 5 *million* new cases of HIV infection occurred.[12] Even if the cost of antiretroviral treatment drops to a $1 a week per person, that's $125 million that must be donated each year for the next several decades, just to prevent HIV in these new cases from progressing to AIDS.

And what about the remaining (estimated) 40 million HIV-infected people? Treating them at the same rate would cost $2 billion more a year, each and every year, for the next few decades. And of course, the $1 a week figure is way too low.

The reality is that most people will not get treated for HIV infection, that $2 billion spent on preventing another 40 million people from getting infected is more cost-effective, *and will save more lives,* than treating those who are now infected.

Given the failure of the present methods, if the present 40 million people infect another 80 million—as could happen as HIV sweeps from Poland across the steppes of Russia and China, down into India—then adoption of an idealistic, patient-centered ethical position would be one of the greatest mistakes in the history of medicine. At first, Farmer's saintly ideal seems noble, but the utilitarian physician-captain has to constantly keep in mind that the opportunity cost, which may be that treating one identified, HIV-infected person with $20 worth of medicine diverts $20 from prevention and thus condemns several children and women to HIV infection. Moreover, this process will repeat tens of millions of times around the globe.

No other disaster on this scale has ever occurred in human history.[13] The saddest part is that, because humans know how to prevent these deaths from occurring and have it in their power to do so, this human tragedy is completely avoidable.

4.7   Farmer and Rawls on Just Medical Care

In "Rethinking Medical Ethics: A View from Below," Paul Farmer and Nicole Gastineau Campos critique contemporary medical ethics from the view of vulnerable, poor people in developing countries. As we might expect, Farmer chastises modern bioethics for either ignoring the dire needs of those dying from AIDS (e.g., by focusing on problems of surrogate mothers, cloning, or live organ donors) or by turning a blind eye in research protocols to the exploitation of the plight of people in developing countries.

Poor Haitians and Africans are guinea pigs who "volunteer" to participate in experiments in which they never understand the real risks. "Medicine, public health, and research are all caught up in a web of unequal relations," Farmer says.[14]

The world's poor suffer the research, while the world's rich garner the medical benefits. Take organ donations. The wealthy receive first pick of organs, while the poor are pressed to "donate" their own organs for money.

Farmer adopts John Rawls's theory of justice with its theme that society should focus the world's medical resources on the neediest. We must "resocialize" and reconceptualize bioethics to exclude no longer those "down below," but to focus on raising them up.

John Rawls, an important American philosopher, argued in his *A Theory of Justice* (1970) that a just, democratic society could be regulated by two foundational principles, the *liberty principle* and the *difference principle*. The first proposed a society giving citizens maximal liberty compatible with equal liberty for everyone else; the second proposed that "differences" or inequalities are only just if they benefit everyone and especially the least well-off group in society.

Rawls combines the deontological ethics of Kant with the social contract tradition of Hobbes and Rousseau. Under a *veil of ignorance* about one's present position in society, one's health, one's race or gender, Rawls argues that self-interested people would choose his two principles.

Rawls and Farmer agree that the training and privileges of physicians are only justified if this unequal system benefits the least well-off. If our scope is the world, the present structure of worldwide medicine does not seem to benefit the poorest and sickest people, and so for Rawls or Farmer, is unjust.

More from Utilitarians

Imagine that there has been a terrible disaster at sea and that 40 million people are treading water, asking to be saved. Another 5 million will join them soon. The world has only so many resources to commit, so what should be done?

One approach is to send out a few luxury ocean liners, like the *Queen Elizabeth II*, and pick up the first ones found, giving them first-class passage back to land. The fortunate, lucky ones picked up in this way will get their own dry, clean beds, food, and friendly support of the crew. Of course, few people will be saved this way, but those who are will not be treated any differently than any other survivor found at sea.

The alternative, utilitarian approach is to quickly identify pockets with large numbers of survivors who appear willing and able to row to land, then quickly airdrop thousands of small boats, equipped with water and emergency rations. In this way, many thousands of people will be able to either row to land or stay alive until freighters and other ships reach them.

We will also need to choose, by air and in advance, exactly where to drop the boats and where to ignore one or two swimmers desperately trying to flag down our planes for a boat. Cruel as it may seem, simply to drop the boats on the first swimmers we see is to condemn too many other people to die.

In exactly the same way, a good utilitarian at the head of the Global Fund Against AIDS will identify those countries willing to do what it takes to suspend the spread of HIV and give them the resources they need to do so. In this way, scarce resources will maximize life in a tragic situation.

So utilitarians such as E. Marseille and others argue that new funds for AIDS in sub-Saharan Africa should be earmarked for preventing new cases of HIV, not for treating people infected with HIV or in the last stages of AIDS.[15] For countries with limited funds for fighting AIDS, these authors argue that "prevention is at least 28 times more cost-effective than HAART [highly active antiretroviral therapy]."

Let us consider another matter. Sometimes, well-intentioned but naïve people create more harm than good. Such could be the case in fighting AIDS. Here are some examples.

In prior decades, HIV-infected patients secured anti-HIV drugs from underground pharmacies, split them with friends who had no access or insurance, undercut clinical trials by discovering the placebo and sharing the real drug, and mixed anti-AIDS drugs with many herbs and other drugs. Unfortunately, such partial compliance allows resistant strains of HIV to emerge.

In Africa, a family must sometimes choose only one member to receive antiretroviral drugs when everyone is infected. Often that person is the male wage-earner. But many African fathers are tempted to share their drugs with their children or their wives, hoping for some benefit for all. Others will mix the good drugs with home-grown remedies, creating conditions for emergence of resistant strains.

This, sadly, is an argument for triage of whole countries with simultaneous saturation-treatment for selected others. Partial or bad treatment of HIV might create a super strain of HIV resistant to all known drugs and, perhaps, one more easily transmissible. For the good of the living and future generations, HIV-infected patients should either get full treatment for their lifetimes or no treatment at all.

Must Farmer and Kantians accept this critique and bow to triage of whole countries? Perhaps not. When a physician happens on a scene after a plane crash, circumstances beyond her control may force her to be a triage officer, but when a patient enters her office (or, in some places, her tent), the patient expects the physician to do everything possible for him. If physicians adopt utilitarian reasoning, they cease being physicians and become health bureaucrats—or worse, *judges.*

Farmer and Kant think a physician should do everything possible for each patient before him and to be that patient's advocate. Beginning and end of story. This means securing for that patient the best antivirals, the best surgery, and the best preventive care. It is immoral to have double standards for rich and poor.

The low esteem in which medicine is held by modern citizens may stem from physicians adopting too many conflicting roles: gatekeepers for health maintenance organizations (HMOs), bureaucrats, researchers, and agents of drug companies (in accepting gifts and monetary inducements).

For example, as Nicoli Nattrass argues, if people testing positive can obtain the best anti-AIDS drugs, voluntary counseling will prevent more new HIV infections.[16] (She argues that if they can't get the drugs, what's the point of getting tested? So getting the drugs encourages testing, which in turn increases awareness of HIV infection, which in turn reduces new rates of infection.) She claims that in middle-class countries such as South Africa, where people receive expensive treatment in hospitals for opportunistic infections caused by AIDS, treating HIV aggressively at the early stages may save a huge chunk of money that would otherwise be spent on end-of-life care in hospitals.

4.8 Placebos with AIDS Drugs on Vulnerable Africans

In addition to the Nuremberg Code, *the Declaration of Helsinki* has been adopted by many professional organizations and contains a list of rights of research subjects.[17] The most important requirement is that in any kind of research, all patients must get the best proven diagnostic techniques and drugs. This

Declaration bans placebos in drug studies when an effective drug already is used in practice.

Despite this Declaration, the randomized clinical trial (RCT) is considered the gold standard of all medical research. An RCT may not benefit an individual patient, especially if it involves a section (or arm) where such patients receive a placebo (a fake, empty drug) to prove that the drug under question really works (in the treatment arm).

Whether it is a new drug or new kind of surgery, the first time an innovation is tried is unlikely to benefit a patient. Despite the deluge of wonderful stories in the mass media about medical successes, progress in medicine comes slowly and most things do not work the first time. Indeed, in a Phase I study, the first stage of studying a new drug, researchers study not a drug's possible therapeutic value (Phase II), but its safety or harm; in other words, they study whether the drug could harm patients.

Whether subjects in the control group receive medicine or standard drugs is controversial. Many established drugs were originally proven effective in contrast with placebos. However, the Declaration of Helsinki requires that subjects receive any standard drug and compare it to any new drug. Drug companies argue that placebos are a simpler, more efficient way of establishing efficacy than comparisons to current drugs. The FDA allows both kinds of studies, but seems to prefer studies with placebos.[18]

The late bioethicist Benjamin Freedman argued that randomized clinical trials (RCTs) are only justified in a situation of *clinical equipoise,* where honest professionals sincerely disagree about the preferred treatment.[19] Bioethicist Charles Weijer builds on Freedman's position in arguing that placebos in RCTs are only justified for first-generation drugs, but after such drugs are established, placebo-controlled trials are no longer justified.[20] For research on subjects with schizophrenia, Weijer argues that placebo controls are only justified when either subjects have failed to respond to all standard drugs or subjects could benefit from a second line of therapy to bolster their first-line, standard drug.

The ethics of placebos in research has already caused a major battle between utilitarians and Kantians over research. What happened is instructive for future battles in this ongoing struggle.

In 1994, a federally sponsored 076 regimen proved that giving AZT (zidovudine) during pregnancy cut transmission of HIV from mother to child by two-thirds.[21] Armed with these results, the next year, CDC, National Institutes of Health (NIH), and WHO adopted a utilitarian strategy to reduce the number of babies born with HIV in Africa. But first they needed to see if a small amount of AZT could prevent vertical transmission (mothers infecting their babies) just as easily and as completely as a large dosage. With this goal in mind, they designed a prospective RCT to prove this, including a control group who received placebos (no treatment).

As the study progressed, executive editor of the *New England Journal of Medicine* Marcia Angell blasted the research and likened it to the Tuskegee Study (see Chapter 8) because African babies were born with preventable HIV infection when a standard treatment existed that could prevent such infection.[22] Angell also charged, correctly, that if done in America, the research would be considered unethical.

Was the study like Tuskegee? Well, it had subjects who were: (1) black, (2) female, (3) poor, (4) illiterate, (5) victims of STDs, (6) without other available treatment, and (7) subjects of a grand experiment run by a huge, distant government bureaucracy—all much like the Tuskegee Study.

Public Citizen, a consumer rights organization founded by Ralph Nader, and its Health Research Group (run by physicians Sidney Wolfe and Peter Lurie), joined Angell's charges.[23] All argued that AZT greatly reduced transmission of HIV from mother to child, that mothers in control groups wouldn't get it, and that withholding it couldn't be justified.

These criticisms sparked fierce rebuttals. Researchers retorted that, even if the research had not been done, because of lack of money, these mothers would never have gotten AZT. So they were no worse off than they would have been "in nature," before researchers arrived.

Angell countered that it had long been established that placebo-controlled studies could not be done on Americans mothers. Once AZT had been shown to prevent transmission of HIV, it became *the standard of care* for all pregnant, HIV+ women. Angell and Nader denied that medical research should adopt a double standard for developed versus developing countries. "If it is unethical to do placebo-controlled trials in America, it should also be unethical to do them in third world countries," they said.

They charged that double standards violated the Nuremberg Code and Guideline 15 of the International Ethical Guidelines for Biomedical Research Involving Human Subjects, which prohibits such double standards.[24] They also cited the Declaration of Helsinki, which required that subjects in developing countries receive not just the best treatment available *locally*, but the best treatment available *anywhere*.[25]

Apologists, including officials in developing countries, replied that ethical imperialists were imposing American standards on African countries. They also emphasized that some local officials had also lost children to HIV.[26]

Philosophically, officials at CDC and NIH implicitly adopted utilitarianism, whereas Angell and Nader explicitly championed Kantian ideals. Angell agreed with Kant and his axiom that people can never be used as a means, as well as his belief that ethical principles are not local but universal. Kantians especially objected to the double standard, where women in the developed countries always get AZT, but women in undeveloped countries got placebos.

The sponsoring agencies, which included those doing research funded by Belgium, Denmark, and France, replied that 300,000 children became infected every year with HIV by perinatal transmission, and that if they could prove—via a placebo-controlled trial—that a shorter regimen could reduce transmission by half, then they could save 150,000 children a year. If delays were caused by the skeptics' criticisms—in putting off proof for a year or more—then such criticisms would cost many children's lives.

Central to the defense of these studies by public health agencies were two more claims: A placebo-controlled trial of HIV transmission could be done faster and with fewer subjects than an AZT-controlled study, and that once good results were obtained, African and Asian governments would give all pregnant, HIV+ women the new, smaller dosage of AZT. (Research with placebos is also discussed in Chapter 8.)

Angell and others argued that placebo-controlled studies were not necessary to prove such results, that retrospectively comparing dosages of AZT to other treatments or to each other could prove the same thing. More important, they strongly denied that, given the poverty of such countries, a proven, reduced dosage would later be given to all pregnant women in such countries. Even a cheap AZT regimen for $80, they pointed out, was 11 times what was normally spent on the average African's annual medical care.

Champions on both sides claimed justice for their side, and this dispute was essentially philosophical, not factual.[27] For utilitarian researchers, the risk-benefit ratio had to differ for poor, illiterate women in developing countries, who otherwise would not get treatment, than for rich people in developed countries. For Kantians, this was the same alleged utilitarian reasoning that led to the Tuskegee Study and to the Nazi experiments: Acquiring new knowledge justifies allowing vulnerable patients to be harmed. Kantians also objected to the view that "they're going to get HIV anyway, so we might as well study them to learn something." As Angell echoed Kant, "People can't be used as a means to a noble end."[28]

On February 18, 1998, CDC suspended the studies, announcing that the experimental, reduced-dosage treatment had been proven effective in reducing mother-to-child HIV transmission, that is, $80 worth of AZT in the last four weeks of pregnancy cut transmission in half.[29] Both sides claimed victory at this early state of the American-sponsored studies.

In the summer of 2004, a similar controversy flared in Cambodia, when 150 prostitutes rejected a randomized, placebo-controlled trial of anti-AIDS drug Viread sponsored by the Gates Foundation, the National Institutes of Health, and the Centers for Disease Control and Prevention.[30] The trial was supposed to focus on at-risk sex workers, and to see if Viread prevented them from getting infected with HIV. Half of them would have gotten a placebo; sex workers objected to the placebo. Obviously, Kantians condemned the trial.

At the end of 2004, the issue of double standards in AIDS research created distrust when it was revealed that the chief of NIH's AIDS division, Dr. Edmund Tramont, had rushed the drug nevirapine into usage in Africa to prevent vertical transmission and had suppressed objections from his staff about the drug's safety.[31] South Africa's ruling party, headed by Thabo Mbeki, accused the United States of using Africans as "guinea pigs."

4.9 Cost of AIDS Drugs

As AZT proved effective, and as new protease inhibitors proved even more so in the 1990s, HIV infection became a manageable disease in developed countries, costing between $10,000 and $20,000 a year to treat with a cocktail of three antiretroviral drugs. But the high cost of these drugs caused a crisis among the Paul Farmers of the world, who argued that millions of HIV-infected people were dying to protect the intellectual property rights of Western drug companies.

In this instance, drug companies faced a powerful coalition of utilitarians and Kantians, all of whom argued against the high cost of these drugs. To the argument that drug companies "deserved" high returns on their investments, critics replied that government-supported research on such drugs did not mean that companies could charge whatever they wanted. Moreover, critics denied that charging cheaper prices in developing countries would create an underground market for such drugs, lowering the prices in developed countries such as America.

During the 1990s, activists chained themselves to bike stands in front of headquarters of drug companies and protested on Wall Street and outside of medical meetings where drug companies hawked their wares. After five years of protest, in which even presidential nominee Al Gore criticized the companies, they backed down and allowed developing countries to manufacture the drugs and sell them at a tenth of the American price.

Even that was only part of the battle, because in order to use the drugs, poor countries needed clinics in remote parts of the country staffed with qualified people, supplied with electricity for refrigerators to house the drugs, and supervisors who would monitor people and make them take the drugs correctly. In short, the developing countries needed the infrastructure of a minimal, modern medical system—not an easy task to accomplish.

On grounds of world security and compassion, the Paul Farmers of the world argued that rich people simply cannot let 100 million Africans die of AIDS, and their efforts provoked some response. By 2005, developed countries, including the United States, had committed billions of dollars to halting the spread of HIV in Africa. Demonstration projects were up and running in South Africa, Zambia, and Angola. Idealistic physicians abandoned lucrative careers in specialties and followed Paul Farmer's example, traveling to Africa and rolling up their sleeves to fight AIDS there. As one of them said, "This is one of medicine's greatest crises. How could we stay at home growing rich while so many of the world's poor are dying? Medicine will be judged later by how it responded to this crisis."[32]

CONCLUSIONS

If John Stuart Mill were brought back to life and read the previous sections of this chapter, he might well remark that, given the urgency of AIDS on the world's stage, something important has been omitted from his defense of utilitarianism and its defense by modern philosophers. That is, like Kantian and virtue ethics, utilitarianism requires addressing the world's AIDS problem in more ways than just individual saints and their heroic battles.

Peter Singer, a modern utilitarian, has led the charge to emphasize that the needs of the starving and dying in the world require a structural critique of life in the developing world. In "Famine, Affluence, and Morality," an article published in 1972, and more recently in *One World,* Singer argues on utilitarian grounds that it is immoral to drive SUVs (which pollute the planet at twice the rate of fuel-efficient cars), eat meat from animals raised in factory farms, and consume extravagant amounts of material goods while people around the world starve and die of AIDS.[33]

His critique of medicine might go even deeper. Commonly, many medical graduates pursue the "ROAD to happiness" where ROAD is an acronym standing for Radiology, Ophthalmology, Anesthesiology, and Dermatology, to which Plastic Surgery could also be added. Given so many people dying of AIDS, can American medicine really justify so many physicians going into these fields, which command incomes of over $300,000 with flexible hours?

Can American society justify the large number of lifestyle drugs marketed directly to customers on television, which drives up the prices of drugs for our elderly and the world's poor, while so little of drug research is directed toward cheap, safe drugs to treat AIDS, malaria, and respiratory infections—the chief killers of the world's poor?

Perhaps most important, once the research for the drug has been done and it has passed clinical trials, the marginal cost of producing extra pills is almost nothing. That is, drug companies can recover their costs and make their profits on people in developed countries and still be magnanimous in either making extra drugs for people in developing countries or letting them make their own versions at cheap prices under license.[34]

Both utilitarians and Kantians can agree that it is a false dilemma that says one must choose between helping many AIDS victims and helping some, especially when 99 percent of the citizens of developing countries help no person at all with AIDS. They might conclude by saying that, with this great crisis upon us, the moral question is not *how* we should act, but *whether*.

It would be nice if this discussion were merely academic, but it is not. The fate of tens of million of people hangs on its answer. It would be nice if ethical controversy were not part of the problem and that the study of ethics could show the way to the solution. However, as seen in discussions of abstinence and vertical-HIV-transmission trials, that isn't true.

Since Tracy Kidder made Paul Farmer famous in 2003, massive upheaval and flooding in Haiti have killed thousands of people and undermined the medical infrastructure that Partners In Health had built. President Aristide was forced to flee, gangs have taken over the country, and for the tenth time in its recent history, Haiti has descended into chaos. Virtually everyone agrees that Haiti is so full of corruption that even its main hospital cannot hire competent nurses or workers because such appointments are handed out as political patronage. Even its remaining hospital lacks drugs, electricity, and doctors.[35] Skeptics wonder whether pouring more money into Haiti, especially for expensive antiretroviral drugs for HIV-infected patients, is not pouring good money down the drain.

On the other hand, Paul Farmer's life inspired hundreds of young physicians to renounce boutique medicine to serve in developing countries. Harvard Medical School started a Division of Social Medicine and Health Inequalities, where 20 physicians bring the best medical care to patients in Siberia, Peru,

Haiti, and poor Boston neighborhoods.[36] And Tracy Kidder's book about Farmer made him so renowned that many charities back his work, enabling him to start a new clinic in remote eastern Rwanda, an area devastated by genocide a decade earlier and with half a million HIV-infected citizens.[37]

Other countries, such as Brazil and Uganda, have made great strides in educating their citizens about AIDS and in preventing new infections. These countries are rays of light, whereas the possibility of multidrug resistant HIV is a harbinger of medical apocalypse. The good utilitarian knows where to put his money.

Nevertheless, Kantians point out there are other values at stake: Giving everyone the best possible treatment may prevent many hundreds of thousands of children from being orphaned and create millions of additional years of life for people living with HIV.

Given the above comment about false dilemmas, perhaps both Kantians and utilitarians can agree with another statement of John Stuart Mill:

> All the grand sources, in short, of human suffering are in a great degree, many of them almost entirely conquerable by human care and effort; and though their removal is grievously slow—though a long succession of generations will perish in the reach before the conquest is completed, and this world becomes all that, if will and knowledge were not wanting, it might easily be made—yet every mind sufficiently intelligent and generous to bear a part, however small and inconspicuous, in the endeavor will draw a noble enjoyment from the contest itself, which he would not for any bribe in the form of selfish indulgence content to be without.[38]

FURTHER READINGS

Farmer, Paul. *AIDS and Accusation: Haiti and the Geography of Blame.* Berkeley: University of California Press, 1993.

Kauffman, Kyle Dean, et al. *AIDS and South Africa: The Social Expression of a Pandemic.* New York: Macmillan, 2004.

Kidder, Tracy. *Mountain Beyond Mountains: The Quest of Dr. Paul Farmer—A Man Who Would Cure the World.* New York: Random House, 2003.

Mill, John Stuart. *Utilitarianism.* 1861. New York: Oxford University Press, 1998.

Nattrass, Nicoli. *The Moral Economy of AIDS in South Africa.* Cambridge, England: Cambridge University Press, 2003.

Partners In Health Web site
http://www.pih.org/index.html

Shilts, Randy. *And the Band Played On: Politics, People, and the AIDS Epidemic.* New York: Basic Books, 1985.

CHAPTER 5

*E*motivism and Banning *Some Conceptions*

This chapter describes ethical issues raised by new ways of creating babies. These methods have emerged over the last 30 years and include artificial insemination, in vitro fertilization, egg transfer, surrogacy, implantation of multiple embryos, and postmenopausal women gestating fetuses to birth. The chapter also discusses reproductive cloning and the ethical theory of emotivism.

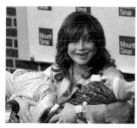 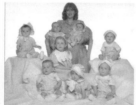 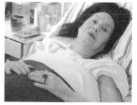

Aleta St. James   Bobbi McCaughey   Adriana Iliescu

*On November 15, 2004, Aleta St. James gave birth to a
5-pound, 12-ounce girl named Francesca and a 5-pound,
3-ounce boy named Gian. Three days later, she turned 57.*

*Raised a Roman Catholic, the unmarried mother claimed
her own grandmother bore her mother when her grandmother
was 53. "My mother grew up fine," and "my grandmother
lasted a long time in her life, and I didn't think that was a
big problem."*[1]

Ms. St. James's twins, delivered by cesarean, developed through in vitro fertilization by implanting eggs from a younger woman that were mixed with sperm from a former boyfriend of hers.

At the time of the births, Ms. St. James became the second-oldest American woman to give birth to twins. In 1998, Judy Cates had twins and delivered at 57.

A few months later, a 57-year-old great-grandmother in Alabama, after having implanted embryos created by in vitro fertilization, gave birth to twins, who respectively weighed 4 pounds and 3 pounds at birth.[2] Rosee Swain and her husband of Fort Payne already had two grown children in their 30s, who gave her six grandchildren. Rosee also had two great-grandchildren, who were a year or two older than her own month-old twins. Rosee hoped the births encouraged other older women to have children late in life. "There are lots of options for older women like me," she said. "Women shouldn't give up hope without exploring all the options."

Many people felt disgust at these older women creating babies. They felt that for them to gestate babies was unnatural, dangerous, and bad for children.

5.1 Background: Assisted Reproduction

Biblical patriarch Abraham and his infertile wife Sarah struggled to produce an heir and he eventually had sex with Hagar, a younger, unmarried woman (a "handmaiden"), to conceive his son Ishmael (Genesis 16:1–4). Patriarch Jacob did the same with his handmaiden Billah (Genesis 30:1–5). Because patriarchal societies valued a male heir to ensure orderly transfer of property and authority, the Bible overlooked these transgressions.

Until the 20th century, infertile couples had to fatalistically accept "being barren" or else divorce in hopes of finding more fertile partners. Medical pioneers J. Marion Sims in the 1860s and Robert Latou Dickenson in the 1930s artificially inseminated wives with husband's sperm (AIH), but ceased trying after condemnation from other physicians and clergy.[3]

Attitudes softened in the 1960s when physicians used AIH to successfully create babies. Using simple procedures, they succeeded without much advance in underlying knowledge. AIH also cost very little.

Unfortunately, AIH couldn't help most infertile couples, whose infertility was caused by older women with less potent eggs or older men with fewer sperm per ejaculate.[4] So physicians tried the next easy step: using sperm of another man (AID), whose identity was usually (but not always) kept anonymous. Some people condemned AID because it produced a child who typically did not know his genetic father. Indeed, the technique may be used to give babies to women who do not want fathers around at all—an especially controversial motive.

Even though another male may raise and legally adopt the child, bioethicists David James and Daniel Callahan argue that it is harmful to intentionally create a child who will lack a connection to his male ancestor.[5] Moreover, when donation of sperm is truly anonymous and when workers destroy records, AID children will never know anything about their biological fathers. "Is this good for the child?" these critics ask.

In the early 1970s, attempts to unite sperm and egg outside the womb inflamed people. This new method was called *in vitro fertilization (IVF)*. Critics glorified unification inside the womb (technically, inside the fallopian tubes) as a mystical event, sanctioned by God and by evolutionary fitness. To them, only perverts depart from anointed couplings.

Louise Brown, the first IVF baby, arrived on July 25, 1978, in a small town in northern England. Physiologist Robert Edwards and obstetrician Patrick Steptoe bathed her mother's uterus with hormones and then used a laparascope (a flexible tube with a fiber optic lens and controls) to implant the embryo. Over nine months, it grew to become Louise Brown.

The first attempts to create a child by IVF were experiments with human embryos (federally funded science today cannot do such research). At first, merely inserting an embryo into the uterus produced no results, because the embryo didn't attach to the uterine wall. Before the first successful IVF birth, at least a hundred embryos created by IVF either failed to implant or miscarried as fetuses.

Before the first IVF birth, alarmist critics such as Leon Kass, Daniel Callahan, and Jeremy Rifkin feared IVF would harm children, families, and society.[6] The Catholic Church asserted (then and now) that the only moral way to conceive children was through sex in heterosexual marriage. Even though they create wanted, human life, Catholics who use IVF are committing a sin.[7]

A downside exists for IVF. Babies conceived through it have approximately twice the normal rate of birth defects, around 4 percent overall instead of 2 percent.[8] According to a 2002 study in the *New England Journal of Medicine,* such babies have an increased risk of Beckwith-Wiedemann syndrome, which causes enlarged organs and cancer in children, and a five to seven times increase in risk of retinoblastoma, a rare cancer of the eye. Nevertheless, all of these conditions are rare.[9]

5.2 Emotivism

In the early 1970s, Leon Kass earned an MD and a PhD in biochemistry. Before he started a residency, the ethical problems created by AID and IVF asserted a powerful pull on him. Thus, the path of his career changed from medicine and biochemical research to ideas and ethics.

The University of Chicago appointed him to its Committee on Social Thought program, an interdisciplinary program and think tank. Over the next 30 years, he championed the wisdom of listening to feelings about natural conceptions, traditional heterosexual marriage, and the problems of technology in medicine. He typically did not extol heterosexual creation so much as condemn deviations from it. Moreover, he characteristically created powerful emotions in his readers by using religious imagery and evocative language to imply that artificial creation of babies was out of control, taking us into dangerous waters, and ultimately against the will of the Deity (although he never directly appealed to God).

Characteristic passages about IVF from Professor Kass in 1979 warned that it would be "foolish to acquire and use the powers" of intervening in human procreation to cure infertility.[10] Once society allows AID, he wrote, clarity about one's origins vanishes:

> Clarity about your origins is crucial for self-identity, itself important for self-respect. It would be, in my view, deplorable public policy further to erode such fundamental beliefs, values, institutions, and practices. This means, concretely, no encouragement of embryo adoption or especially of surrogate pregnancy.[11]

For Kass, IVF and AID lead via a "wedge logic" (slippery slope) to other tools to cure infertility, such as embryo transfer and surrogacy. From there, humans will slide down the slippery slope and soon be using

> "... any available technical means" to cure infertility, including "artificial wombs," and will soon need "to decide whether human beings will eventually be produced in laboratories.... Once the genies let the babies into the bottle, it will be impossible to get them out again.[12]

Twenty years later, in "The Wisdom of Repugnance," Professor Kass used even stronger language to condemn human reproductive cloning and to explain why we should listen to our emotions:

> In crucial cases, however, repugnance is the emotional expression of deep wisdom. ... The repugnance at human cloning belongs in this category. We are repelled by the prospect of cloning human beings not because of the strangeness or novelty of the undertaking, but because we intuit and feel, immediately and without argument, the violation of things that we rightfully hold dear. Repugnance, here as elsewhere, revolts against the excesses of human willfulness, warning us not to transgress what is unspeakably profound. Indeed, in this age in which everything is held to be permissible so long as it is freely done, in which our given human nature no longer commands respect, in which our bodies are regarded as mere instruments of our autonomous rational wills, repugnance may be the only voice left that speaks up to defend the central core of our humanity. Shallow are the souls that have forgotten how to shudder.[13]

In the above quotation, Kass moves from using emotional language about allegedly disgusting things in order to persuade in ethical argument to actually extolling appeals to disgust as wisdom. So he advises us to listen to our feelings of revulsion about human cloning, as well as to feelings about other reproductive technologies, and to respect the "yuck factor."

Most people on the planet share Professor Kass's feelings about cloning humans. But what exactly should we make of his claim about the role of emotion in ethics? Indeed, what exactly is his claim? As we saw in Chapter 1, sometimes our feelings are good moral guides, but sometimes not. Moreover, some people claim that ethics is only about feelings and nothing else. This theory, known as *emotivism*, has had many champions in the history of ethics. We shall discuss emotivism throughout the rest of this chapter.

5.3 Paradoxes About Conception

As we have seen, critics of assisted reproduction often argue that children created in new ways are harmed. In contrast, champions of new ways of making babies reply that, no matter what risks are taken, existence is better than nonexistence, and therefore no child is harmed in being created in a new way. What are we to make of these claims?

As said, a child created by AID could be said to be harmed because he will not know his male ancestor. On the other hand, if AID is the *only* way he could exist, that harm does not seem to outweigh the disvalue of not existing. If AID were not used, there is no person who could possess the disvalue of not existing, so it is also difficult to see who is harmed, if anyone, if the embryo-that-will-become-the-child is never created.

This raises a problem in bioethics: How should we compare nonexistence with existence? Or to compare nonexistence with a possible existence that carries some risk of harm?

In thinking about this problem, it seems wrong to say that any kind of life is better than no life. Is being born blind, deaf, and paralyzed from the neck down better than not living at all? Maybe not. We certainly want to be careful in taking risks with the health of fetuses and babies because they are so innocent and easily harmed.

One way to try to clarify this problem is to ask if a new way of originating babies has an overall compensating benefit that makes taking a risk worthwhile. This seems to have been so with AID and IVF babies. At least a hundred thousand IVF babies have been born in America, as have thousands of AID babies, almost all of whom were wanted by their parents, who usually had good incomes. Even if a few had birth defects, the normal existence of another hundred thousand wanted children compensates for this harm.

Kinds of Harm and Their Referents

Another kind of problem concerns parents who could have prevented harm to their baby but did not. Suppose parents

wanted a deaf child and chose an embryo with a genetic dispo-
sition to deafness. Can we say they have harmed their resulting
child when otherwise this particular child would not have been
born?

It is important to distinguish between different meanings
of "harm." Like the concept of good, the concept of harm covers a broad range of meanings. In law school, such meanings
are covered in one of the major courses, *torts* (Latin for "harm").
For our purposes here, we can distinguish three broad meanings of harm.

In the first way, both a baseline and a temporal (time) component are necessary, so that a change occurs that makes someone worse off. *Baseline harm* requires an adverse change in someone's condition. With baseline harm, someone who doesn't yet
exist cannot be harmed, because he has no baseline from which
change can occur.

The second way of defining "harm" compares a present
deficiency with what normally would have been. In this *abnormal harm,* someone is injured by being brought into existence
with some defect that could have been avoided by taking reasonable precautions. Here, the event or omission that causes
the defect is the cause of harm.

Third, "harm" may be defined as a life of total pain and injury, such that no hope exists of relief. Perhaps this is the lot of
many pigs raised in industrial factory-farms, confined their
whole lives and squashed together for maximal profits in tiny
metal pens with their tails cut off. Let us call this third harm
total harm. To some of its critics, cloning a child would be so bad
for the child as to constitute total harm.

Preventing abnormal harm underlies the belief that parents should do everything possible to have healthy, unimpaired
babies; that anything less than the maximal effort is blameworthy; and that it is wrong for a woman to take risks with a future
person's intelligence or health. In this sense, deaf parents harm
their children when they only implant embryos genetically dis-
posed to be deaf.

These concepts matter legally. Total harm in the law is
called *wrongful life.* In such cases, lawyers claim that the lives of
some babies are so miserable that their very existence is a tort.
In contrast, *wrongful birth* assumes abnormal harm, and claims
not that the child's life is totally miserable, but that the child
has been damaged by being born less than normal, and that a

physician's action or omission caused the relevant defect. Courts have almost always rejected wrongful life suits because courts have rejected the implication that killing a baby can benefit it.

These two concepts of harm can be applied to new conceptions. With baseline harm, a person created by a new form of assisted reproduction cannot be harmed because otherwise he wouldn't exist. According to abnormal harm, a new conception could harm a baby if it caused some defect or deficiency that a normal baby would not have had. Finally, new conceptions would rarely, if ever, be so bad as to qualify for total harm.

Wronging vs. Harming

For utilitarians or consequentialists, what matters about new kinds of human creation is that babies are not harmed. On the other hand, virtue theories focus on the state of mind or motives of prospective parents. Virtue theorists ask how a good person would act, and, whether it is AID, IVF, surrogacy, or cloning, they ask, "What would a good mother do? What kinds of risk would she take?"

This is a useful perspective because it emphasizes that, even though a child might not be *harmed* by being brought into existence (where he would not exist otherwise), a mother can still be *wrong* in bringing him into existence. That's because "wrong" here is divorced from consequences to the child and instead married to the motives of the mother in conceiving a child. To take a more mundane example, if a mother conceives a child not because she wants a child but to try to force a wealthy man to marry her, then the child who comes into existence is not thereby harmed, but the mother is wrong to bring the child into existence for this motive.

Starting vs. Stopping Lives. South African philosopher David Benatar nicely distinguishes between a *life worth continuing* and a *life worth starting*, arguing that judgments about the former are made at a much higher threshold than the latter.[14] In other words, we need much stronger justification for ending a newborn's life than for not starting a new life. This distinction recognizes the de facto importance in procreative ethics that we place on birth.

Why do we place so much importance on birth in establishing a baseline? One reason is that the parents have nurtured the fetus for nine months and made plans for its birth. Another is that women often suffer depression after delivery and courts are reluctant to sanction any infanticide at such a time. Another is the protective mechanism that occurs in interacting with visible newborn babies, whom humans and other animals instinctively desire to nurture. These reactions are muted with hidden fetuses.

So why do we have a much lower standard for not starting a human life than for ending the life of an impaired newborn? Part of this answer is that many mishaps occur in starting a new life, such that we are uncertain about whether it will be born at all: Half of embryos created sexually fail to implant in the uterus and some fetuses miscarry.[15] New forms of conception, such as in vitro fertilization, carry high rates of failure. Finally, factored into this judgment is the belief that for almost all births, some life is better than none, and that any newborn's life is likely to fall in this category rather than into total harm.

Emotivism and "Brainwashing" Couples

Critics worry that because the American government does not regulate assisted reproduction in private clinics, prospective parents may be exploited. (In England, the Human Fertilisation Board must approve new kinds of conceptions.) Only 25 of 100 infertile parents using IVF bring home a baby. As such, they may be talked into using eggs from younger women, an expensive, even-less-probable option.

Do Americans now falsely hope scientists will cure infertility, disease, aging, and death? For Daniel Callahan, medicine will never cure these age-old problems, so we should accept our limitations.[16] Is society telling women they can only be happy as mothers? Will young women imitate celebrities having babies without husbands or conceiving very late, as actress Julia Roberts did in having twins at age 37?

Famous women who had children in their 40s and 50s, such as Joan Lunden, Geena Davis, Cheryl Tiegs, and Jane Seymour, hide from the public whether they used eggs from young women. By giving the impression that their children were conceived from their own eggs, they falsely imply to younger women that they can wait until their 40s or 50s and also conceive. For example, Rosee Swain, who encouraged young women not to give up hope of having babies and to explore "all options," did not reveal if she used donor eggs to conceive her twins at age 56.

Emotivists such as Leon Kass warn against a culture where prospective parents become consumers and can select traits of future children. Other critics worry about "brainwashing" women. Note that such criticisms implicitly attack autonomy in reproductive ethics, the idea that a woman is self-governing. To paraphrase John Stuart Mill in *On Liberty,* "Over herself, over her own body and mind, the individual is sovereign."[17] Note also that when Kass appeals to emotions to justify why others say parents shouldn't be able to use new methods to have children, or when critics say women are brainwashed into wanting children, they almost always exempt themselves from the same charges. So Kass should allow rejection of his views by those who feel his views to be repugnant. Similarly, the brainwashing criticism can boomerang on critics when champions of autonomy retort that such critics *themselves* are brainwashed into fearing new reproductive technologies.

In 1997, an Iowa couple, Bobbi and Kenny McCaughey, used Pergonal (a purified preparation of hormonal go-nadotropins) to help Bobbi superovulate. As a result, seven or more of her eggs released from her ovaries and traveled down her fallopian tubes. At this point, physicians artificially intro-duced sperm from her husband Kenny, and soon thereafter, seven embryos began to gestate. When told of the high number of embryos growing, the couple refused to consider reduction (abortion). They were told that one or more babies might be severely disabled. If that happened, the couples asserted, it would be God's will.

When first reported on national television, reporters (especially NBC's Ann Curry) adopted the mode of the miraculous claiming how wonderful it was that all babies were born alive and appeared normal. At the time, no one wanted to hear from physicians who specialized in such births and who claimed that some of the children would later have cerebral palsy, but that it would take years for it to show up.

5.4 Multiple Embryo Implantation

The McCaughey case illustrates a case where a couple took drugs and used techniques of assisted reproduction to create multiple embryos. In some such cases, many of the embryos successfully implanted, producing quadruplets, quintuplets, sextuplets, or even (in this case) septuplets.

The great ethical issue here is that the more fetuses share a uterus, the greater the chance of birth of one or more children with a lifelong, severe disability. Among the disabilities associated with multiple implantation are cerebral palsy and several forms of retardation.

It is also true that the greater the number of embryos implanted, the greater the chance an infertile couple has to bring home *at least one* baby. In some cases, physicians implant four embryos but only one successfully gestates to birth, which means that if they had implanted only one, it could have been one of the ones that failed to gestate.

Infertile couples often pray for pregnancy and may consider any reduction of a multiple pregnancy to violate their "gifts" from God. Given the choice before conception of how many embryos to implant, they may implant the maximal number to have the best chance of success, taking multiples as a bonus.

Because most states do not require insurance companies to cover IVF, which averages $12,500 per attempt in 2005 in the United States, infertile couples with limited means may try to maximize their chances of birth in one cycle by taking the risk of multiple births and risking a child with a major disability.[18] In Louisiana, where state law once required insurance companies to cover one attempt at IVF and only one, many couples risked multiple implantation. By mandating such coverage, the Louisiana legislature undoubtedly didn't understand that it had indirectly created more disabled babies.

It appears that the McCaugheys were not given one choice by their two physicians; that is, after seven eggs released, they were not told, "Since you don't believe in reduction, it might be better to wait until next month when so many eggs aren't released." During the next cycle, perhaps only two eggs would have been released and then, after fertilization, at most only twins could have been born.

The appeal to God and the role of human choice in the McCaughey case should be scrutinized. To say "it's up to God" how many babies come about is misleading because the Mc-Caugheys *chose* to take drugs to artificially stimulate release of many eggs, something that wouldn't have happened naturally. It wasn't God's will but the choice of the McCaugheys that so many eggs were created, released, and fertilized at the same time in one uterus.

Another problem with attributing too much to God concerns Jane Simeone, a Pentecostal woman from Marana, Arizona, who in 1997, after hearing the McCaugheys attribute their success to God, prayed that all her triplets would survive. When two did not, Simeone felt rejected by God and, in turn, rejected God: "After what I've been through, I just can't believe," she said, adding, "Maybe he does miracles for other people, but not for me."[19]

No matter what kind of new form of assisted reproduction is under discussion, the major ethical focus should be on what is best for the conceived child. Of course, that is not the only value, for the good of the parents is also important. At times, we might even agree that a small risk of injury to the prospective child can be taken to help prospective parents avoid the pains of childlessness.

Critics of the McCaugheys' decision said that in this case, if God was clear about anything, it was that the McCaugheys were not intended to have kids. They also said that if a couple took a fertility drug, and it resulted in too many conceived eggs, they should be willing to reduce the embryos for the good of the children born. In other words, a couple shouldn't run the risk of having severely disabled kids and then say that, if disabled kids are born, it's God's will. Virtue ethicists claim that they should be thinking about how to produce good, healthy children, not just the most children.

Besides, why isn't it God's will for couples to *think* and be compassionate toward their future children? Why does God's will have to be equated with, after certain questionable human decisions have been made, accepting everything that happens? Indeed, if you're going to be a religious fatalist, why use modern medicine at all?

During their fourth birthday in 2001, the McCaughey septuplets lagged in development (true for all preemies) and were not all potty trained.[20] *Joel suffered seizures, for which he gets medication. Nathan had spastic diplegia, a form of cerebral palsy that requires Botox injections to paralyze his spastic muscles; he also needs orthopedic braces. Alexis had hypotonic quadriplegia, a different form of cerebral palsy, which results in weak muscles. Alexis also had trouble walking and learning to talk. In addition, for four years she had an indwelling feeding tube.*

Another child, Natalie, required a feeding tube during these years. Although Bobbi and Kenny McCaughey homeschooled their children, the task of homeschooling Nathan and Alexis, who were developmentally delayed, was too great, so Nathan and Alexis attend a school for kids with cognitive disabilities, at public expense.

After spending a year on the road on a self-reported lucrative speaking tour, requests for talks later declined, so Kenny stayed at home for a few months, helping Bobbi with the kids. But then he grew restless and wanted a job outside the home. Explaining why he wanted to leave, he said it had nothing to do with not wanting to help raise eight kids at home but that "it goes back to biblical times, you know, when the man went out, did hunting; they did their things to supply the bread for the family."[21] *So he took a job on an assembly line producing metal parts, leaving Bobbi and an older child at home to care for the seven kids.*

In 2004, Nathan, the sixth of the septuplets, had surgery at Gillette medical campus in Minnesota to relieve hypertight muscles related to his cerebral palsy.[22]

5.5 Sex Selection

Some of the techniques useful in assisted reproduction allow choice of whether a newborn is male or female.[23] Because X chromosomes carry more DNA and weigh more than Y chromosomes, MicroSort, a modified flow cytometer, can separate heavier from lighter sperm with 90 percent accuracy.[24] Although officially intended for use in preimplantation genetic diagnosis, MicroSort is used in China and India to create firstborn male babies, making gender selection less expensive and more available to millions there.

Using in vitro fertilization and MicroSort, a private clinic outside Washington, D.C., in Fairfax, Virginia, has helped hundreds of couples create 400 babies of the sex of their choosing. Its rate of success for creating boys is 75 percent; for girls, 90 percent. It charges $3,000–$4,000 per attempt.

Sex selection has already created problems in China, the Republic of Korea, and India. Families prefer a firstborn male child because females leave the family, whereas males must care for elderly parents. Use of MicroSort will intensify rates of sex selection in Asia and India, which to date have relied on sonograms. (After the sonogram detects a female fetus, some families abort in hopes that the next child will be male.)

As a result of past policies, women are now in demand in China, where 20- to 44-year-old never-married men outnumber their female counterparts 2:1; young females there are sometimes kidnapped and sold into marriage. *Science* magazine predicts that in 2020, one million excess Chinese males will enter the matrimony market in China.[25]

Many bioethicists consider sex selection wrong in Asia because it causes the death of many female fetuses, but what about sex selection in middle-class America to create balanced families? Is a tool employed in China for bad results okay in America among middle-class families?

Critics don't think so. Georgetown philosophy professor Alfonso Gomez-Lobo says, "From an ethical point of view, all this is quite unacceptable."[26]

Communitarian bioethicist Michael Sandel argues, like Leon Kass, that sex selection "runs the risk of turning procreation and parenting into an extension of the consumer society. Sex selection is one step down the road to designer children, in which parents would choose not only the sex of their child but also conceivably the height, hair color, eye color, and ultimately, perhaps, IQ, athletic prowess, and musical ability. It's troubling."[27] Boston University lawyer and bioethicist George Annas concurs, saying, "It's the first step toward the concept of a designer baby."

Sandel also worries about parental expectations: "Consider the father who wants a boy in the hope of having as a son the athlete he had never been. Suppose the son isn't really interested in sports. What sorts of expectations will burden a child who was designed with a certain purpose in mind?"[28]

Not everyone sees the slippery slope around every new procreative corner. "The overall concern that we have one foot over the edge of the slippery slope is overstated because of the limited role that individual genes play in complex human traits," replied Kathy Hudson, director of the Genetics and Policy Center at Johns Hopkins University.[29] As for one fertility physician, all he thinks is, "My job is to help people make healthy babies, not help people design their babies."[30]

On January 18, 2005, 66-year-old Adriana Iliescu gave birth to a healthy daughter in Bucharest, Romania. This sensational case made headlines around the world because Iliescu immediately became "the world's oldest mother." Previously, she had undergone fertility treatments for nine years.

Asked why she had created a child so late, she replied, "You only live once." Asked whether she wanted to be an example for older women, she replied, "No. I'm a warning to younger women that they should conceive when they can when they're young." Asked why she didn't try assisted reproduction at an earlier age, she replied, "Under the previous Romanian regime, it wasn't available and we had forced abortions."[31]

At the delivery, an additional, 1-pound, 8-ounce twin of the healthy girl baby was stillborn. Both babies were delivered by cesarean section.

Ms. Iliescu, an unmarried professor of literature, reportedly had two abortions in her early 20s. An author of books for children, she became pregnant using an egg of a younger woman, secured anonymously, and sperm from an anonymous donor, to create the implanted embryo. She said, "I believed all my life that a woman has a right to give birth . . . no matter how old I was."

Adriana Iliescu was healthy and was medically and psychiatrically tested before the procedures—facts that even critics acknowledge. For most critics, the sole issues were her age and the good of a child born to a woman who, under other circumstances, might easily have been a grandmother.

She didn't believe she was too old. "I'm a dynamic person. Within 48 hours of the birth, I was running up and down the hospital's hallways. I do Swedish gymnastics every morning."

Asked what she thought her daughter would later think of her, she replied, "She will know I was a personality, a university professor, an exceptional woman."

*The Romanian medical association and Orthodox
Church in Romania immediately denounced the birth and
called for a ban on assisted reproduction for women above
normal reproductive ages.*

*"Another case does not have to exist," ran a statement
by the Romanian Professional Association of Medical
Doctors [Colegiul Medicilor], in all the major newspapers in
Romania.[32] The Association called for a law that would
forbid assisting older women to conceive children artificially.
It also asked that assisted reproduction cease in Romania
until the new, proposed law went into effect.*

*In the months following the birth, a 62-year-old nanny
helped Professor Iliescu with the baby at home. As for her final
feelings on criticisms of the birth, Professor Iliescu quoted an
old Romanian proverb, "Eat the apple that falls in your
garden and don't ask where it came from. Eat it and you
will be happy."*

5.6 Age of Parents and the Good of the Child

Our culture has a double standard for men and women as parents. In the Bible, the patriarchs Abraham and Jacob were old
men when they conceived with their handmaidens. Senator
Strom Thurmond began a family at age 66 in 1968 after marry-
ing his second wife Nancy Moore, a former Miss South
Carolina, who was then 22. They had four children together.
Senator Thurmond died in 2003 at the age of 100. (At the time
of his death, his children were all adults and he and his wife had
lived apart for several years.) Likewise, actor Clint Eastwood
began a new family at age 65, Tony Randall at age 78, and nov-
elist Saul Bellow fathered a child at age 84 (he died in 2005 at
age 89).

Although the occasional feminist blasts these ancient men
for creating babies, old men seem to escape the condemnation
that has been heaped on older women. The American Medical
Association did not start a petition to ban assisted conception
for men over 75, nor did the American Jewish Federation criticize Saul Bellow for imitating Biblical patriarchs. But imagine
the chorus of indignation that would have ensued had an
84-year-old, American Jewish woman given birth!

Let us turn from old-men-versus-old-women to the general issue of whether elderly people should have kids at all. Thanks to assisted reproduction, more and more older people are having more and more kids. In 2002, women between the ages of 45 and 49 gave birth to over 5,000 babies, and women aged 50 to 54 gave birth to over 200 babies.[33] These rates represent a doubling of numbers in one decade. The same kind of figures hold true for men. In 2002, men aged 50 to 54 created over 20,000 babies, an increase of 6,000 babies over a decade before. The same is true in the United Kingdom, where births to women over 40 almost doubled between 1981 and 2001.[34]

It is widely assumed that children benefit from having younger, rather than older, parents. One recent book by a physician argues that, compared to children born to men under 25, children born to men over 35 have increased risks of schizophrenia and Down syndrome (and the older men are twice as likely to be infertile).[35] And we know that risk of Down syndrome increases as a woman ages, with significant risks after age 35.

Is it good for a newborn child to have parents who are almost eligible for Medicare? Who are unlikely to be alive at the child's graduation from high school? The most important reason why elderly people shouldn't create babies is that children need parents who are alive, healthy, and energetic while they are growing up.

Although no one thinks such tables apply to them, mortality tables used by insurance companies are correct: The chances that a 65-year-old woman or man will live another 20 years in a healthy, energetic way are low; most will succumb to cancer, heart disease, or neurological disorders. And how many of these older parents are rich enough to provide enough money for future care and education of these new children? How do they know their own medical care and custodial care in a nursing home won't eat up all their savings? Should a child be created to be a future nursemaid?

On the other hand, some elderly parents are well-equipped to handle child-raising, as evidenced by the fact that many grandparents raise grandchildren when their children die, are imprisoned, sent off to war, or simply abandon them. Elderly parents are almost always richer, more mature, more stable, and wiser than teenage parents. They may also have more time to give children and may not be as caught up in ambitions about their careers or in stormy relationships.

5.7 Hume, Kant, and Aristotle on the Emotions

In the history of ethics, three famous philosophers staked out three famous positions on the role of emotions in ethics. The first, Scottish philosopher David Hume, lived during the Enlightenment and was generally a skeptic about the role of reason in life and concluded that its efficacy was largely illusory. Hume did not think that reason alone could prove the existence of God or discover truths of science, much less discover objective, eternal truths in ethics.

In ethics, Hume thought that our values entirely come from our emotions or feelings (Hume used the 18th-century term "sentiments"). Reason is limited to discerning how to satisfy the goals given to us by our feelings. Hume put it dramatically: "Reason is, and ought to be, the slave of the passions."

Hume made several important claims. First, claims about ethics are essentially claims about how people feel. Such feelings can be educated or shaped, but they are always the real basis of moral judgments. Second, passions or emotions dictate the goals or ends of life. That the life of a married man with two children is better than the life of a bachelor cannot be decided by reason itself. Reason can only tell us, if we decide to be a bachelor, how best to do it. Finally, Kant's claim (see below) that morality is essentially rational is but a fantasy and obscures the true causes of our moral judgments.

Perhaps reproductive ethics best illustrates Hume's thesis. Certainly arguments about abortion sometimes seem only to illustrate how people on each side feel. When it comes to new ways of creating children, people commonly react with fear and disgust. This happened when "test tube babies" such as Louise Brown first started. When scientists announced the birth of the cloned lamb Dolly in 1997, the possibility of cloning humans became real and most people feared it.

As we have seen, Kant held the opposite of Hume and argued that if a person acts from feelings, that person will *not* be acting morally. For Kant, people can only act morally when they act rationally, and that means acting out of respect for the moral law. For Kant, what feeling indicates and what duty indicates are not the same. Frequently, doing the right thing requires acting *against* feelings.

In short, Kant distrusted feelings. He thought they were governed by our lower nature, a nature determined by causal forces. In contrast, our rationality is the seat of our personhood and also the seat of our free will. Only decisions that stem from this seat of personhood for Kant are moral. Actions that stem from feelings are simply those that have been determined by how we have been conditioned and socialized, but that have nothing to do with our true selves.

In between Hume and Kant, surprisingly, is a philosopher who lived two thousand years before us, Aristotle. For this ancient Greek, a properly educated young man would be raised to feel honor, shame, and pride "at the right times for the right reasons in the right ways." He would have the traditional Greek excellences or virtues of self-control *(sophrosyne)*, courage *(andreia)*, and practical judgment *(phronesis)*.

Most of us know a person who matches Aristotle's ideal: people whose feelings match their rational judgment and act morally with passion "for the right reasons at the right time in the right ways." In other words, the person is intelligent but also passionate about her causes, such that when the two are fused together, she is a real force to counter. So for Aristotle, good people should not experience conflicts between their feelings and their duty; ideally, the two should run together, reinforcing each other.

Aristotle envisioned a static society with each person knowing his place, a society that had to be both militaristic and hierarchical, with leaders who could make decisions in case of attack. In such a society, it might be possible to train young men how to feel "the right thing at the right time in the right way." However, in our modern, complex society, which has inherited many different ethical traditions and which has many kinds of people, it is more difficult, but perhaps possible, to raise children to feel the correct feelings at each time.

Martha Nussbaum, trained in ancient philosophy and a virtue theorist teaching at the University of Chicago law school, defends the role of emotion in ethics. For her, one's emotions are judgments about the value that other people or events have to that person.[36] To get mad about infidelity is to judge that fidelity matters in a relationship. To feel joy in one's soccer or debate team winning a championship is to express a judgment that such winning is desirable.

Nussbaum doesn't think that our emotions are *simply* rational judgments. Instead, they are largely formed in infancy and childhood, so there is a role for therapy and rational insight in helping us find new ways of judging; that is, of feeling, and of abandoning destructive ways inherited from bad childhoods. Obviously, the relation between emotions, reason, and ability to change in therapy is a complex subject, but Nussbaum at least has taken the subject to the public.

5.8 Surrogate Mothers and Compensating Gametic Donors

Fertilization of embryos outside the womb made surrogate mothers possible, where a woman other than the egg donor could gestate an embryo to birth, either for pay or voluntarily.

According to the Organization of Parents Through Surrogacy, a nonprofit agency that tracks such statistics, about a thousand babies have been born in America through surrogates.[37] On average, surrogates are paid $20,000 (plus medical expenses and travel) and have already conceived children of their own.

Well-known celebrities, such as former *Good Morning America* host Joan Lunden, at late ages used surrogates to have babies. At age 54, Lunden used donated eggs and her husband's sperm to create twins, born in 2005. Lunden hired a wet nurse for the twins and also had a teenager from a former marriage for a nanny. When she was 52, supermodel Cheryl Tiegs and her fourth husband, Rod Stryker, had twins in 2000 by a surrogate mother.

Several hundred women had helped infertile women create babies when in 1986 biochemist Bill Stern and pediatrician Elizabeth Stern hired Mary Beth Whitehead for $10,000 to bear a child created by his sperm and Whitehead's egg through artificial insemination. At birth on March 27, 1986, at Monmouth County Medical Center in Long Branch, New Jersey, Mrs. Whitehead bonded with Baby M, also known as Melissa Stern, and refused to give her to the Sterns. When Mr. Stern threatened legal action, Mrs. Whitehead fled with the baby to

Florida but, after a national search of some high drama, was discovered and returned to New Jersey for trial.

At this trial in 1987, Judge Harvey Sorkow upheld the legality of the contract, said it did not constitute baby selling, required Whitehead to hand over the baby, awarded Whitehead $10,000, and decided it would be best for the baby never to see Mrs. Whitehead again. On appeal in 1998, the New Jersey Supreme Court unanimously reversed his decision, declared Mrs. Whitehead the legal mother with full visiting rights, and invalidated surrogacy contracts.

Mrs. Whitehead later became a well-known critic of surrogacy, and feminists, who believed not only in bonding but also that women were naturally superior to men in nurturing children, supported her. Such feminists, sometimes called *social feminists,* part ways with traditional *merit feminists,* who sided with Elizabeth Stern and thought that women should be held accountable for contracts they signed. Ironically, merit feminists saw social feminists as sexist.

Six states (Michigan, New York, Washington, Utah, Arizona, and New Mexico) reacted to the Whitehead/Stern case by criminalizing commercial surrogacy. Arkansas, Florida, Ohio, Virginia, Nevada, New Hampshire, and California legally recognized it. In many states, laws about surrogacy either do not exist, are based on one particular case, or are contradictory.

Controversial cases make news; successful cases do not. A case of the former was Jaycee Buzzanca, a.k.a. "the child with 5 parents," born in March 1995 from a paid surrogate. Entangled in a divorce between the parents who hired the surrogate, Jaycee was conceived from sperm and egg other than from the parents who hired the surrogate. A California appeals court ruled in 1998 that the parents who had hired the surrogate were legally responsible for him.

Another controversial trend is surrogate mothers bearing babies for gay couples. One company in California matches gay couples to surrogates and has helped arrange over 300 births to gay and lesbian couples.[38] For complex reasons, gay couples get along better with pregnant surrogate mothers than heterosexual couples and are more willing afterward to have the surrogate involved in the child's upbringing, causing some surrogates to prefer to work with gay couples.

Many people, especially elderly people, have bad feelings about surrogacy. They worry that mothers are drifting away from natural motherhood and use surrogates for convenience.

Let us now consider egg transfer. Because so many women in North America lack children, and because eggs of young women increase chances of successful in vitro fertilization with a husband's sperm, young women get paid to transfer their eggs. Originally, volunteers supplied eggs, but altruism doesn't meet the demand. In 1993, the American Society for Reproductive Medicine (ASRM) suggested a flat fee of $2,500 for egg donation, but payment since has soared.

Women get paid more than men because egg retrieval is more complicated than obtaining sperm. A woman takes drugs daily for a month or more to induce superovulation, after which eggs are aspirated with a long thin needle inserted through the vagina into an ovary and guided by ultrasound imaging. According to one such woman, each time an egg is sucked from an ovary, "it feels like someone kicked you there."[39] Use of the drugs may slightly increase the risk of uterine and ovarian cancer, especially in women who have precancerous conditions and who use the drugs extensively.[40]

In the winter of 1998, a New Jersey Assisted Reproduction (AR) clinic advertised that it would pay young women $5,000 for a month's worth of eggs. This was double the approved rate of $2,500. A year later, an ad ran in a newspaper at Princeton University and at other Ivy League universities, stating that an anonymous couple was offering $50,000 for a "woman over 6 feet tall and with SAT scores over 1450 who was willing to sell her eggs."[41]

Such stories create powerful feelings in people. They falsely make people feel that "GATTACA" or Nazi eugenics was just around the corner, that baby-boomer parents are out of control, and that few women are having babies in traditional ways. Such stories created a reaction against all biotechnology, including genetically modified food and stem cells, creating the feeling that led one critic to title his book, *Enough!*[42]

Emotivism, Again

In the 20th century, Hume's emotivism was given a more careful expression by philosopher Charles Stevenson, who argued that moral disagreements are not about facts but about differences in attitude.[43] According to Stevenson, when people say

"Cloning is wrong," they think they are referring to something objective (i.e., the wrongness of cloning), but really they are just expressing a negative reaction to cloning, something that could be expressed as, "Cloning! Yuck! Boo!"[44]

When he became chair of President George W. Bush's newly formed Bioethics Council in 2001, Leon Kass argued that feelings of disgust toward human cloning should be honored by making attempts to clone humans (as babies or as embryos) a federal crime.[45] The Bush administration similarly tried to persuade the United Nations to criminalize all forms of cloning worldwide.

The problem in general with emotivism and in particular, with Kass's use of it in bioethics, is that some of our feelings are downright shameful and shouldn't be used to guide morality. Indeed, some of the very conservatives who glorify feelings in condemning cloning also accept the view that humans by nature are sinful. The terrible racial violence in Serbia or the Congo shows what can happen when racist feelings, ordinarily suppressed by morality, surface and go unchecked by moral principles.

The other problem with emotivism and Kass's use of it in bioethics is that people who accept this theory don't accept its implications for their own judgments. Kass is not just arguing that he *feels* cloning is wrong; he is arguing as if it's *rational* to view cloning as wrong, and that *reasons* should be given why it should be made illegal. But why should reasons be given, why should we read his reasons or try to give our own, if everything is just a matter of honoring our feelings? Indeed, isn't arguing for this position self-contradictory?

Hundreds of years ago, many white Christians ridiculed Jews, the Irish, Africans, homosexuals, Asians, and Native Americans. Many despised such people and referred to them with racist, derogatory names. Gradually, moral progress occurred through a slow, painful process over hundreds of years of education, debate, reasoning, maturation, and political struggle. Today, we would be embarrassed by a presidential candidate like Theodore Roosevelt who referred to Chinese as "yellow niggers" or by Henry Ford who, when he ran for president, cursed the evil of "Jew bankers" and who made similar kinds of remarks about black Americans and Catholic "papists."[46] People back then, who listened with approval to these candidates for president, had strong feelings about new ethnic immigrants to America—feelings that Roosevelt exploited—but that does not mean, then or now, that appeal to such feelings counts as moral justification.

5.9 Reproductive Cloning

Announcement in 1997 of the birth of Dolly, created by cloning, aroused strong feelings against originating humans the same way. Dubbed the "Bioethics Story of the Decade," cloning has dominated bioethics and politics ever since. A broad coalition of Catholic bishops, Southern Baptist leaders, environmentalists, and social conservatives attempted to make it a crime in America to originate a baby this way. Similar efforts occurred in the United Nations. To date, these attempts have failed.

Many of our feelings about human cloning stem from lurid descriptions of cloning in science fiction or in scary films such as *Jurassic Park*. Language referring to "escaping clones" or "the clone" prejudices our feelings, causing us to imagine such people as zombies or mutants. And when an eccentric cult, the Raelians, falsely claimed to have created a child by cloning, it greatly increased the associated "yuck" feelings.

Nevertheless, when cloning is safe to try, a child created by cloning is best thought of as a later-born twin of an ancestor's genes. About half of the person we are probably comes from the environment (including nutrition during gestation and how much our parents nurtured us in the first two years of crucial brain development), the other half from genes (how genes are expressed also depends on environmental inputs). So a later-born twin of the author, born not in 1948 but in 2018, would have a vastly different upbringing and enter a very different world than did the author, and hence, would be a substantially different person.

Reproductive cloning differs from embryonic cloning. The former aims to produce a baby, the latter, only the entity that looks (at 14 days old or younger) like a tiny golf ball. Cloned embryos are used in medical research to create stem cells but, if allowed, could be implanted in willing women to create babies with the help of fertility clinics.

People make many objections to human cloning. Some claim it violates human dignity or condemns a child to a future determined by parental expectations. Others worry about cloning's effect on the gene pool or that family dynasties of cloned children will exacerbate innate differences between people. Still others believe that humans should forgo creating life or choosing kinds of humans because all this is best left to God, whose invisible hands work through the genetic lottery at conception or through the inner springs of evolution.

Most of those objections are speculative, question-begging, or factually suspect.[47] But one good, real moral objection exists: Cloning would likely create a child who would be physically or mentally abnormal in some way, and according to the abnormality standard, harmed. At the present time, evidence based on animal models indicates that attempting to gestate a child from a cloned human embryo would result in miscarriage during gestation or a child with a significant risk of early death or a lifelong impairment. At this time, that is a knockdown argument against attempting to originate a human being by cloning.

Does that mean that we should never attempt to clone a baby? No. When Christiaan Barnard performed the first heart transplant in 1967, Louis Washkansky's immune system rejected the heart. Not until some 10 to 15 years later, when cyclosporin was discovered and proved to selectively inhibit immune rejection, did heart transplantation become clinically reasonable. It was then on its way to becoming a routine operation.

Medical research normally proceeds by experimenting on animals to improve human life. One day, most mammals will be able to be cloned safely and in large numbers. When scientists can do so safely with primates such as chimpanzees and gorillas, then it may be safe to try to create a human baby this way.

In the meantime, we might study cloned human embryos and see what goes wrong or right in embryonic development. At least, we might do so with private funds, for no federal funds at present can fund work with cloned embryos.

CONCLUSIONS

This chapter has discussed both new ways of making babies and the ethical theory of emotivism, and tried to sketch some of the standard criticisms in ethics of emotivism. It has indicated that feelings about new conceptions can be unreliable guides to the morality of these ways of making babies. At first, we are shocked and disgusted at something new and worried that innocent babies may be harmed. Over time, we see that the babies and children are not harmed and, like the first time we see the aftermath of heart surgery, we become desensitized to the new thing as it becomes normalized.

This certainly happened with IVF babies and, to a lesser extent, with AID. (To some critics, AID is worse because in most cases of IVF, the child knows his genetic ancestors, who are also the parents who raise him, but not so with AID.)

To most people, cloning is a paradigm case where emotional disgust should reign supreme. But time will tell whether such disgust is merited. If objections about safety are met, and when children can safely and regularly be created by cloning, then the main objections will appeal to feelings of revulsion, to alleged violations of dignity, and to speculation about the psychological health of the child. At that future time, that may not be enough to ground a good moral judgment against cloning.

Another example where appeal to feelings is powerful is when women around 60 create, bear, and raise babies. Many of our feelings here may be out-of-date. As fiftyish law professor and bioethicist Lori Andrews says, "I see nothing wrong with postmenopausal women having children using egg donation and hormonal stimulation. In fact, I think that clinics that won't do it are being discriminatory because they will do IVF for a couple with a man in his seventies, so the argument that the woman is too old isn't persuasive to me."[48] Given that healthy women today can easily expect to live until their mid-80s, healthy, wealthy women can have happy children, especially if they have other relatives ready to take over, should they die early.

In any case, if this discussion of reproductive ethics has shown anything, it is that our initial feelings about new developments are unreliable guides to good moral judgments. What we eventually decide based on reasons about each new reproductive technology may differ greatly from our initial feelings about it.

When it comes to feeling in ethics, we must be careful what we are discussing. When discussing emotivism as an ethical theory, supporters often cite very emotional issues in ethics such as abortion, cloning, and reproductive ethics. But ethics casts a much broader net than this list implies.

Take bioethics. One of its most pressing issues is health care for the working poor. Nearly 40 million Americans lack any or decent medical coverage. Although they work and pay taxes, their employers don't buy group medical coverage for their employees.

Understanding and fixing this problem is a complex process. It's hard to get people excited about the problem or fixing it. But that does not mean it is not an ethical problem or an important ethical issue to understand.

What is true is that emotivism fails miserably as an ethical theory when it comes to complicated issues like a just national health-care policy. If few emotions attach to a subject, what has emotivism to offer?

Outside bioethics, many other ethical issues require thought and study to understand. For example, subsidies by American taxpayers to American farmers keep prices low for sugar, cotton, and corn, undermining the efforts of farmers in developing countries to sell these crops to local markets and become self-sufficient. Proving that claim requires study and discussion, and passion doesn't take you far along the road of that study or discussion.

Whether it be global economic justice, starving people in Darfur, sweatshop labor in the Philippines, environmental racism, or understanding practices in finance that hurt and exploit vulnerable people, there is much in ethics that cannot be understood simply by appealing to a "yuck" or "yeah!" emotive response.

Overall, people always feel that new methods of human reproduction may harm babies, harm traditional parenting, or society. Historically, most of those feelings have been unfounded, as new ways of creating babies were mostly just new tools for helping infertile couples.

New conceptions also cause passions to boil partly because commentators use emotionally inflammatory language, such as "test-tube babies" and "escaping clones." Such language rarely enlightens the debate.

On the other hand, giving reasons does work to justify good moral judgments. In this chapter, it was argued that reproductive cloning right now is too dangerous and therefore not in the best interests of future children. A similar argument was put forth that implanting more than two embryos with assisted reproduction was not in the best interests of resulting children. In these two cases, reasons convince us that regulation of these practices would be a good thing.

So we can condemn a case that appeared on *Good Morning America* in April 2005 in which a surrogate mother revealed she was carrying five six-month-old fetuses for a couple who had paid her $15,000. Again told as a wondrous story, no one asked her or the couple why they hadn't reduced the number of implanted embryos and why they were risking creation of children with disabilities.

In ethical theory, philosophers such as Hume and Stevenson held that condemnations of abortion or cloning were nothing but expressions of feeling. However, emotivism fails as a theory of ethics because it does not explain how people can overcome their feelings by use of evidence and reflection.

It may also be true, as Martha Nussbaum implies, that we will one day have a richer theory of emotions, one which can better inform us about how educated emotions should work in ethics. But a lot of work remains to be done in psychology and ethics for us to arrive at that theory.

In bioethics, Leon Kass and popular writers such as Dean Koontz have tried to elevate emotional disgust to justification, but this move fails because emotional disgust is too often just the expression of how we have been conditioned.[49] Moreover, disgust is one of the baser emotions, hardly one that we want to elevate to national law or public policy. Many Americans last century were conditioned to accept racial segregation and to condemn homosexuality, but rational debate has since created progress in these areas.

The late Pope John Paul II, who once taught in Polish universities as a philosophy professor, remarked in his last book that uncritically taking the Bible as literally true was a kind of "intellectual suicide."[50] In the same way, we could also say that taking emotivism to be a true theory in ethics is a kind of intellectual suicide: It leaves no room for giving reasons or for looking at evidence.

FURTHER READINGS

Nussbaum, Martha. *Upheavals of Thought: The Intelligence of Emotions.* New York: Cambridge University Press, 2001.

Peters, Phillip C., Jr. *How Safe Is Safe Enough: Obligations to the Children of Reproductive Technology.* Oxford, England: Oxford University Press, 2004.

Plotz, David. *Genius Factory: The Curious History of the Nobel Prize Sperm Bank.* New York: Random House, 2005.

CHAPTER 6

Terri Schiavo: When Does Personhood End?

This chapter discusses a famous case in medical ethics, perhaps *the* most famous case, that of Terri Schiavo. Her case involves the question of when medical treatment should be stopped for a being caught in the twilight between personhood and death. What criteria should be used to make this decision? When families disagree, who should make the decision? What is the proper role of the courts? [1]

Like all cases in this book, details of this case are progressively revealed amidst discussion of the issues. As we shall see, a perfect storm of powerful forces and ambiguity came together to create sensational coverage of this case by the media. Furthermore, this case is partly a medical mystery and it is very difficult to determine exactly what happened to Terri and why she collapsed.

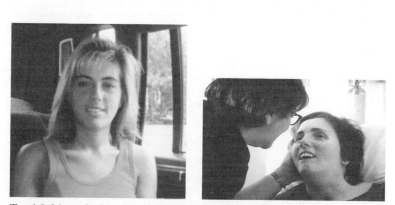

Terri Schiavo, before her collapse, and, above right, after

Terri Schiavo grew up a shy, overweight child in a suburb of northern Philadelphia. In high school, she never felt pretty and wore glasses with huge frames, which gave her a nerdy look. The eldest of three children, she avoided dances at her all-girls Catholic high school; she didn't go to her senior prom. At one point during her senior year in 1981, her parents said that this 5-foot-4-inch woman weighed as much as 250 pounds.

Between high school and college, she decided to become a new person. She went on a NutriSystem diet and lost 100 pounds. Soon thereafter, she enrolled in Bucks County Community College outside Philadelphia. A few months later in 1983 and at age 19, weighing around 140, she met Michael Schiavo, a handsome blonde, tall man, the first boy she had ever dated or kissed.[2]

On their second date, Michael asked Terri to marry him, and after dating for five months, Terri became engaged.[3] Seven months later, they married in 1984 in the Catholic church of her family's parish. They spent their honeymoon in Disney World.

Just before the wedding, Terri got a job as a field representative for Prudential Insurance Company. Michael worked as a manager of a McDonald's.

In 1986, her parents, Robert and Mary Schindler, retired and moved to a condominium they owned in St. Petersburg, Florida. Shortly thereafter, Michael no longer had a job and the couple asked if they could live with Terri's parents in Florida, who agreed. Michael got a good job there managing an expensive restaurant, Agostino's, and Terri got a transfer from Prudential. While Terri worked 7:30 AM to 3:15 PM, Michael worked nights. They saw each other on weekends.

The two couples lived together for several months until the parents bought a house, leaving the condo for the young couple. In 1988, Terri and Michael moved to their own apartment.

About this time, Terri and Michael tried to have a baby, but Terri had trouble getting pregnant. She consulted an obstetrician because of infrequent periods and for fertility treatment.[4]

The Schindler family and Terri's friends at work paint Michael as very controlling. They also emphasize that

Michael had expensive tastes and that Terri's family had more money than Michael's.

At this time, Terri weighed about 110 pounds. Although she appeared to eat and drink normally, in retrospect friends think she may have suffered from anorexia nervosa. As a way of keeping her stomach feeling full and dieting, she also drank several gallons of iced tea each day. Michael Schiavo's brother, Scott, saw her in a bikini shortly before her collapse and said that her skin seemed "to hang off her like sheets."[5]

A close friend of Terri's, Jackie Rhodes, later testified that Michael and Terri had fought and that Terri had thought about getting divorced.[6] Terri's brother Bobby, who lived nearby in Florida, also said the same.

6.1 Cessation of Personhood

One of the master philosophical questions in this case concerns criteria of personhood. We can put this question in several ways: Who is a person and who is not? What is the difference, if any, between being a *human,* a member of a biological species, and a *person,* a being with a right to life and intrinsic moral value?

Much of the controversy in bioethics over the past half century has centered around expanding and contracting *the circle of personhood.* If we think of normal adults as the core of this circle, then as we expand outward to its margins, we encounter more and more controversy about who counts as a person: A 2-day human embryo? A 14-week human fetus? A 98-year-old man in late-stage Alzheimer's disease? A comatose patient? A baby born without any higher brain (an anencephalic infant)? What about presently nonexisting, but merely future humans, such as our grandchildren's grandchildren?

In these controversies about personhood, battles concern both the start and end of personhood. This chapter concerns the latter.

One way to start defining criteria for personhood is to clearly define what is *not* a person. Since that is a very large class of things, a more practical approach is to define when a person *ceases* to be a person. Finding such a definition at first glance might seem easy, but the history of bioethics shows that it is not. Indeed, the Schiavo case has made it even more difficult.

In the following discussion, we will consider whether a person ceases to be a person when in a coma, in a persistent vegetative state (PVS), in a minimally conscious state, and under contemporary criteria of brain death. Before starting, it will be good to emphasize what is at stake in finding a good definition of cessation of personhood.

Legally, what is at stake is that, after a person is gone, cessation of care no longer brings a possible charge of murder, manslaughter, or neglect. What is also legally at stake is giving vulnerable, incompetent patients every chance to get better and to be protected by the State. Such protection matters when not every family or physician seeks maximal protection for vulnerable patients. Such protection matters in an age of limited financial resources and of almost unlimited ability of medicine to prolong the life of a person-absent body. Socially, what is at stake is that physicians and families can begin to be comfortable in accepting that the person is gone and that further efforts are futile. Ethically, what is at stake is that when personhood ceases, no person exists to be harmed by nontreatment. Moreover, when a person no longer exists, no patient's rights are violated by removal of treatment.

On Saturday, February 24, 1990, Terri went to an afternoon Catholic mass with her parents. She then ate dinner with her parents and left around 8 PM. She complained about a yeast infection and bought some medication for it. At 8:30 PM, she called her mother, complaining of discomfort from the infection and saying she didn't feel well in general. Her mother told her to apply the medication and just "go to bed," adding that they would see a gynecologist in the morning.

Michael usually came home after midnight from his job at Agostino's and Terri, because she had to be at work at 7:15 AM, would almost always be asleep. Things appeared to have been no different on this night.

At 5:52 AM on Sunday, February 25, 1990, St. Petersburg paramedics responded to a 911 call from Michael Schiavo, who reported that he had been awakened by a "thud" in the hallway of their apartment, where he found his wife not breathing and unresponsive on the floor. Upon arrival, paramedics found that Terri had no heartbeat, no respiration, and no blood pressure.

Over the next 42 minutes, they repeatedly tried to resuscitate her. Her heart restarted several times but had the wild beat of ventricular fibrillation. Indeed, it must have stopped altogether several times because paramedics defibrillated her seven times and gave her several doses of epinephrine, Narcan, and lidocaine. During this period of 40 minutes or more, they never succeeded in getting her blood pressure to detectable levels.

The police arrived at 6:30 AM. Their report indicated no signs of a struggle in the apartment, no signs of trauma on Terri's head or face, and no bruises. Police questioned Michael, her parents, and her brother extensively about possible drug use. They found several medications in the drug cabinet, two prescribed for Terri, but did not list what they found.

The paramedic report states that Terri "was unresponsive the entire time" and "was unresponsive upon arrival" at the hospital at 6:46 AM.[7] Blood tests showed a potassium deficiency, hypoglycemia, a low albumin (protein) level, and no traces of illegal drugs, and the lowest possible level of alcohol (from a glass of wine the night before). A CAT scan at the hospital showed no "midline shift of the brain," a measure indicating no obvious injury to the brain caused by violence.

At the hospital, Terri never regained consciousness, never spoke to anyone, and never showed alertness. Her coma had begun.

The investigating police asked Robert Schindler if he thought Terri's coma could have anything do to with Michael or domestic violence. "No. No way," the father told the officer.[8]

Over the next three days, Terri "coded" (i.e., her heart stopped beating) several times, but each time physicians brought her back. They cut a tracheostomy and breathed her on a ventilator. They inserted a PEG (percutaneous endoscopic gastronomy) feeding tube.*

Physicians eventually stabilized Terri and removed the ventilator. The physicians, her husband, and her parents were mystified as to what had happened to her.

---

*When a patient lacks the reflex to swallow, a PEG tube is placed through the abdominal wall into the stomach, allowing a nutritious, slushy mixture to feed the patient. PEG tubes are sometimes inserted to buy time after an emergency, with the implicit understanding that they may be temporary and removed later. Once attached, feeding tubes can be emotionally difficult for people to remove. Years later, removal of the feeding tube became the central issue of this case.

Two months later in April, her husband Michael transferred Terri from the hospital to a rehabilitation center. In May, and with no objection from her parents, he became her legal guardian. In September, her parents took her to their home to care for her, but were overwhelmed by the task and returned her to the center.

In November 1990, about nine months after her accident, Michael and the Schindlers raised $50,000 at a "Terri Schiavo Day" to fly her to California for a two-month experiment with a "thalamic stimulator implant" in her brain. When this failed, Terri returned in January 1991 to the Mediplex Rehabilitation Center in Brandon, Florida. For the next six months there, months 11 to 17 into her coma, three shifts of workers worked 24 hours on rehabilitating Terri.

For two years after her collapse, Michael devoted himself to Terri's care. He quit his job. He visited her almost every day. Prudential paid Terri's salary for two years, which Michael lived on, after which Social Security disability payments began. Terri also had life and medical insurance through her job at Prudential.

According to one person's later testimony, Michael at times was very demanding about Terri's care. A former nurse (who also later married into the family of Michael's future girlfriend) said that nurses around Terri remarked, "He may be a bastard, but if I were sick like that, I wish he was [sic] my husband."[9]

In July 1991, Michael transferred Terri to Sable Palms, a skilled care facility, where neurologists continued to test her and where speech, occupational, and physical therapists worked on her for two more years, from 1991 to 1993.

6.2 Background: Brain Death and the Quinlan and Cruzan Cases

Terri Schiavo's collapse put her in a coma, but what does that mean? "Coma" is vague, covering everything from extended sleep to permanent unconsciousness. While we don't say a person goes into a coma when he goes to sleep, if he failed to awaken for four days, we would. At the very least, a coma disrupts the body's natural sleep/wake cycles.

Some people awake from comas. Minor head injuries, allergic reactions, and surgery may disrupt consciousness. While comatose, the brain may be healing.

Even if patients are not legally brain dead, some comas cannot be reversed and amount to death. The late philosopher James Rachels said a person's *biography* may be over, even though his physical *life* is not.[10] To say one's biography is complete is to say that all the significant mental, personal, social, and emotional markers in one's life are over: In writing the obituary of this life, here is where it would end, with a final sentence perhaps stating that "the body lingered for another three years, during which the patient never regained consciousness."

Even in medicine, "coma" is vague. Some physicians use "coma" to represent a state of the brain that occurs just prior to death. Others use "coma" in a much looser, broader sense, one consistent with a recovery. In either case, comas should not be confused with brain death.

First described in medical literature in 1959, *brain death* did not become an operational criteria until 1968, shortly after surgeon Christiaan Barnard transplanted Denise Darvall's heart into Louis Washkansky.[11] The question had then arisen as to whether Denise Darvall had really been dead before Barnard removed her heart. Technically, she had not because her heart was healthy and beating when surgeons prepared her for the transplant (otherwise the heart wouldn't have been a good candidate for the transplant).

For thousands of years, death had been defined by cessation of breathing and heartbeat. When breathing stopped, cardiac *anoxia* (lack of oxygen) soon began, followed by *ischemia* (lack of blood flow to an area), followed by cessation of the heart, and then by ischemia to the brain, which destroys brain tissue very rapidly. This series of events describes traditional, *whole-body* death.

During the 1960s, physicians began to use ventilators, which allowed respiration of brain-damaged patients. Such machines could maintain brain-damaged patients indefinitely, especially if they had a swallow reflex and could eat. Use of such machines meant that medicine needed a new standard of death, specifically of *brain death,* to determine when a healthy heart could be removed from a body.

Note that people don't have to be declared brain dead to die. Today, most people who die are declared dead by the traditional whole-body standard. People are only declared brain dead who have healthy hearts and terrible head injuries, who might be candidates for organ transplants, and whose hearts can be maintained after declaration of brain death to permit transplantation.

An ad hoc committee at Harvard Medical School in 1968 developed *the Harvard criteria of brain death*, which included un-awareness of external stimuli, lack of bodily movements, no spontaneous breathing, lack of reflexes, and two isoelectric (nearly flat) electroencephalogram (EEG) readings 24 hours apart. These criteria required a loss of virtually all brain activity (including the brain stem, and hence breathing).[12]

No one declared dead by the Harvard criteria has ever re-gained consciousness. Standard in all states, these criteria were meant to be ultraconservative and preempt any criticisms about premature taking of organs from nondead patients.

The *cognitive criteria of brain death* falls on the opposite end of the spectrum. These criteria identify a core of properties of per-sons, assume that beings without such a core are no longer per-sons, and include reason, memory, agency, and self-awareness. When a person is dead according to the cognitive criteria, his or her biography is over.

For example, in neurological disorders such as Alzheimer's or Lewy body disease, brain cells deteriorate at a high rate, so that after a dozen years, only a shell remains. According to the cognitive criteria, a patient with Alzheimer's disease in its final stages, such as former President Ronald Reagan in his last years, is dead and it is not wrong to remove a respirator from such a patient and let his body die.

The cognitive criteria have the greatest potential to gener-ate organs for transplantation. So far, however, these criteria have been considered too controversial and too vague to be adopted by any state, although countless families in fact act on them when they agree to reduce treatment to speed a patient's death.

During the 1960s, another invention dramatically changed medicine: Feeding tubes began to be used, allowing a body to be kept alive even though the person inside had long since ex-pired. These developments explain a widely heard comment that "medical technology has moved faster than our wisdom." Over-all, respirators and feeding tubes showed patients' bodies could exist long after their biographies had ended, and moreover, that neither the traditional whole-body definition of death nor the newer Harvard definition of brain death could define how biographical death could be recognized.

Michael Schiavo and Terri's parents stopped living together in May 1992. About that time, Michael started dating other women. That August, Michael received a settlement from the malpractice case.

Michael and his attorneys argued that the obstetrician should have diagnosed Terri's eating disorder and potassium deficiency, and that the latter had caused a heart attack, which in turn had caused her coma.

Michael won. The jury said Terri was 70 percent to blame and the obstetrician, 30 percent. After legal fees, Michael got $750,000 from the hospital for a trust fund specifically for Terri's care and $300,000 (after legal fees were subtracted) for loss of her companionship. If Terri died, Michael inherited the trust money.

Michael and the Schindlers then fought over money. The Schindlers claim that Michael had discussed with them using the money to build an addition to their house to provide 24-hour-a-day nursing care for Terri. Both sides agree they fought over money. Michael says the Schindlers wanted part of the money for their own needs. After this dispute, relations soured between the three adults.

In 1993, several neurologists told Michael that Terri no longer had any chance of meaningful recovery, and Michael agreed to their request for a "Do Not Resuscitate" (DNR) order for Terri. Her parents violently disagreed and Michael later rescinded the order. After this, Michael never authorized any more therapy or rehabilitation for Terri.

Evidently at this point, the Schindlers began to believe that Michael wanted Terri dead, that Terri was still very much alive, and that Michael had various bad motives. Tensions between him and the family and Terri's friends now came to a head.

The Schindlers then tried to remove Michael as Terri's guardian, but a court-appointed special guardian investigated and recommended against them. The guardian reported that Michael had acted appropriately toward Terri. A court accepted this view and kept Michael as Terri's guardian.

As described earlier, one serious form of coma is called *persistent vegetative state* (PVS). PVS is a phrase implying deep unconsciousness that is usually irreversible. Three neurologists testified that Terri Schiavo was in PVS.

In 1976, a 21-year-old woman named Karen Quinlan overdosed on drugs and became a PVS patient: She was unconscious, but her eyes occasionally opened and sometimes she seemed to laugh or cry; in this condition, her eyes were *disconjugate* (i.e., at the same time, they moved in different, random directions). Despite eye movements, she was also *decorticate* (i.e., her brain could not receive input from her eyes). Because she had slow wave but not isoelectric electroencephalograms, she was not brain dead.

The New Jersey Supreme Court in 1975–1976 in the Quinlan case set a precedent and allowed removal of a *respirator.* Fifteen years later in 1990, and after she had been in PVS for seven years, the Nancy Cruzan case in Missouri went before the United States Supreme Court and involved her parents' request for removal of her *feeding tube.*

Missouri law required the high standard of *clear and convincing evidence* of Nancy's desire not to be kept alive—a standard that straddles the most difficult standard of *beyond a reasonable doubt* and is more demanding than *preponderance of evidence* (which applies in most states). The U.S. Supreme Court found Missouri's law constitutional, so the Cruzans were not allowed to discontinue the tube (they later did so after they acquired enough evidence to meet the Missouri standard, and after removal of the feeding tube, Nancy's body expired).

The Cruzan case concerned the kind of law a state could pass to protect incompetent patients. Practically, "clear and convincing" evidence could be met by having an advanced directive (popularly known as a "living will").

But what exactly is PVS? Neurologists believe that consciousness has two components: *wakefulness* (arousal) and *awareness.* So PVS patients such as Karen Quinlan or Terri Schiavo can be described as wakeful but not aware.

Physicians and nurses who work with patients in PVS know a remarkable fact: *Patients' biographies can be over, yet they may have open, moving eyes.* Families find this fact hard to bear and, although it was well documented during the Quinlan and Cruzan cases, ordinary people don't understand it.

Clinically, long-term PVS is a new kind of death. Some commentators call it "upper brain death," but that is confusing. The most accurate thing to say is that no person who was truly in PVS for at least three years has ever returned to consciousness.

Legally, long-term PVS has not yet been recognized as a kind of death, perhaps because it is uncertain how long a person may be in PVS and reawaken, and also because some people may be misdiagnosed as in PVS when they are actually in a slightly higher state.

Six years before the Schiavo case made headlines, a family battled in Virginia over disconnecting the feeding tube of former news anchor Hugh Finn. Virginia's governor then set a precedent for undermining the courts in such family matters, allegedly to give "everyone a time out." He also set a precedent for allowing disgruntled relatives to appeal to the media to pressure the governor to overturn an end-of-life decision by a spouse who had been given permission to do so by judges after legal hearings.[13]

> *Four more years passed, during which Terri's condition did not improve. During this time, Michael became certified as a licensed respiratory therapist, supposedly in order to help care for Terri.[14]*
>
> *In March 1997, Michael hired George Felos, a Florida lawyer who specialized in right-to-die cases. Michael would pay Felos at least $380,000 out of Terri's estate before the case finished.[15]*
>
> *In May 1998, eight years after Terri's collapse, Michael asked a court to allow removal of the PEG tube so that Terri could die. The Schindlers retorted that their daughter would have wanted to live and that Michael wanted her money.*

The Media and Bioethics

This presence of open, moving eyes mattered in the Schiavo case because the Schindlers used a videotape of Terri made in 2002 to plead their case, and this video clip played countless times on Web sites and on television.[16] The 2002 clip of her with her mother, to whom her eyes seemed to respond, is perhaps the most widely seen picture/videotape in the history of bioethics.

When the tape was shown on television, hardly anyone ever mentioned that the tape was three years old and did not show her then-current state.[17] Moreover, when it was shown, few commentators emphasized that the clip had been carefully chosen from hours and hours of videotape, almost all of which confirmed Terri's *non*responsiveness. To make an analogy, imagine a slot-machine player in a casino plays a machine 200 times and the casino videotapes the whole thing for a commercial. Of course, the only segment likely to be shown is the 1 time in 200 when the gambler wins.

For the first time, most Americans saw that a PVS patient could have open, moving eyes. They saw that such a patient could be declared legally hopeless and have a feeding tube removed by a judge, even though she appeared to respond to her mother's voice. That was hard to take. Upon learning the above, some people flatly denied that she was in PVS because, to them, "vegetative" meant no semblance of motion, eye movement, or response. Others hoped that long-term PVS patients could regain consciousness. People trusted what they saw on television over what neurologists said.

Widespread uncertainty by the public about exactly what the videotape of Terri implied created controversy that intensified. On top of this, the image of a vulnerable young woman who seemed to be responding to her mother's voice moved people deeply.

In many ways, the Schiavo case was a case of media ethics and of the limitations of the media. Although reporters tried to present both sides, the 2002 video was too powerful. On a scale of 1 to 100 in persuasiveness, the video was a 100 and a neurologist talking unemotionally on television was a 5. As an ethics professor from the University of Missouri's famous school of journalism said of this case, "Cable-television news is a triumph of intensity over reason."[18]

The problem of course was that, given the clip shown, Terri didn't *look* like she was dead. Because there had been no video of Karen Quinlan or Nancy Cruzan, the public didn't realize we had been there before. Nor had the public seen patients in PVS in long-term-care facilities.

Given this powerful piece of evidence, many people wondered: Why not err on the side of life? Why not give her the maximal chance to recover? Why not give her parents custody and let them take care of her? Especially if it wasn't clear what she would have wanted done in such a situation.

Although the Schindlers lost in the courts, they appealed to the mass media, which in some sense enjoyed the controversy because it helped ratings. The Schindlers released a videotape of Terri to the national media, appeared on the *Oprah Winfrey* show to plead Terri's case, aggressively fought Michael Schiavo every step of the way, and vehemently attacked his personal motives. In contrast, Michael may have been mistaken in believing that the public would accept the decision of the judges who heard the case and in not releasing more representative video of Terri's state to counter the video shown by Terri's parents.

Few physicians or neurologists went on television to explain facts to the public, and as the case intensified, even those who did couldn't stay on every day for weeks and weeks, the way the Schindlers and their other daughter and son did. Although the public could view an EEG and CAT scan of her brain, no one knew how to interpret them and television journalists did not refer to them. For the most part, physicians tended to their own patients and families and, naturally, feared getting swamped by the growing crisis over how, and whether, Terri's life could be ended. Consequently, few physicians ever spoke to the public about the case.

Although the oft-shown videotape seemed to show Terri responding to her mother's voice and tracking a balloon, Judge Greer and the three neurologists found that Terri did not consistently react the same way to her mother and that her tracking of the balloon was a random, nonrepeatable act. During other videotapes, where the Schindlers gave her more than a hundred requests, Judge Greer found that she responded to none of them.

Nearly two years after Michael Schiavo's initial request to have Terri's PEG tube removed, Judge George Greer ruled in 2000 that the tube could be removed. He ruled that clear and convincing evidence existed that Terri would not have chosen to live under such circumstances. The Schindlers appealed, which took a year, but they lost. They appealed again, this

*time to the Florida Supreme Court, which denied their appeal
in April 2001.*

6.3 Families, Criteria of Personhood, and Character Issues

So when does a being stop existing as a person? In popular culture, some people believe that a uniform (perhaps metaphysical) event marks death, probably one with physical manifestations and perhaps as the counterpart of a similar event at the beginning of life. Some people would describe these events as the entrance and departure of a soul. Of course, the occurrence of such metaphysical events cannot be proven and, even if they do occur, seem to have no physical manifestations. So in medical ethics, after relevant medical facts are discussed, the definition of death is not so much a matter of discovery as a *decision* that families and their physicians must make.

If declaring that an incompetent PVS patient is dead is a decision, and not a discovery, then we can predict that good, well-motivated relatives will disagree about such decisions and the ethical criteria used in making them. If it's a decision that declares death and not recognition of a medical fact, then various interests will need to be weighed and weighed carefully indeed, using some larger worldview or ethical standard.

In this case, the Schindlers weighed the various interests this way: They were willing to expend a vast amount of their own and public monies to give Terri a tiny chance of recovery. They believed this is what she would have wanted. Her husband Michael weighed these interests differently, accepting the view of skilled specialists that Terri had no chance of recovery, and wanting to move on with his life.

One key element of dispute concerns whether clear and convincing evidence existed of Terri's wishes. Michael reported in 1994 a conversation where he said he remembered hearing Terri, many years before when the two of them were alone watching television, that she wouldn't want to live on artificial nutrition. The Schindlers denied ever hearing her say anything like this. Regardless of these opposing assertions, is a spouse's recollection of a conversation many years before, especially if contradicted by her parents, really "clear and convincing" evidence? Such a statement might meet "preponderance of evidence," but it does not rise to the higher standard of "clear and convincing." Score one massive legal point for Terri's parents.

More important, several of Terri's friends, as well as a woman Michael later dated, said that Michael had told them after Terri's collapse that he had "no idea" what Terri would have wanted.[19] It does not appear that Judge Greer made any real efforts to use substituted judgment and discover what Terri would have wanted. He seems to have decided that in such cases the spouse had the right to decide.

Other families have come to different decisions than the Schindlers. The Quinlan and Cruzan families went to court *against* their hospital and state government and sought to discontinue life support of their young daughters. On the other hand, in the case of Helen Wanglie in Minnesota, Helen's husband went to court to force public officials to continue his wife on a feeding tube and fought neurologists there such as Ronald Cranford (who testified in the Schiavo case) who thought continued care for Mrs. Wanglie was medically futile.

Standards of personhood used in making these judgments also matter. Failure to meet the vague cognitive criteria is essentially a matter of judgment. On the other hand, being declared dead by neurological criteria is almost entirely a matter of fact.

At heart, this case was a family dispute. Physician Timothy Quill, famous for his acceptance of physician-assisted dying, opined in the *New England Journal of Medicine* that "The Schiavo case raises much more challenging questions [than the Cruzan case] about . . . how to proceed if members of the immediate family are not in agreement."[20] Everybody watched across the world, thankful that their family wasn't having a similar dispute on international television.

Let us think about families in a different way. One of the ways we think about ethics is in terms of the character of the people involved. One of the major ways that ethical theory conceptualizes ethics is in terms of such character and its related traits. Virtue theorists emphasize general moral character in terms of moral integrity, good will, virtue, or personal responsibility, or specific traits, such as courage, compassion, self-control, or loyalty.

It is difficult to evaluate virtue and vice, especially in bits and pieces seen from afar on national media. In the Schiavo case, some people placed great emphasis on the behavior of the parents and the husband. To many people, the parents appeared in the media to be sincere, vulnerable, idealistic, and compassionate. In contrast, they saw the husband as self-serving and hard-hearted.

The Schindlers appeared more sympathetic on television than Michael. As retirees, they seemed to have much more time to talk to reporters and go on television than Michael, who had to work. Perhaps, too, Michael felt uncomfortable talking about his relationship with a new woman, a relationship started after physicians had told him that Terri had no meaningful chance of recovery.

Also, Americans tend to emphasize sexual behavior in thinking about virtue. Some thought that Michael should not have moved in with another woman or had two children with her. These actions were interpreted by some people as evidence of his bad character. Because he was neither as idealistic nor as emotional as the parents, and seemed to be angry at the way he was portrayed by the parents and their supporters, some viewers opined that he didn't care about Terri. The same viewers dismissed evidence that the Schindlers initially wanted money from Michael and dismissed Michael's becoming a respiratory therapist, his taking Terri to California for treatment, and his dogged efforts to get excellent treatment for her for the first four years.

None of these impressions may be accurate. Judging virtue requires intimate knowledge of a person's motives, habits, plans, and actions, and it is difficult to make correct judgments when participants are embroiled in a high-profile case tried on television.

Even if the Schindlers have better character than Michael Schiavo, the character of the parties in this case matters little to the underlying medical reality that concerned whether Terri had any meaningful chance of recovery. The consensus of neurologists and specialists in rehabilitation medicine was that she had no such chance.

Overall, the most striking aspect of the Schiavo case was the intractable dispute between Terri Schiavo's family. Some people speculate that her parents could not accept her death, that both her husband and her parents sought money from the malpractice award, and that personal animosity between the husband and parents fueled this case.

Unfortunately, none of these charges can be proved, and most lack evidence. The most charitable way to think is that the core of this issue is a genuine philosophical dispute about criteria for ending a person's life, expansion of the concept of disability, and society's obligations to protect vulnerable patients.

One can also empathize with Michael Schiavo, without thinking him motivated by money or bad intentions. Few of us know how we would act if called upon to act in a saintly way for more than a decade toward a being whom we believed to have been dead for at least a decade. Is it saintly or foolish to persist in keeping alive the shell of a former person, one whom neurologists say died a decade before? As one person said, "Most men would have walked away and said, 'See ya later.' If I were Terri and he were my husband, I would be so thankful that he stood by me until the end to let me go to a better place."[21]

Still, it is puzzling why Michael didn't divorce Terri and let the Schindlers take over Terri's care. Perhaps he was too committed—in battles in the courts and with the Schindlers—to ever give up. Perhaps he was correctly defending Terri's true wishes. But for many people, he didn't seem like that kind of person, so the mystery remains about his true motives.

At one point toward the very end of the case in 2005, the Schindlers offered to let Michael have all the remaining money from the malpractice award and any money from book or movie deals, if they could just take over Terri's case, but he refused.

As we shall see below, the Schindlers made the extraordinary claim on television and in court that Terri's coma may have been caused by violence and abuse by Michael. An autopsy after her death proved that no such abuse occurred.

Charging Michael with abusive behavior and, in effect, abusive behavior that killed Terri was a horrendous charge to make, especially since Michael had lived with Terri's parents for many years. Perhaps at the time the parents really believed it, but one can also understand why afterward Michael was so bitter toward them. Once the parents had made this claim, in court and on television, they burned their bridges behind them, cutting off any possibility of future reconciliation with Michael.

The Schindlers later testified that they would never remove Terri's feeding tube under any circumstances, even if she had asked them to, orally or in writing. They said that if she developed gangrene and all her limbs had to be amputated, they would still keep her alive, even against her will. That is, there were absolutely no circumstances under which they would let their favorite daughter die.[22]

> *After obtaining in 1998 a copy of a report on a bone-scan of Terri done in 1991, the Schindlers tried to introduce it in November 2002 as new evidence, claiming that Terri's coma was caused by trauma and not anoxia. They implied that Michael may have abused Terri and that this alleged abuse could have caused her neurological damage.*
>
> *They also claimed that Terri was not then in PVS and that they had new witnesses claiming that Terri would really have wanted to live under her new conditions. A second appellate court allowed five physicians to examine Terri, two obtained by Michael, two by the Schindlers, and one by the court itself.*

What Caused Terri's Problems?

Terri Schiavo may have suffered from bulimia or anorexia before her heart attack. People with such eating disorders may suffer from an imbalance of potassium.

According to documents filed in the first legal appeal, a three-stage imbalance of potassium could have led to a heart attack, which caused anoxia and Terri's subsequent brain damage. Many diets today contain too little potassium; the average American woman consumes less than half of the 4700 milligrams a day considered to be adequate.[23] Among other medical conditions, chronic lack of potassium can cause heart attacks and strokes. Moreover, blood tests for potassium can be normal even when real symptoms occur from chronic potassium insufficiency. As a result, physicians often fail to diagnose a chronic lack of potassium.

The claim that Terri Schiavo, first, had a heart attack because of a potassium imbalance and, second, that the heart attack caused her long-term coma was disputed by her parents and by Michael Baden, a New York forensic pathologist.[24] In 2004, Baden examined a 1991 bone-scan report that only became available to the Schindlers in 1998. Baden, first, claimed that "it is extremely rare for a 20-year-old to have a cardiac arrest from low potassium and no other diseases" and, second, that Terri "had no other diseases."

The original radiologist, W. Campbell Walker, said that the 1991 bone-scan report was requested to "evaluate for trauma" based on a suspected "closed head injury." He also noted on the report Terri's "history of trauma" and apparent injuries to ribs, vertebrae, ankles and knees. Appearing on Fox News Channel's *On the Record with Greta Van Susteren,* Dr. Baden concurred with Dr. Walker's assessment of bodily trauma.

But what caused the trauma? Dr. Baden said, "The trauma could be from an auto accident, . . . a fall, . . . or some kind of beating that she obtained from somebody, somewhere." In other words, it could have been from a beating by her husband, from a fall inside a hospital, or from some other, unknown event.

However, this reasoning is not credible. If Terri had arrived at an emergency room with this kind of trauma, surely Michael would have been reported (as required by law) to authorities for domestic violence, battery, or possible manslaughter. Nor would the hospital and its physicians have settled a malpractice case or allowed Michael to become Terri's guardian.

Chances of Awakening from PVS

Although most patients who have been in PVS for over a year never wake up, on rare occasions, some do. In one well-known study, 7 of 434 adults with traumatic head injuries who were in PVS for more than a year made good recoveries and regained consciousness, some with normal quality of life.[25] These seven recoveries warn against any quick judgment that a patient's condition is irreversible. Should PVS befall some people, they would want to be given this 7/434th chance of recovery. Several other studies have shown that, although few patients ever emerge from PVS, some people do within the first year, and once in a thousand times, after 3 years.[26]

No case exists of anyone emerging from PVS of 4 years' duration. In Terri Schiavo's case at the end, when activists shouted the contrary at cameras, she had been in PVS for *15 years,* and hence, according to clinical evidence, had no chance of returning to normal consciousness. Physicians who have seen her CT scan said that her brain, instead of being filled with normal brain tissue, then only contained cerebrospinal fluid, an indication of gross neurological damage and vegetative status.[27]

Whether anoxia or trauma caused the coma changes the prognosis. More patients seem to emerge, especially in the first few months, after coma caused by trauma than by anoxia. "It's the difference between taking a blow to the brain, which affects a local area—and taking this global, whole-brain hit," asserted New York bioethicist Joseph Fins in explaining the difference.[28] Because she had no blood pressure for over 40 minutes and because her heart often wasn't beating during this time, anoxia probably caused Terri's coma.

Whether or not Terri was really in PVS was crucial in this case, because several cases have been documented over the last decades where patients have emerged from some kind of deep coma of many years. In other words, patients have on rare occasion emerged out of comas that were not as severe as PVS.

Consider what happened in four cases of long-term comas. First, after an automobile wreck in Arkansas, Terry Wallis emerged from a coma of exactly *19 years,* his first word being "Mom."[29] Second, in 1996, ex-police officer Gary Dockery of Tennessee emerged out of his coma of *8 years* to talk for a few hours to his family, after which he lapsed back into a coma and died a year later in April.[30] Third, Patricia White Bull became comatose while giving birth to her fourth child and could not speak, swallow, or move much, but suddenly awoke *16 years later* to full consciousness on Christmas Eve, 1999. Fourth, Sarah Scantlin of Kansas in 1984 went into a coma after a car accident and emerged *21 years later.*[31]

Ethically, the fact that anyone at all comes out of a long-term coma is crucial because it changes the prognosis from a certainty to a probability. Families who want emotional closure on a case prefer to hear physicians say that the patient has "no" chance of recovery. The emotional weight changes when a patient has a "tiny" chance of recovery rather than "no" chance.

A review of these cases reveals an interesting conceptual disagreement among neurologists. Some claim that any patient who emerges from PVS was not really in PVS. But this is a nonfalsifiable, circular argument: If you awaken, you weren't in PVS. If you never awaken, you were in PVS.

A year later in the fall of 2003, having exhausted all appeals in Florida, the Schindlers appealed in federal court for a ruling to prevent removal of Terri's feeding tube. The Schindlers appealed to the public through the media, and several physicians publicly joined their side, including a pathologist and a physician who hoped to try exotic "coma stimulation" therapies.

Lawyers for Florida Governor Jeb Bush, a Catholic, filed a brief on the side of the Schindlers; Governor Jeb Bush praised the parents in the media for defending their daughter's right to life. President George W. Bush praised his brother's stand.

The Advocacy Center for Persons with Disabilities filed a lawsuit claiming that removal of Terri's PEG tube was abuse of a person with disabilities. The antiabortion group, Life Legal Defense Fund, helped the Schindlers hire lawyers, eventually paying bills of $300,000.

Physicians Disagree About Treatment

Three neurologists, including distinguished neurologist Ronald Cranford, who had examined Nancy Cruzan, testified that Terri was in PVS (Cranford substituted "permanent" for "persistent" to emphasize the irreversibility of her condition). The Schindlers cited Terri's ability to swallow saliva as evidence that she was not in PVS; Cranford rebutted and testified that such swallowing was controlled by primitive functions of her brain stem.

Dr. William Mayfield, a pioneer in the field of medical radiology and a founder of the American College of Hyperbaric Medicine, testified that he believed that hyperbaric oxygenation therapy (HBOT) would have benefited Terri. Neurologist Ronald Cranford, who examined Terri in 2002, retorted, "Increase the blood flow to dead tissue, and what do you get? Dead tissue."[32]

Another physician who championed HBOT was William Hammesfahr, who testified for the Schindlers that Terri was not in PVS and would respond well to the hyperbaric treatments that were his primary business. Hammesfahr, who seemed eager to appear on television, presented himself as an unappreciated genius, like Dr. Ignaz Semmelweis, who was far ahead of the medical community and, hence, a pariah. (Semmelweis was the 19th century Austrian physician who came to believe that his colleagues were spreading childbirth fever by not washing their hands and going from birth to birth. He was ostracized by his fellow physicians for this claim, even though it was correct.)

The three neurologists found Hammesfahr unprofessional and noted that he required cash in advance for his hyperbaric treatments and had published no articles documenting the amazing successes he claimed from using his hyperbaric chambers.

Critics also claimed that Mayfield and Hammersfahr stood to gain money by the treatments they recommended and that such treatments had no published proof of benefit. Moreover, Mayfield and Hammersfahr represented extreme, marginal positions in the medical community. The overwhelming medical consensus was that Terri had died long ago, that she had no chance of returning to any normal conscious state, and that dragging on the controversy was two steps backward from the Cruzan case in moving toward an enlightened national policy about ending care for comatose patients.

At the last moment, a neurologist affiliated with the Mayo Clinic in Jacksonville, Florida, William Cheshire, visited Terri in her room and opined that Schiavo "may" have been in a minimally conscious state, although he did not extensively examine her.[33] Cheshire was director of the Center for Bioethics and Human Dignity, a Web-based (virtual) bioethics center and passionate critic of assisted suicide.[34]

Another disagreement among these physicians concerned what Terri's movements meant. Ability to respond to a squeeze or pinch is consistent with PVS. In the Cruzan case, when neurologist Cranford examined Nancy, her lawyer William Colby described what happened:

> Cranford next grabbed hold of Nancy's stiff right leg and tried to bend it straight. Nancy grimaced. Then he reached for the soft skin on the inside of the upper part of her right arm, and held the pinch. Slowly, as if she were a robot, Nancy's head lifted off the bed and turned. Her face locked on her father's for about ten seconds, before she lowered just as slowly to the pillow.[35]

Despite being there and witnessing this phenomenon in this case, Dr. Cranford insisted that Nancy Cruzan's biography was over, that no one was conscious within the reflexes of her body, and that further treatment was futile.

6.4 A New Category of Consciousness?

During the Schiavo case, some New York neurologists proposed a new category of *minimally conscious state* (MCS) for patients in long-term comalike states, a new category between the only two previous ways of classifying such beings as either *comatose* or *vegetative*.[36] Neurologists Nicholas Schiff, Joy Hirsch, and Joseph Giacino, along with seven other co-authors, proposed this new category after working with brain-damaged patients at several facilities around New York City. To cause even more confusion in the public, their claims were often reported on the front page of the *New York Times* rather than in the best journals of neurology.[37]

Through an intense program of stimulation, they enabled one or two patients to return to a minimally conscious state (MCS). Using scans of blood flow to the brain, they identified dozens of patients with this potential, and one or two were able to remarkably improve.

Controversy surrounds these claims. Alan Shewmon, a famous pediatric neurologist, calls the new category "an inaccurate name for an invalid concept." Shewmon argues that there is no scientific or philosophical way to distinguish between minimal consciousness and full consciousness, implying that consciousness is something one either has or does not have, like saying you can't be a little bit pregnant.

But maybe that's the wrong analogy. Why can't a light bulb be, not on or off, but bright or dim? Why can't consciousness be a gradient? Terri's defenders retort that people are minimally conscious all the time—in sleep, or after injury—and what is important is the potential for recovery of consciousness. If it's impossible to prove any difference between minimal consciousness and consciousness, it also must be impossible to *disprove* a difference. So if Terri was in MCS, she might at times feel something. After all, the brain does not get injured in neat taxonomic lines.

The potential for recovery of such a patient is probably best when maximal efforts are made *in the first few months* after injury. This potential diminishes as the years increase. At the beginning, physicians should always act as if the brain-damaged person is minimally conscious, but after many years (15 years for Terri), chances of recovery approach zero.

Terri's electroencephalogram (EEG) was flat and her CT scan showed severe atrophy in her cerebral hemispheres. Vasodilators would not have helped, as a Schindler-friendly physician suggested.

Dartmouth neurologist James Bernat agreed, but understood why laypeople rallied behind Terri. "Just looking at a videotape of someone propped up in bed, with their eyes blinking and so on, it looks like they're aware," he said.[38] They are awake, he said, but not aware. With an intact brain stem, their eyes can still follow things, but only slightly to the left or right. For a diagnosis of persistent vegetative state, "there really has to be zero evidence of any responsiveness that suggests awareness."

> *In the fall of 2003, the Florida legislature passed a special bill,* Terri's Law, *that allowed the governor to issue a one-time stay of a judge's order to remove a feeding tube in certain cases where a patient is in PVS. After its passage, Governor Bush immediately issued such a stay.*
>
> *Michael and the American Civil Liberties Union appealed in state court and won, but the governor appealed to a mid-level appellate court. In June 2004, the Florida Supreme Court agreed to hear arguments as to whether Terri's Law was constitutional on direct review.*

6.5 Religious Issues

As the case received greater coverage in the print and visual media, different groups took stands on the case. Within the Christian community, and especially within the Catholic Church, people disagreed about the ethics of removing artificial nutrition and hydration (ANH) from Terri Schiavo.

Perhaps after having seen the videotape of Terri on international television news, and referring to her case, Pope John Paul II said in 2004 that ANH was to be considered ordinary, as opposed to extraordinary, care. He specifically said that removal of feeding tubes from patients in PVS was "euthanasia by omission."[39] In 1957, Pope Pius XII had told a group of anesthesiologists that they were not obligated to provide extraordinary care to dying patients.

The *Cruzan* decision allowed feeding tubes to be removed for PVS patients at the request of legal surrogates. Prior to John Paul II's comments, feeding tubes had been routinely removed from PVS patients in Catholic hospitals. Although the pope's comment was not delivered *ex cathedra* as official Catholic dogma, the new remark cast doubt on that practice, as well as on the role of advance directives in Catholic hospitals. Several Protestant leaders and some U.S. Catholic bishops also denounced Michael Schiavo's attempt to have Terri's feeding tube removed, saying it was murder.

In contrast, Father Kevin O'Rourke, one of the leading Catholic medical ethicists in North America, argued that providing ANH was indeed extraordinary care and should not be used to prolong the life of PVS patients. He noted that both Catholic ethicists working in hospitals, as well as doctors and nurses there, followed a much more liberal standard that allowed removal of life support from patients in PVS.

Father John Paris, a leading Jesuit bioethicist and professor of ethics at Boston College, noted that the pope's remarks targeted a specific audience and predicted they would have little impact in America. "I think the best thing to do is ignore it, and it will go away," Paris said. "It's not an authoritative teaching statement," he said.[40]

Catholic hospitals were thrown into confusion by the pope's remarks about the Schiavo case. They had been removing respirators and feeding tubes for a decade. What were they to do now? Would people fear dying in a Catholic hospital? In the end, they elected to redouble their efforts to have every patient sign an advanced directive and assign durable power of attorney. Lacking such documents and in such hospitals, young trauma patients could end up like Terri Schiavo.

On another front in this fight, lay Catholics and evangelical Christians flexed new political muscles. Bobby Schindler, employed as a science teacher in a Catholic high school, started accepting money in 1989 from Assemblies of God.[41] James Dobson's Focus on the Family issued daily news updates on the case. The ultraconservative Family Research Council emailed its subscribers with headlines such as "Terri Communicates" and included links for donations. Gary McCullough, a bearded Floridian who often escorted Mary Schindler to a microphone, owned Christian News Wire, whose clients include antiabortion organizer Randal Terry.[42]

Before this case, Catholics and Catholic hospitals had great flexibility about withdrawing feeding tubes. The Schiavo case changed that. Now Catholic patients and their families can ethically remove life-sustaining care under very few conditions.[43] The case also had other effects. A director of education for the Catholic Diocese of Birmingham said that the Catholic Church now refuses to recognize the diagnosis of a vegetative state, saying that "a person is never a vegetable."[44]

6.6 Disability Issues

As interest grew in the Schiavo case, advocates for people with disabilities began to take notice. While the Quinlan and Cruzan cases had never been conceptualized as involving discrimination against these persons, the last decades have witnessed the growing influence of *disability culture*, leading to interest of disability advocates in the Schiavo case.

Charleston disability rights lawyer Harriet McBryde Johnson charged that "Ms. Schiavo has a statutory right under the Americans With Disabilities Act not to be treated differently because of her disability. Obviously, Florida law would not allow a husband to kill a nondisabled wife by denying her nourishment. Because the state is overtly drawing lines based on disability, it has the burden under the ADA of justifying those lines."[45]

Advocates for disabled persons see American culture as one that systemically prejudices Americans against people with disabilities by extolling the ideals of youth, health, beauty, wealth, cleanliness, maximal functioning, and intelligence. Such advocates abhor the invidious messages given by television shows emphasizing scantily clad young women and men doing physical feats.

They criticized also the indirect *rationing* that occurs when the medical system does not provide enough financial and medical resources for people with disabilities to function on their own. Such advocates also criticize the idea of encouraging persons with disabilities to exercise their right to die only when a stingy medical system has made their lives so miserable that the only autonomous decision left for them is to give up and die.

One new issue arising from the Schiavo case was that it was the first one where a patient who was severely cognitively impaired was claimed to be *a victim of discrimination against disabled persons*. Since passage of the Americans with Disabilities Act (ADA) in 1990, denial of medical resources to a person who has disabilities because he is disabled violates federal law. However, the ADA has never specified end-of-life cognitive deterioration (which also would include Alzheimer's disease) as a covered disability.

A central ethical issue about disability concerns how much protection is owed to a vulnerable, incompetent person with disabilities by the State, especially when such protection is measured in money. How much public money is that person owed, especially if without that money, that person dies? A thousand dollars a month? A million dollars a year?

Many people wrongly believe that medical insurance, Social Security, or Medicare cover care for patients in long-term nursing homes; they don't. Given that state governments or families cannot be expected to spend a fortune on medical care for a patient in PVS, what is a *reasonable standard of care* for such expenditures? When does falling below that level constitute *structural discrimination* against persons with disabilities?

Most states have limited Medicaid budgets for care for patients who are poor (Medicaid is a state medical program matched by federal dollars and that varies in coverage from state to state). Most families have limited savings for medical catastrophes. When does rational allocation become discrimination? Newborn babies with severe disabilities may cost a million dollars. If a state allocates no money for their care, is that discrimination?

When governor of Texas, George W. Bush signed a law allowing hospitals to disallow treatment in futile Medicaid cases, and a week before the finale of the Schiavo case, a 5-month-old premature baby named Sun Hudson died in Texas Children's Hospital in Houston when physicians followed this law.[46] Disability advocates also excoriated the hypocrisy of Congress intervening in this case when Republicans had been cutting the Medicaid budget that "keeps many millions of [disabled] people alive."[47] Florida Republican Senator Mel Martinez passed out a memo to his colleagues, saying that Schiavo for them was a "great political issue" that would help them in upcoming elections.[48]

Groups such as Not Dead Yet, the World Association of Persons with Disabilities, the National Spinal Cord Injury Association, and Joni and Friends opposed removal of Terri's feeding tube. Of course, to claim that Terri Schiavo is a victim of discrimination against persons with disabilities assumes that she is still a person and could emerge from her coma. That is exactly what disability advocates and her parents claimed. Given the increasing acceptance that a patient in PVS for a decade cannot revert back to consciousness, Terri's advocates increasingly *claimed that she was not in PVS at all but in a state of minimal consciousness.*

6.7 Virtue Ethics: The Many Faces of Compassion

Before the patients' rights movement of the 1960s overthrew paternalism, physicians made end-of-life decisions for families and thereby protected them from the agony of making these decisions on heart-wrenching, unfamiliar grounds. Because families sometimes find it difficult to accept the death of a previously vibrant young daughter or son, such paternalism in retrospect seems compassionate. The new autonomy of patients and their families burdened them during times of crisis when they were unprepared to decide.

Let's talk a little about the virtue of compassion in this case. Suppose we give Terri's parents their premises and see what follows: Assume that some small part of her mind is still intact in some strange slipstream between normal consciousness and death. That is, assume she sometimes is in a so-called minimally conscious state. What follows then?

Would not most people abhor such a life? Abhor the thought of inhabiting 15 years inside a body in which they could not scratch an itch, express a wish, or perform any human act? No one knows what might be going on in such a mental remnant. Whatever destroyed the original mind might have left it in disarray, such that Terri's mental life was an endless nightmare.

If Terri could have awakened for 15 minutes and could have understood her condition, what she looked like, and what the case was doing to her family, can anyone think that this shy, weight-conscious woman would have wanted her brain-damaged, disfigured body exhibited to the world this way?

There is no doubt that Terri's parents cared so deeply about their daughter that they could not let her go. The question is: Was this the highest form of compassion?

6.8 The Politicization of the Schiavo Case

The essential question faced by the Florida Supreme Court concerned whether Terri's Law was constitutional. In September 2004, the Court ruled 7–0 that it was not. It based its decision upon two constitutional canons: the separation of powers and the unlawful delegation of authority. "It is without question an invasion of the authority of the judicial branch for the Legislature to pass a law that allows the executive branch to interfere with the final judicial determination in a case," wrote Chief Justice Barbara Pariente.[49]

Even if it were constitutional, the case summary suggests that the law would still be suspect since the "Legislature provided the Governor unconstitutionally inadequate standards for the application of the legislative authority. . . ." The judges ruled that Terri's Law also failed to provide any level of standards or limitations on the governor's power to issue a stay.

In December, Governor Bush appealed the case to the U.S. Supreme Court. Two months later, this Court declined to get involved.[50] Activists predicted the imminent "brutal murder" of a "purposefully interactive, alert, curious, lovely young woman who lives with a very serious disability."[51]

In February 2005, 15 years after the case began, Judge Greer ordered the feeding tube removed. The Schindlers filed a variety of desperate motions to delay the removal. A Florida appellate court denied them all.

Then, extraordinarily, the U.S. Congress became involved. House Majority Leader Tom DeLay subpoenaed Terri to appear before a House committee to put her under the federal program that protects such witnesses. Judge Greer ignored this subpoena.

In the Senate, Senator Bill Frist, the physician, worked with President George W. Bush to have Congress pass a federal version of Terri's Law, which it did. President Bush flew back during a congressional recess to sign a bill passed at midnight by a vote of 203 to 58.[52]

Like everyone else, Senator Frist (a physician) watched the edited video clip on television. Although he never visited Terri, he remarked to a national audience that Terri "did not seem to be" in a persistent vegetative state. In reaction, one of his critics fumed, "It's quackery. It'd be hilarious if it weren't so grotesque, how his presidential ambition and pandering to the right wing is clashing with his life's work."[53] Congressman Dave Weldon, also a physician and a Republican, agreed with Senator Frist about Terri's condition.

Congressmen Frist and Weldon had one problem: The federal government could not order a physician to insert a feeding tube. The only thing it could do is order a federal judge to review the case, once again, which was done. Federal judge

James Whittemore reviewed the case in two days and concluded, like two dozen judges before him, that nothing was amiss and that previous courts had made no errors. An appeal to the U.S. Court of Appeals in Atlanta, as conservative a group of judges as any in the country, came to the same conclusion.

Basically, the entire legal system was increasingly frustrated that half of the country and the media seemed not to trust its most basic processes. It was not going to reverse itself now, no matter what the political pressure to do so. And yet substantial doubt remained that Michael Schiavo had met the standard of clear and convincing evidence.

During March, media exposure escalated, producing what *Newsweek* later called "a public spectacle airing nonstop on cable and playing on front pages around the world."[54] People traveled to Pinellas Park, Florida, to hold prayer vigils for Terri while activists addressed them. Michael and his lawyer, George Felos, received death threats. A former girlfriend of Michael, a disgruntled nurse (who had been fired from Terri's nursing home), said on national television that Michael had cursed Terri and couldn't wait for her to die.

A juggernaut for Terri ensued: Soon, four Schindlers, plus recovered coma patients, odd physicians, activist monks, Patrick Mahoney, director of the Christian Defense Coalition, and anti-abortion activist Randal Terry campaigned on television, radio, and the Internet to "save Terri." The events gave new meaning to the oft-heard phrase "media circus."

Barbara Weller, an attorney working for the Schindlers, said that she had seen Terri trying to talk. Protestors called Judge Greer a "judicial murderer" and Republicans blasted the "imperial judiciary." The Rev. James Kennedy urged Governor Jeb Bush to ignore the federal judges.[55] The FBI arrested a man offering $250,000 to kill Michael Schiavo and $50,000 for the death of Judge Greer. Two people were arrested trying to break into the hospice.

Commentators repeatedly said that Terri's starving made her "suffer terribly." Physicians in palliative care repeatedly denied that terminal patients suffered when feeding tubes were removed and emphasized that no person was left to suffer in this case.[56]

On March 18, the last appeal failed to the U.S. Supreme Court (which had already twice refused to the review the case) and physicians removed Terri's feeding tube for the last time. Palliative care physicians predicted it would take about two weeks for Terri to die. After 13 days, while protestors prayed and rallied outside, Terri's body expired, on March 31, 2005.

The case had an anticlimax. Governor Bush ordered state attorney Mark McCabe to investigate an alleged gap 15 years before between the time Terri became unconscious and the time Michael called 911. McCabe investigated and found nothing suspicious.[57] After McCabe's final report, Governor Bush finally "declared an end to Florida's involvement in the matter" in July 2005.

6.9 What the Autopsy Showed

Chief Medical Examiner for Pinellas County, Florida, Jon Thogmartin, MD, released Terri's autopsy on June 13, 2005. It answered some questions and left others as mysteries.

First, he cleared up the mysterious bone scan of 1991 introduced by the Schindlers in 1992 with the claim that Terri's coma had been caused by trauma, possibly by Michael. Here is what happened: When Mediplex admitted Terri in early 1991, her physicians there ordered a bone scan to rule out degenerative changes in her bones. The bone scan was done at nearby Manatee Memorial Hospital. There, the bone-scan form *erroneously* listed Terri Schiavo as a case of "closed head injury" and said "the patient has a history of trauma." Thogmartin writes, "It appears that with little or no knowledge of the admitting diagnosis or clinical situation of Mrs. Schiavo, Manatee Memorial staff and radiologists completed the report."[58]

The coroner writes that it is true that the bone scan showed a compression fracture of the spine, but it was *due to osteoporosis*, a common condition in paralyzed patients. Moreover,

> In summary, any rib fractures, leg fractures, skull fractures or spine fractures that occurred concurrent with Mrs. Schiavo's original collapse would almost certainly have been diagnosed in February, 1990, especially with the number of physical exams, radiographs, and other evaluations she received in the early evolution of her care at Humana Hospital-Northside. During her initial hospitalization, she received twenty-three chest radiographs, three brain CT scans, two abdominal radiographs, two echocardiograms,

one abdominal ultrasound, one cervical spine radiograph, and one radiograph of her right knee. No fractures or trauma were reported or recorded. . . . By far the most likely explanation for the bone scan findings in Mrs. Schiavo are prolonged immobility induced osteoporosis and complicating H.O. in an environment of intense physical therapy.[59]

In sum, there was no evidence of trauma or abuse by anyone. Michael was wrongly accused of killing Terri. Everyone misunderstood what the 1991 bone scan revealed and how it had originally been mistakenly labeled.

The big surprise of the autopsy was that "Mrs. Schiavo's heart was anatomically normal without any areas of recent or remote myocardial infarction. Her heart (including the cardiac valves, conduction system and myocardium) was essentially unremarkable." That was big a surprise because, although the cause of her heart attack was debatable, few of Michael's supporters doubted that she had had one.

Now we know that neither trauma nor a heart attack caused Terri's coma. Probably, we will never know exactly what happened to her heart. Two crucial pieces of evidence are that she may have consumed as much as one gram of caffeine a day and that she had hypoalkemia. Perhaps this combination, after the extreme weight loss, stressed her heart too much that night.

According to reports filed by paramedics or police on the night of her original collapse, no other drugs were found in her system.

Another surprise was that the autopsy showed no clinical evidence of bulimia, especially the kind of wear on the enamel of the back teeth that is often caused by this condition. Despite the fact that the malpractice suit was settled on the assertion that Terri had an undiagnosed eating disorder, the coroner's report showed no evidence of this disorder.

However, it still could be true that 15 years before, she was anorexic. Certainly her low potassium level, the fact that her weight dropped over a hundred pounds in a few months, combined with her drinking large amounts of iced tea, are evidence for this hypothesis.

The autopsy also revealed that Terri Schiavo was not in a minimally conscious state. In fact, she had massive brain damage. "Mrs. Schiavo's brain showed global anoxic-ischemic encephalopathy resulting in massive cerebral atrophy. Her brain weight was approximately half of the expected weight. Of particular importance was the hypoxic damage and neuronal loss in her occipital lobes, which indicates cortical blindness. Her remaining brain regions show severe hypoxic injury and neuronal atrophy/loss. No areas of recent or remote traumatic injury were found."[60]

Finally, without the PEG feeding tube, she would have died. "Oral feedings in quantities sufficient to sustain life would have certainly resulted in aspiration." Aspiration of food in such patients is a serious, even lethal, complication, causing infection, choking, and possible suffocation.

CONCLUSIONS

Many clinical details of this case remain murky for the public. Both parties in the court debate convinced themselves that the other side had bad motives. The constant cameras of the media made everything worse, as did outlier physicians pushing their for-profit remedies like snake-oil salesmen and paid lawyers and physician-politicians who made "video diagnoses" in neurology.

Mark Fuhrman, the former Los Angeles police detective involved in the O.J. Simpson murder trial, was allowed by the Schindlers to investigate the case and given complete access to the family. Although he used all his investigate resources and access, he could find no evidence that Michael had done anything wrong.

Looking backward, it is easy to see how the case became so adversarial and how it spiraled out of control. First, what caused Terri's collapse was mysterious. Second, Michael's previous relationship with his wife, her parents, and her friends may have had problems. Third, the parties probably had different ideas about what to do with the malpractice award. Fourth, and emotionally very important, Terri's movements in PVS seemed to laypeople to indicate some remnant of self inside. Fifth, the parents and husband disagreed about the relevance of expert testimony by neurologists. Sixth, Judge Greer granted Michael the right to remove the feeding tube on flimsy hearsay evidence, not nearly enough to be "clear and convincing" and contradicted by testimony from Terri's parents and friends.

Outsiders made things worse. Not understanding the history of the false report of abuse and trauma on the 1991 bone scan, outside experts guessed that something malevolent had happened to Terri, making Terri's advocates suspect a cover-up by Terri's husband and the courts. Outside physicians, pushing their own exotic, for-profit schemes, exploited gullible parents and friends. Outlier neurologists, pushing a new category of consciousness not in medical journals but on the front pages of *The New York Times,* also didn't help any.

When the parents went to national media, especially in an age of fierce competition among cable news stations for sensational topics, the floodgates opened. Because politicians on the national scene love media attention, and as Florida Senator Mel Martinez predicted, U.S. senators, congressional representatives, and even the president got involved.

In the end, the snippet of video of Terri seeming to respond to her mother, which aired across the planet for months, trumped all evidence, all legalities, all rational arguments, especially for Terri's parents' supporters. The video pulled the emotions hard, such that almost everyone wondered whether some snippet of intact consciousness might exist in Terri's body.

In the end, who could not empathize with the desperate parents who did not want their cherished daughter to die? And questions linger as to how the "clear and convincing" standard was initially met, why Michael resisted letting the parents care for Terri, or how she became deficient in potassium (if she really was).

Finally, three facts remain: (1) Being without blood pressure and a beating heart for most of 40 minutes ended Terri's biography; paramedics and ER physicians resurrected her body and used the technology of modern medicine to maintain it for 15 more years. (2) Michael did not kill or physically abuse Terri and indeed for the 3 years after her collapse made almost superhuman efforts to rehabilitate her. (3) Like a custody dispute over a child or a grandchild, this case essentially was a *family dispute* about stopping a relative's end-of-life care, but one that got dragged into much larger forces that almost no one could control.

FURTHER READINGS

"Between Life and Death: The Terri Schiavo Story," A & E films. Excellent 50-minute summary of case, with good pictures of Terri in various stages of her life and pictures of Patricia White Bull and Terry Wallace, coma patients who awakened after many years. http://store.aetv.com/html/search/index.jhtml?search=Terri+Schiavo+Story&x=12&y=6

Buchanan, Allan. *Deciding for Others. The Ethics of Surrogate Decision-Making.* New York: Cambridge University Press, 1990.

Colby, William. *The Long Goodbye: The Deaths of Nancy Cruzan.* Carlsbad, CA: Hay House, 2002.

Downloadable video of Terri Schiavo http://www.glennbeck.com/news/09092003-1.shtml

Fins, Joseph J. "Rethinking Disorders of Consciousness: New Research and Its Implications." *Hastings Center Report* (March–April 2005), pp. 22–24.

Legal issues about Schiavo case http://abstractappeal.com/schiavo/infopage.html http://www.sptimes.com/2003/11/02/State/How_Terri_s_Law_came_.shtml

Michael Schiavo's statement http://news.tbo.com/news/MGA9DXB31MD.html

Other Web sites about Schiavo case http://www.apfn.org/apfn/Terri_doctor.htm

Pence, Gregory. *Classic Cases in Medical Ethics,* 4th ed., Chapter 2, "Comas." New York: McGraw-Hill, 2004.

Plum, Fred, and Jerald Posner. *Stupor and Coma.* New York: Oxford University Press, 1982.

Quinlan, Joseph, and Julia Quinlan, with Phyllis Battelle. *Karen Ann: The Quinlans Tell Their Story.* New York: Doubleday, 1977.

Terri's Fight Web site http://www.terrisfight.org/times.html

Time line in Schiavo case http://www.miami.edu/ethics2/schiavo/timeline.htm

CHAPTER 7

A re Genetic Abortions Eugenic?

This chapter discusses a new kind of abortion, one done after genetic tests have revealed retardation or other disability in the fetus. Although this kind of genetic abortion has been done before, it was usually done late in the second trimester, around 24 weeks. What makes this kind of abortion different, and potentially much more common, is new technology that allows testing in the first trimester, before the woman shows pregnancy and where the fetus is much less developed. Geneticists can also test for more diseases and conditions than ever before, potentially allowing thousands of women to test fetuses in the first trimester. For the first time, widespread genetic testing may not be the stuff of science fiction but an inchoate norm in medical practice.

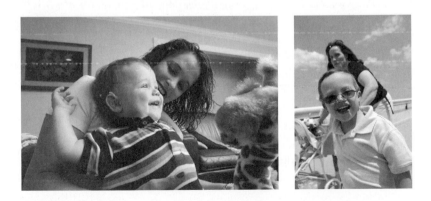

Alice and John Dryer always considered themselves to be antiabortion and religious people. Alice, 35, worked as an accountant in a large practice and John, 36, worked as

an accountant with his own firm. They knew that pregnant women over 35 were at increased risk of having a fetus with Down syndrome, and also knew that people with a family history of Down syndrome had increased risk. Even though one of their ancestors had Down syndrome, when Alice became pregnant, they did not really consider themselves at increased risk.

At 15 weeks, Alice's obstetrician asked her if she wanted to schedule an amniocentesis on her fetus at 18 weeks.[1] "At age 35, you have a small extra risk of having a fetus with Down syndrome," he said. Alice said she didn't think she would undergo the test, but said she would still go home and discuss the test with her husband.

7.1 Down Syndrome

Down syndrome is a chromosomal abnormality discovered by Langdon Down in 1866. A person with Down syndrome has 47 chromosomes in each cell rather than the usual 46. The extra chromosome is chromosome 21. *Trisomy* refers to an extra chromosome; hence the syndrome is also called trisomy-21.

Down syndrome always causes mental retardation and a characteristic facial appearance, and is often accompanied by cardiac or intestinal problems. In the early 1970s, physicians told parents that although the eventual intelligent quotient (IQ) of a person with Down syndrome could not be predicted at birth, IQ usually ranged between 25 and 60. However, some severely impaired individuals would have IQs below 25. By definition, normal IQ is scaled to be 100.

In the 1950s, some surgeons refused to perform life-saving cardiac surgery on babies with Down syndrome. At the time, society commonly placed them in state institutions with few programs to stimulate their intellectual growth. Such institutions often had abysmal standards of care.

During the last 50 years, a Copernican revolution has occurred in thinking about people with Down syndrome. Many earlier studies of IQ were made on those who were institutionalized. This sampling bias failed to take into account the higher IQs of people with Down syndrome who lived with supportive families.

At present, although most people with Down syndrome will have IQs below 70, less than one-third (some studies say only 10 percent) will have IQs lower than 25 (profoundly retarded and untrainable).[2] Most people with Down syndrome who receive good early care, maximum stimulation, and support will have IQs between 50 and 70.

What does this imply about quality of life for a person with Down syndrome? IQ is a measure of intelligence, of course, and academics and physicians often associate intelligence with happiness. However, it is an unwarranted conclusion to infer that people with IQs between about 50 and 70 must be unhappy, unless we simply define unhappiness in those terms.

Given reasonable stimulation, love, and supervision, most people with Down syndrome will, to use a phrase made important in ethics by philosopher Tom Regan in another context, "have a life."[3] Almost every person with Down syndrome will have a narrative history, and lives that will go (to use another famous phrase from Regan) "better or worse for them." Under almost any criteria of quality of life, most people with Down syndrome would not be better off dead.

Note the mention of early care, stimulation, and support. The prognosis for Down syndrome varies with treatment: For example, early stimulation can raise IQ, whereas custodial care will lower it. At birth, we cannot predict whether a baby with Down syndrome will be at the low or high end of the IQ range; consequently, the best interest of these babies is maximal treatment. Whether maximal treatment best benefits their families is another question.

Alice's physician outlined why she might want to consider amniocentesis. "We can now test for about a dozen genetic conditions. For $2,000, we can test your fetus for 40 common causes of mental retardation. Even if you are against abortion, a positive test allows you to plan for a developmentally challenged baby.

"We also have noninvasive tests that can test for Down syndrome and other abnormalities by using fetal ultrasound and simple blood tests to diagnose abnormalities. Again, a positive result does not imply you would abort but may help you plan for a special-needs child."

When a close friend gave birth to her second child with cystic fibrosis, Alice changed her mind and called for an appointment.

This case raises several important questions in bioethics. First, when does a human fetus have such moral value that it should not be aborted? More generally, what criteria allow us to separate nonpersons from persons? In Chapter 6 about Terri Schiavo, we raised this question about cases at the end of life and now we raise it about cases at the beginning.

Different questions concern a choice against the life of a fetus specifically because it has Down syndrome. Does the moral justification of this kind of abortion differ from that of abortion in general? As science increasingly creates prenatal tests for genetic disorders, parents can have more choices against certain disorders that their fetuses carry. Does allowing parents to abort their fetuses based on such information constitute prejudice against existing people with Down syndrome? When many similar tests become available and many parents use them, will this be a new eugenics movement?

7.2 *Roe* v. *Wade* and the Legalization of Abortion

In January 1973, the *Roe* v. *Wade* decision by the United States Supreme Court ruled it unconstitutional (and hence illegal) for states to ban abortions before fetal viability. *Viability* here means the ability of the fetus to live on its own outside the womb. Then and now, the real-life criterion of such viability is good fetal lung function.

It is a common misunderstanding that *Roe* v. *Wade* simply legalized abortion with no thoughtful analysis. In fact, the written decision of *Roe* v. *Wade* nicely illustrates philosophical reasoning. In general, this decision describes and compares two competing *interests* in the context of abortion.[4]

"Interest" is an important legal concept referring to a being's sphere of concern. A person normally has interests that his property be protected from theft, that his good name not be damaged by libel, and that his body not be damaged by medical malpractice.

In *Roe* v. *Wade*, the Supreme Court decided, first, that a mother has an interest or right to control her body and her reproductive choices; second, that the interests of the *embryo* (first 9 weeks) expand as it becomes a *fetus* (9 to 39 weeks), and finally a *baby* (at birth). In other words, a fetus at 38 weeks has more of the interests of a person than at 13 weeks, and a fetus at 13 weeks has more interests than an embryo at 8 days.

The language of "interests" is a legal way of discussing moral value or standing. Translated, the Court decided that the moral value of a human mother is that of a full person, but that of an 8-day human embryo is minimal. As the embryo grows to become a fetus, its moral value grows. At birth, its moral value or standing matches that of its mother.

This analysis implies, as the Court ruled, that during the first two trimesters (weeks 1–13 and 14–26), the mother's interest outweighs that of the fetus and that abortions can be justified. Of great importance to ethical reasoning, the analysis implies that as the moral value of the fetus increases, the reasons needed to justify aborting it become more demanding. This is why using a morning-after pill to prevent a 2-day-old embryo from implanting in the uterus requires much less justification than a very late-term abortion of a fetus at 37 weeks.

The concept of viability is vague (with no sharp boundaries), and in 1973, the Court said that it is "usually placed" at about 28 weeks but "may occur earlier, even at 24 weeks." In a later decision, it ruled that the physician performing the abortion could make the decision about viability, not a legislature or judge.

Later decisions denied states' ability to give a parent of a teenage girl, or the father of a fetus, a veto over a woman's decision to abort. In contrast, provided there was a system for case-by-case judicial appeal, states could pass laws that require notification or consent of one parent about a minor's abortion. Many states passed such laws.

Roe v. *Wade* also controversially permitted states to allow abortions in the third trimester (although no state passed a law allowing them). State laws must allow abortions in any trimester to protect the health or life of the mother. For this reason, so-called "partial-birth abortions" must be allowed to protect the life or health of the mother, although critics dispute whether such third-trimester fetuses really threaten the mother in the required way.

A high-resolution sonogram showed a high likelihood that Alice's fetus had Down syndrome. At 18 weeks, she had further blood tests, and at 21 weeks the results came back that her fetus definitely had Down syndrome.

After Alice and John discussed it, they were suddenly not so sure that they would keep their fetus. Alice knew that she would have no trouble raising a child with Down syndrome, but John hated the idea. Alice already worried that, if they had the child, their marriage would be in jeopardy.

"To be honest," John tells her, "I can't handle a Down kid, much less a Down man who's my son and 40 years old. Maybe I'm not cut out to be a saint."

7.3 Choosing Against Pregnancy vs. Choosing Against Abnormality

In this case, the Dryers *chose* to be pregnant and they *wanted* a baby; what they didn't want was a baby with Down syndrome. In this way, we can say they were not choosing as is the case with abortion, against having a baby at the present time, but choosing not to have *any* baby with Down syndrome. The late bioethicist John Fletcher once emphasized that a big difference exists between choosing against pregnancy, where a completely healthy fetus may be aborted but which may not be wanted, and choosing against a serious genetic disease, where the couple wants a fetus and hopes to bring it to term.[5] The Dryer case raises the question of whether an abortion for genetic reasons is more or less justifiable than an abortion for not wanting any baby at all.

Some people believe that choosing against a serious genetic disease comprises one of the cases where abortion is most justified. Not every family can handle raising a child with special needs and most families want the right to choose the number and kind of children who make up their family. For bioethicist Fletcher, two choices really do differ dramatically: one is simply choosing against any and all human fetuses, the other is choosing against an unlucky fetus that occurred and trying again for a normal one.

7.4 Abortion and Personhood

One of the ethical issues raised by this case is the general issue of the rightness or wrongness of abortion. Opponents of abortion consider it wrong because they see abortion as killing a person. Supporters of choice believe that other considerations may justify termination of *this* pregnancy.

So what is a person? In the context of abortion, bioethicists usually distinguish between a *person* and a *human being*. Although a fetus is human, it does not meet certain criteria of personhood, and since a fetus is not a person, it does not have a right to life. In this sense, "human" is a factual, biological term whereas "person" is an evaluative term, implying a right to life.

Probably, the most intuitively plausible of these arguments is offered by philosopher Mary Anne Warren. Warren offers a *cognitive criterion of personhood* and holds that a human fetus does not meet this standard.[6] According to Warren, to be a person is to be able to think, to be capable of cognition. What separates a normal, adult person from, say, a mouse, is certain capacities for reasoning, reflective self-awareness, communication, agency (motivated action), and consciousness of the external world. Warren does not think that any one of these capacities alone is sufficient for cognition; rather, these capacities define the core criterion. For Warren, a being lacking *all* of these capacities does not meet the cognitive criterion, and is not a person.

Before it develops a brain, a fetus possesses none of these characteristics. When exactly does such a brain develop? The answer depends on what is meant by "a brain." The ability to react to pain probably begins around 18 weeks and more cognitive abilities begin around 25 weeks. According to the cognitive criterion and practically speaking, first-trimester abortions performed around 10–13 weeks, when most abortions have been done historically, are justified because no person is killed.

Let us examine some issues concerning this *cognitive criterion*. To begin with, it can be objected that the criterion does not represent an adequate definition because it includes some nonpersons and excludes some persons. The cognitive criterion does seem to admit to personhood some beings that we don't naturally regard as persons; there is good evidence, for instance, that apes communicate, are conscious, may reason, and may be self-aware, yet we don't usually consider them persons. However, that may be just because we don't understand the implications of the cognitive criterion and are accustomed to a less defensible view.

For critics, a problem of the cognitive criterion is that it does not protect vulnerable human beings whose cognitive capacities are absent. Such patients include former President

Ronald Reagan in the late stages of Alzheimer's disease and Terri Schiavo in a persistent vegetative state. Advocates of the cognitive criterion, such as Princeton bioethicist Peter Singer, accept these implications.[7] Nor does the cognitive criterion protect *potential* persons, such as human fetuses or embryos.

Of course, *the whole point* of the cognitive criterion is to provide a standard for when we should not protect human beings, when it is permissible to let them die, or when it is permissible not to gestate them. The weakness that critics find in the cognitive criterion is a strength to its supporters.

Some conservative Christians advocate a *genetic criterion*, arguing that when sperm and egg meet and merge genomes, a genetically unique being is created (unless, of course, the zygote divides into identical twins). In its DNA, with a woman willing to gestate it, the resulting embryo has all the potential to be a full person.

However, having the potential to *become* a person is not the same as *being* a person, as we realize when we consider the thousands of frozen embryos stored around the world. Another problem with the genetic criterion is that it collapses the distinction between being human and being a person. Yet something can be a member of the human species and have no moral value as person. For example, a dead human has a unique set of genes but is no longer a person. These implications seem to refute the genetic criterion. Being a person must be something more than having human genes.

In 2004, the President's Council on Bioethics debated potentiality and personhood in discussing medical research on human embryos. The Council's chair, Leon Kass, argued that these embryos' potential for personhood conferred moral value on them. A dissenting member of the Council, Dartmouth neuroscientist Michael Gazzaniga, disagreed, making the analogy that "Even though a Home Depot may contain the supplies to build a dozen homes, when a Home Depot burns down, we do not say that a dozen homes were destroyed."[8]

A third possible criterion for personhood (in addition to the cognitive and genetic criteria) is the *neurological criterion*. This is actually a minimal, operational version of the cognitive criterion; it defines a person as a human being with a detectable brain wave, and claims that a human without such a brain wave is not a person. This simple standard would be applicable across many issues of medical ethics; it would, for instance, recognize as persons both third-term fetuses with developed brains and adults in persistent vegetative state.

> *Now the Dryers had to make a decision not only to have an abortion but whether to have a late, second-term abortion. The physicians told them that they must decide within 2 weeks because after 23 weeks, most physicians would consider the fetus viable and would not perform an abortion. The couple agonized about the decision and, during their process of deliberation, Alice mentioned their dilemma in a Sunday school class at church. She also said that, because the fetus had Down syndrome, they would probably decide to terminate the pregnancy.*

The Perspective of Disability Advocates

Disability advocates argue that allowing parents to abort a fetus because it has Down syndrome is wrong. To them, it makes prejudice against people with disabilities into moral justification. This is the wrong message to send in public policy because it says to people who are deaf, have Down syndrome, or spina bifida, that they are not valued as much as people without these conditions. In a time of scarce medical resources, when it is already difficult to get adequate help for such people, they believe that this is a terrible set of values.

Disability advocates argue that blindness, deafness, neural tube defects, and Down syndrome are not diseases, but valuable, different ways of existing that add diverse, new viewpoints to our society. In other words, having these conditions is not a problem; instead, the problem is society's reaction to these conditions.

The Scriptural Basis of Prohibitions on Abortion

Although the Catholic Church and conservative Protestant religions have opposed abortions for some time, it is important to distinguish between such teachings and original Scriptures. In the New Testament, neither Jesus nor Paul nor the Apostles discuss or condemn abortion. Hence, those seeking a scriptural basis for condemning abortion turn to the Old Testament.

The usual passage cited is this passage in Jeremiah 1:5: "Before I formed thee in the belly, I knew thee; and before thou camest forth out of the womb, I sanctified thee, and I ordained thee a prophet unto the nations." Now this passage in the context of its chapter is clearly about the life of the prophet Jeremiah and his destiny having been fixed by God before he was born. It is not about abortion and cannot be interpreted to be about abortion without the wildest stretches of license.

Moreover, other passages in the Old Testament seem to imply that abortion is not murder. In Exodus 21, men who are fighting and accidentally knock down a pregnant woman, causing her to miscarry, are only fined, not charged with murder. In Deuteronomy 22:21, Leviticus 21:9, and Genesis 38:24, pregnant women who conceived while not married are to be stoned, even though the stoning will also kill the fetus inside.

These biblical facts create an awkward dilemma for people who want to base answers in bioethics on the Bible. Such people want to avoid the subjectivism and relativism of a pick-and-choose approach, where readers shop for what they like and reject the rest. But most people who adopt this attitude believe that abortion is wrong. So one of their most fundamental moral beliefs is not based on the Bible. On the other hand, they usually reject other biblical commands, such as the one at the end of Mark (16:18) for believers to handle poisonous snakes.

7.5 New Genetic Tests, Disability Advocates, and Eugenics

For 40 years, alarmists have breathlessly predicted a new wave of eugenics as soon as geneticists began to take the first steps toward predicting many genetic diseases. Most of this was sensationalism, so the public grew weary of the hype, leaving many new books predicting the genetic apocalypse gathering dust.

In 2004, such developments finally began. These developments started profound changes in how parents think about their future babies. Understanding the significance of these changes requires a little background.

In the previous analysis of *Roe* v. *Wade* about moral value and the age of the fetus, we observed that the decision analyzed moral value as increasing with age of the fetus; a near-term fetus having much greater value than a two-day-old embryo.

This analysis reflects the actual behavior of physicians who perform abortions: Many are comfortable with early abortions, but not with third-term abortions. Most physicians would also be comfortable inserting an intrauterine device (IUD), or prescribing a morning-after pill, which prevents embryos from implanting, and which (on some definitions) is an abortion. On the other hand, very few physicians will perform third-term abortions when the fetus is near birth, even if the mother's health or life is at risk. (If the fetus was wanted, it could be delivered by cesarean at this time.)

Until recently, abortions for genetic reasons had to be performed around 23 weeks because that was when results came back from amniocentesis. Before 23 weeks, the amniotic sac around the fetus was not big enough to safely insert the needle to withdraw fluid for testing. When results showed a genetic condition such as Down syndrome, couples were faced with the decision to terminate a planned pregnancy at a very late date.

Another test, called chorionic villus sampling (CVS), samples fetal cells derived from the placenta at about 10 weeks of gestation. Because both CVS and amniocentesis cause slightly increased risks of miscarriage ($1/100$ and $1/300$, respectively), some couples avoid them.

Amniocentesis, followed by abortion, has been a difficult choice for many couples. Even when they chose abortion, couples are traumatized because they really wanted a baby; because the abortion had to be so late, the mother has bonded with the fetus during 23 weeks of gestation. For almost six months, the couple's thoughts had been on the expected baby. Many couples also felt it wrong to abort because the fetus had a genetic disease. Finally, whatever decision the couple made, they ended up feeling guilty.

Despite the claims of alarmists, most couples are sensible about such choices: They do not abort because a fetus lacks blonde hair or blue eyes (assuming medicine could now test for these traits, which it cannot). In general, the more severe the defect, the greater the reluctance of couples to carry the fetus to term. For example, a fetus with neurofibromatosis or Huntington disease will often be aborted, but one with Turner syndrome (which can be treated by hormone replacement therapy, although even successful treatment leaves such adults infertile) will not.

By 2004, high-resolution sonograms showed prospective parents remarkable pictures of first-trimester fetuses: As early as 15 weeks, some fetuses had human faces and appeared to be smiling. Antiabortion advocates showed these pictures to women contemplating abortions. Unnoticed amongst this clamor was the fact that the very same sonograms could show the neural tube defects of spina bifida or the characteristic translucent area at the back of the neck of a fetus with Down syndrome.

In the same year, physicians used a high-resolution sonogram and three simple blood tests to determine if a first-trimester fetus has increased risk of Down syndrome or other genetic conditions.[9] This new testing has several important aspects.

First, according to *Roe* v. *Wade's* analysis of moral value, an earlier abortion can be done when the fetus has less moral value than a late, second-trimester fetus. Because less weighty reasons are required to justify a first-trimester abortion than a late, second-trimester abortion, and because abortion to avoid genetic disease is considered by many people one of the best possible reasons for an abortion, such abortions seem most justifiable.

Second, because the abortion is at the end of the first trimester, family, friends, and neighbors need not be aware of the pregnancy. If the mother or father has a familial history of genetic disease and wishes to have the option of an abortion for genetic reasons, they can keep the pregnancy quiet. That is important.

Because many people fear the condemnation of others for personal acts such as abortion, this new development allows for private abortions. If no one knew a woman was pregnant, the intervention described in this chapter's case could not occur.

Third, genetics labs have developed a reasonably priced test for 50 conditions that cause mental retardation. Baylor College of Medicine, and its associated Quest Genetics, now can screen fetal cells for more than 450 conditions, including deafness and dwarfism.[10]

Fourth, all these tests can be done with no additional risk to the fetus of miscarriage. For Down syndrome, sonograms measure Nuchal Translucency (NT) of fluid at the back of the fetal neck. This result is combined with measurements of maternal blood levels of three substances—alpha-fetoprotein, human chorionic gonadotropin, and estriol—as well as the woman's age, to give a 90 percent detection rate of Down syndrome and a 97 percent detection rate of trisomy-18, another genetic cause of retardation.[11]

These tests also allow today's women or couples to test a first-trimester fetus for cystic fibrosis, the most common genetic disease among white couples, and, after a positive test, undergo an early abortion. Other couples abort after learning their child would have Fragile X syndrome, another genetic cause of mental retardation. It is also true that some couples receive the same news and decide not to abort.

Predictably, disability advocates contend that such genetic testing will create a new, *grassroots eugenics,* resulting in a massive number of deaths of fetuses that carry genes for undesirable genetic conditions. Antiabortion advocates fear that such testing will add a new legitimacy to first-trimester abortions (when most abortions of healthy, unwanted fetuses are already performed).

Reacting to a case like the Dryers', one Christian writer asks, "Can people really do this? Abort their baby while *knowing* it is their baby? And to do so for no other reason than a minor health problem? . . . What right have we to decide if a baby has a right to live?[12] Commenting on a decision to abort a fetus with Down syndrome, the Christian writer asks, "Did no one tell this woman that this was not a decision that was hers to make?" She ends by predicting a new slippery slope leading to a new kind of eugenics.

> One day at their church during an adult Sunday school class, the Dryers were surprised when a group of members from their church "ambushed us" (in Alice's words). One earnest woman exclaimed, "Alice! Please don't kill your child with Down syndrome." Another said, "We hope you won't be selfish." Two parents brought along their adult Down son.
>
> The members who confronted the Dryers later said they felt they needed to do an "intervention" for the sake of the baby. "Our intentions were good," they said.
>
> The Dryers felt hurt and rebuked by the semipublic attack on their personal decision and felt the church members had no right to coerce their decision.

7.6 Eugenics

What was the eugenics movement and why was it so bad that any reference to it stops conversation and the possibility of ethical justification? Contrary to popular belief, the eugenics movement did not start in Nazi Germany; in fact, its center was on Long Island, New York. It was based on a smidgen of fact and many incorrect, alarmist inferences from that smidgen.

In 1859, Charles Darwin published his famous *The Origin of Species*, defending the evolution of humans from primates and using concepts such as competitive advantage and survival of the fittest. Because they contradicted the biblical story of creation of Adam and Eve, Darwin's ideas took decades for educated people to accept.

In the late 1880s, Darwin's cousin Francis Galton invented the term "eugenics" (literally, "good birth") and championed maximal births by the most "fit" people and sterilization or voluntary abstinence of "unfit" people. By 1905, eugenic organizations had sprung up in Europe, Japan, and Scandinavia, but especially in Cold Springs Harbor, Long Island. American politicians and geneticists urged "eugenic marriages," sterilization of the unfit, and worried that the "breeding stock" of America was under attack from incoming hordes of Irish, Italian, Chinese, and African immigrants, who (without birth control) tended to have large families.

Because of these ideas, 31 states passed laws allowing involuntary sterilization of "mental defectives," and by 1941, 36,000 Americans had been sterilized.[13] In Nazi Germany, where Hitler gave these ideas greater reinforcement, more than 225,000 people were sterilized for perceived mental illness or perceived inheritable physical disabilities. In addition, the Immigration Restriction Act of 1924 severely limited entry into the United States of people from "inferior" lands such as Asia, Africa, southern Europe, and Ireland, while simultaneously encouraging immigration from England, Germany, Switzerland, and Scandinavia.

As medical historian Daniel Kevles emphasized in his classic, *In the Name of Eugenics*, most of the early ideas of eugenics were based on racism and false ideas. Early geneticists did not know that mental retardation can be caused not only by inherited conditions but by chromosomal breakage later in development.[14]

They did not know which human traits were based on genes and which on the environment (or the interaction of both). They did not completely understand dominant and recessive genes, and the principles of population genetics, so they miscalculated how long it would take to eliminate genetic conditions from the population. Most egregiously, they did not understand, or care about, the degree of state coercion necessary to control reproduction in millions of people and the consequent violation of procreative liberty of millions of couples (later, when China limited its couples to having only one child, the world discovered the severe measures needed to accomplish this result).

By 1935, the geneticist Hermann J. Muller said that eugenics was "hopelessly perverted," a cult for "advocates for race and class prejudice, defenders of vested interests of church and State, Fascists, Hitlerites, and reactionaries generally."[15] Another leading geneticist of the time, and a founder of modern, statistical genetics, J.B.S. Haldane, said that "many of the deeds done in America in the name of eugenics are about as much justified by science as were the proceedings of the Inquisition by the Gospels."[16]

After World War II, eugenics was discredited based on its bad science and its association with the Final Solution of the Nazis. The Final Solution, of course, dealt with the "problem" of breeding of unfit people. For the Nazis, the "solution" was the Holocaust, the deaths of 6 million Jews, gypsies, homosexuals, and others whom the Nazis judged to be genetically unfit.

Eugenics secretly continued in Scandinavia, for example, in Sweden, where citizens with low intelligence or gross physical defects were forcibly sterilized over four decades; amazingly, the practice only ended in 1976.[17] Similar secret eugenic sterilizations occurred during the same decades in China and Australia.[18]

Separating Eugenics from Parental Choice

The past eugenics movement was evil because it was founded on state coercion, because it had false views of how to eradicate genetic disease, and because it was racist. Let us refer to this as Eugenics with a capital "E."

What opponents today decry as "eugenics" is not the above movement where some women and couples were forced to abort their fetuses or where many were sterilized. Instead, people *voluntarily* choose to abort to prevent genetic disease, not based upon false information about their fetuses but upon reliable data. In one study in Australia, the number of babies with Down syndrome has dropped by half in mothers younger than age 35 (note: Australia provides free medical care to all its citizens, making such testing easy.)[19] Let us call this "eugenics" with a lowercase "e."

Is this new eugenics wrong? Some say it is for two reasons. First, when the Dryers choose against having a child with Down syndrome, they send a message to existing people with Down syndrome that their lives are not worth living and that their parents should have aborted them. They argue that a just public policy cannot both support parents choosing against undesirable genetic conditions and also not devalue the lives of existing people with these genetic conditions.

Second, they believe that only God, not people, should have the right to choose to kill a fetus because it has a genetic disease. Some echo the Catholic Church in condemning birth control pills and intrauterine devices (IUDs), rejecting the idea that women should be able to control when and if they become pregnant.

Such criticisms inflame pro-choice women:

> A child psychologist from Atlanta who terminated a Down syndrome fetus earlier this year said she was outraged by people who told her, "If you have to have a perfect baby, you shouldn't be a parent." "I was like, 'What?'" said the psychologist, who is 35. "I've always been pro-choice, but now I'm pro-choice with a vengeance. Don't tell me I have to have a baby with Down syndrome because you say so."[20]

Remember that the big question overall is whether giving parents more choices about not having children with genetic conditions is tantamount to a new eugenics movement that will result in fewer resources for, and discrimination against, people living with disabilities.

Alice Dryer's sister, Carol, age 49, and her husband, Dave, age 54, belonged to an organization of parents who supported people with Down syndrome, mainly to support her close friend, Beth, who had an affected teenager, Mike. However, and in part because of her extensive, intimate knowledge of

*this condition, when Carol herself became pregnant,
she knew that her age and family history put her fetus at
increased risk for Down syndrome. Carol and Dave knew
they did not want to carry a fetus with Down syndrome,
but at the same time, they did not want to "send the wrong
message" to Beth and Mike.*

*Because of her work with people with Down syndrome,
Carol was also aware of the new tests that allowed diagnosis
of Down syndrome and other causes of mental retardation in
the first trimester. This meant Carol knew she could test her
fetus and, if positive for Down syndrome, have an abortion
before her pregnancy showed.*

*Carol's fetus tested positive for Down syndrome and,
after several days of hesitation, she and Dave decided upon
a first-trimester abortion for this pregnancy. After doing so,
she tried to get pregnant again, hoping this time for a
normal fetus.*

"It's Not Our Right to Choose"

Lurking beneath the opposition of some people to genetic
abortions is the view that people really shouldn't have the right
to make these kinds of choices, that the very possibility of
choice is evil and wrong. What is the source of this view?

Ultimately, it may be a religious view, stemming from a belief that an omniscient, omnipotent God or Allah has designed
the world and has a plan for it. In that plan, things happen to
people for a reason, and part of being happy, as well as gaining
eternal life in heaven, is to discover and accept that plan. So,
for example, a pregnant teenage girl may say to herself, "If God
didn't want me to be pregnant, I wouldn't be."

Similar attitudes see God as dictating infertility and some
believers skeptically eye the current fanaticism of infertile
couples to conceive. In the same way, God is seen as having a
reason for creating a fetus with Down syndrome. For a woman
or couple, it may be a test of faith, or to help them grow in ma-
turity, or to make their other children less selfish, or to make
them realize they cannot cope with this child alone and need
the help of a large church.

One way antiabortion advocates define an absolute value
is to say that no competing value can ever be strong enough

to justify a judgment not to act according to that value. To be resolutely pro-life is to assert that humans must always choose to implant an embryo with a severe disability or always choose to gestate a fetus with a genetic disease. Humans lack the right to make such choices; allowing such choices goes against God's plan for us.

This is a fatalistic view. It minimizes the role of human free will in life, not only in being saved but in everyday morality. The girl who is pregnant and says "It's God's will" ignores her own complicity in the sexual act that led her to be pregnant (in all cases except rape).

The extreme opposite view denies God's existence and thinks girls become pregnant because they have unprotected sex. Period. And some couples have babies with Down syndrome because the mothers over age 35 have chromosomes that start to break down (haploid gametes, containing one-half of the new child's genetic complement, are more prone to error over age 35, hence the extra one in trisomy-21). Or babies are born with genetic conditions because of bad luck in the genetic roulette of reproduction. To say parents shouldn't try to eliminate bad results, if they have the chance, is nonsense.

A possible compromise exists between these extremes. According to most theists, free will is necessary for true salvation: A person must freely accept God's offer of salvation, submit to God's plan, and then Grace results. This view implies that God has given humans free will for a reason.

If so, there is also evidence that such free will figures prominently in morality and reasoning: Sometimes we need to figure out what is the right thing to do in medicine (hence this book!) or the right way to treat our family members. But if this is so, why wouldn't there be a place for choice and reasoning in matters as fundamental as creating families? Why shouldn't medical advances, such as in vitro fertilization, be seen not as *thwarting* God's will, but as *manifesting* it? In other words, why not see new ways to make children as gifts from God to the infertile? Why not see new ways of choosing children also as gifts?

In the same way, one can see medical advances as gifts from God, giving humans new choices to avoid ancient curses, creating happier children and a better world. In this way, more choices in genetics about children are compatible with people as thinking, choosing, compassionate believers.

7.7 Genetic Testing, Malpractice, and Insurance Companies

It is one thing to speculate that increased parental choice about fetal genetic testing will create grassroots eugenics, but it is another to see it from the perspective of a physician threatened by lawsuits. The two together—high parental expectations of a normal child and threats of malpractice suits—might make testing of fetuses for genetic disease into a norm, with the consequent abortion of substantial numbers of fetuses found to be carrying genetic disorders.

But how likely are malpractice suits resulting from not offering genetic tests of fetuses? Several parents have indeed sued physicians in this way. In *wrongful birth* suits, some action by physicians is alleged to have made the resulting baby less than normal, and hence harmed. The most common kind of wrongful birth suit involves anoxia (lack of oxygen) at birth, which may cause cerebral palsy or a vegetative state. Another kind of suit results from a failure by a physician to inform parents about a test that might have led to a decision not to carry a fetus to term.

In New Jersey, parents of a baby with Down syndrome sued pro-life obstetrician James Delahunty, who they say discouraged them from pursuing amniocentesis when a sonogram showed a fetus with a thickened skin on the back of the neck (a sign in utero of possible Down syndrome).[21] The jury awarded the couple nearly $2 million and found Dr. Delahunty guilty of "failing to recognize, appreciate, and failing to discuss the results of the tests, particularly ultrasound" with his patients. The large award stemmed partially from Dr. Delahunty's combative behavior in the courtroom.

At least 27 states allow parents to sue for wrongful birth, although Michigan and Georgia recently disallowed such suits. In 1999, the Georgia Supreme Court ruled that a couple with a child born with Down syndrome or other impairments could not sue their physician for failure to perform amniocentesis or other prenatal tests.[22]

In France, anything connected with eugenics is deeply associated with the Nazis. An uproar occurred when a court ruled in 1995, after 13 years of litigation, that parents of a child born to a mother with German measles (who was not offered an abortion) were entitled to compensation for wrongful birth. In two subsequent French cases, damages were awarded to parents of children with disabilities who argued that if they had known prenatally of the disability, they would have aborted.

Critics in France assailed these results, saying they had established a "right not to be born," had begun a new eugenics program, and would make malpractice premiums soar. In protest, the French association of obstetricians held a work slowdown. In 2002, the French legislature responded and made wrongful birth suits illegal.[23]

Another important case concerned Karen Coveler of Houston, Texas, who at 34 had earned a doctorate in genetics and whose physician, even though she requested "all the DNA tests she could to determine if she was at risk of passing on a genetic disease," did not offer her a test for a genetic cause of deafness, which her son had, leaving him deaf at birth.

Physicians don't offer similar tests for breast cancer and mental retardation because they make a cost-benefit moral judgment that (1) the genetic condition was not too bad, (2) that the risk of this condition was low, and that (1) and (2) did not justify an abortion.

Another important reason why physicians don't offer such tests is that their professional societies fear such testing will become a norm (i.e., offering the test will soon become *the standard of care*, such that it is *malpractice* not to offer it). Fear of such lawsuits prevents physicians from offering more scientifically sound, new tests for genetic conditions.[24]

For example, controversy abounds over testing for Fragile X syndrome, a common cause of mental retardation, and one that is not routinely offered to parents unless a family history exists of this condition. Even though some have estimated the number of couples at risk for Fragile X is twice the number at risk for cystic fibrosis, the American College of Obstetricians and Gynecologists (ACOG) does not recommend the test be given to most prospective parents, even though it does recommend such testing for cystic fibrosis.[25] One critic suggests that ACOG does not do so because, if it were recommended, patients would have a better malpractice claim against ACOG members who did not offer to test when a child with Fragile X was born.[26]

Let us look at another issue about genetics, insurance companies, and ethics. To understand any practice in bioethics, it helps to understand the financial incentives and penalties that support it. Consider tests for genetic conditions.

On the one hand, those who hold patents on human genes and on genetic tests favor widespread testing because such testing may make them money. On the other hand, companies that sell life insurance and medical insurance fear that people will take such tests without their knowledge. Such covert testing could result in *adverse selection* into their policies: Unhealthy people will buy their policies and healthy people, whose premiums are needed to subsidize sick people, will not.

California once tried to ban companies from requiring a test for HIV before selling life insurance, but the companies then refused to sell life insurance in California because if they continued, they predicted they would be quickly bankrupt. So California's legislature relented.

To avoid adverse selection, insurance companies want to know who has taken a genetic test before issuing a policy. The danger of allowing them to know is *genetic discrimination.*

Today, most insurance companies are for-profit. A for-profit company wants the maximal amount of premiums coming in while paying out the minimal amount for claims. It does not want to insure people with genetic diseases; rather it wants to insure as many people as possible who carry no genetic diseases. Legislatures will need to strike a balance between keeping such companies in business while not allowing them to discriminate against those who need coverage.

For newborn screening, the implications are similar. Genetic diseases in children cost billions of dollars a year. In a 2004 study, an underlying disorder with a significant genetic component was found in 71 percent of children admitted to a children's hospital for over a year.[27] Any regional children's hospital sees hundreds of children daily who suffer from genetic diseases and who come for surgery, drugs, and therapy. If all such children could have been screened in the womb or as embryos, and healthy embryos/fetuses substituted, and if the same premiums were paid by parents, insurance companies would save billions of dollars a year.

So, financially, and assuming parents may abort, it is to the financial advantage of for-profit insurance companies to pay for preimplantation diagnosis (PID) of genetic disease in embryos, genetic testing during the first trimester, and newborn screening. What will be a fine line to walk, both in ethics and the law, is to not go from *encouraging* parents to take such tests to *requiring* them to test as a condition of keeping coverage.

Consider now a dilemma about all this. Sometimes it seems that medical insurance companies are the bad guys in bioethics. In the above analysis, we saw how for-profit companies may encourage genetic screening to reduce the number of children born with genetic disease, and their exposure to risk. Now suppose federal or state law bans insurance companies from paying for genetic tests. What happens then?

Critics will say that genetic testing is only available for the rich. Working people cannot afford to pay $2,000 for a battery of 50 tests to screen out mental retardation. Practically speaking, if medical insurance does not cover such screening, only well-off couples will use it.

Economic status is already associated with health (i.e., poverty is associated with disease and early death).[28] Some economists estimate that genetic disease causes two-thirds of the serious conditions treated in children's hospitals. Having a child with a serious genetic disease may cause a couple or woman to drop out of the middle class into poverty (due to time lost from work in taking the child to see physicians), so eventually, the parent may quit work or get fired.

Paternalism and Different Worldviews About Genetic Testing

Some obstetricians regret that ACOG recommended testing for cystic fibrosis and are happy that their hospitals don't offer testing for Fragile X. "I just feel that some people are not ready for some of the information," one said.[29] That attitude is the classic paternalistic attitude of physicians.

Karen Coveler was incensed that she was not offered the test for deafness, especially when she learned that her child's chance of being deaf was greater than his chance of having many of the genetic conditions for which she was in fact offered a genetic test. Coveler wanted the opportunity to make the decision about her child herself and was mad that a physician took it away.

Not to offer a genetic test because one is personally opposed to abortion raises a key problem in the physician–patient relationship: What should an ethical physician say to patients about such services when he or she thinks that such services are evil? The basic answer involving medical professionalism is that, while one is not obligated to perform such services oneself, one must mention them and mention someone else who will do them. Is this a workable solution?

This is a problem in medicine for several reasons. First, there are many practices and behaviors that many physicians find repellent, offensive, or downright evil: clitorectomies in Africa, Jehovah's witnesses not allowing themselves or their children to have blood transfusions (more on this in Chapter 10), avoidance by conservative Mormons and Christian Scientists of medical care for their families, and hope for miracles for dying patients when such hope means subjecting patients to painful, futile medical procedures. In addition to these, physicians disagree about physician-assisted dying, physicians creating life through in vitro fertilization, surrogate mothers, and artificial insemination. Still others believe all abortions are evil.

Second, we don't want physicians to be amoral, unfeeling robots. Many great physicians say it's their passion that keeps them going through the difficult times. But physicians care deeply about many different things in medicine: care for the poor, hatred of pharmaceutical companies, feminism, abortion, geriatric medicine, and wanting to achieve a breakthrough. So the problem occurs when physicians passionately support people with disabilities and oppose abortion but find themselves counseling pregnant women who are good candidates for genetic testing. Can we find a compromise?

Let's consider why courts have not allowed parents to let their child die rather than having a blood transfusion or emergency medical services. In these cases, the courts reasoned that the life of the child was more important than protecting religious freedom, and second, that children differ from adults. Adults can sacrifice their own lives, but children may grow up and decide not to be a member of the same religion. Hence, the courts found a way to preserve the lives of children in health care until they can become adults; then, if they wish, they can refuse medical services based on their own beliefs.

Reasoning the same way, we can begin by noting that forcing a couple to have a child against their will is a very bad thing. If a physician didn't believe in contraception and deliberately gave placebos (sugar pills) rather than birth control pills to female patients, we would consider the doctor evil and guilty of malpractice. But condemning parents to have *any child* against their will is not that different from condemning parents from having a child *with Down syndrome* against their will, especially if the parents in both cases have the power to prevent the birth. So both are equally wrong.

Moreover, in the first case, the freedom of religion of parents must be balanced against the good of the child, but with physicians, there is a lesser good in the balance, their personal ethics. Although we want physicians to have their own personal ethics, patients realize that the ethics of a physician may differ from their own, and for that reason, patients reserve the right to make personal decisions about their bodies and families.

In the end, if we ask, "What is medicine *for?*" the answer involves patients going to physicians for help in getting medical care. Almost always, patients want to avoid disease, dysfunction, and death, and physicians help them as best they can.

To raise again the value of autonomy in patient's lives, we note that few patients see physicians *as physicians* for help about which religion is best, which denomination offers most hope for salvation, or whether abortion is wrong. Generally, autonomous adult patients have developed their own views on these matters and don't go to physicians for advice about such issues.

For all these reasons, a physician opposed to genetic abortion still must mention to patients that this option is open to them and if they want the test, to refer them. If he or she just can't manage to do so, then the physician should avoid these kinds of situations. This is what medical professionalism is all about.

Medical Tools Can Be Used in Many Ways

After high-resolution sonograms were introduced to monitor development of normal pregnancies and to detect genetic abnormalities, groups opposed to abortion realized the potential of the same machines to show powerful images of the young fetus. For example, a "pregnancy counseling center" in Bowie, Maryland, offered a young woman pregnant at six-and-a-half weeks, who inquired about abortion services, a picture of her fetus to check its viability. When the woman heard the fetal heartbeat and saw the images, she decided she could not abort it.[30]

Conservative Christian groups such as James Dobson's Focus on the Family and the Southern Baptist Convention have raised millions of dollars to give such clinics ultrasound machines, which cost about $25,000 each. A group that tracks success of pregnancy centers says that use of such machines jumps their success rate from 70 percent to 90 percent in dissuading women from abortions. About 3,000 such pregnancy counseling centers exist in America, whose primary purpose is to dissuade women from having abortions.

Some of these pregnancy centers partner with adoption agencies. Adoption agencies cannot explicitly charge for babies, which would be illegal baby-selling, but they can charge substantial sums for arranging the adoption. Standard fees for healthy white babies go as high as $50,000.[31]

Preimplantation Diagnosis (PID)

Many alarming things have been written about preimplantation diagnosis (PID) as a kind of new eugenics. This is an excellent example of why alarmist predictions must be taken with a grain of salt and why, in ethics and elsewhere in life, *the scale of the problem* must always be considered.

In this case, PID may be used in conjunction with in vitro fertilization (IVF), where sperm and eggs are mixed in a Petri dish to form human embryos and then inserted in the womb. While the embryos are outside the womb, a single cell can be taken from each embryo and subjected to genetic tests for diseases such as cystic fibrosis or Huntington's disease, and only healthy embryos will be implanted.

Most couples would rather have a healthy child than one born blind, deaf, or with a major disability. Despite any bad message sent to adults with these conditions, couples using PID are in reality going to choose healthy embryos—especially because the only couples likely to pay for PID are those who fear having a child with a genetic disease.

Once questions of scale arise, PID does not seem like such a large question for public policy and certainly does not imply a new eugenics. The numbers tell the story: IVF is expensive (about $12,000 per attempt) and few states require insurance companies to cover it. Second, it commonly fails: Of 100 couples trying IVF, less than 30 will take home a baby. Finally, of those 30 couples, it will be a rare couple who will use PID.

One of the largest and most successful infertility and genetics institutes has done PID on only 600 couples over the last two decades.[32] If we add this figure to all the smaller clinics, most of which don't do PID, then maybe a few thousand couples at most have used PID over the last decades. Of these, maybe a third identified a genetic disease and elected not to implant that embryo.

Eliminating genetic disease from a few hundred babies a year in America is not going to affect significantly the gene pool of 300 million Americans. Why is that? Because the numbers are so large. Over 4 million babies are born in America each year.[33] With so many births passing along so many genes, the small numbers of PID-related births won't affect the huge genetic mass of the 4 million babies. In statistical terms, this is an example of the law of regression to the mean. In ordinary terms, the genes of one baby in 20,000 get washed out among those of all the others.

7.8 Newborn Genetic Screening

In contrast to PID, newborn screening may affect *tens of millions* of babies and is of a categorically different scale than PID. Similarly, the new, noninvasive tests during the first trimester of pregnancy could affect, not hundreds, but millions of babies around the globe.

Presymptomatic genetic testing may be used for other reasons than to abort a fetus with an undesirable genetic condition. It may also be used for early intervention at birth to try to prevent death and retardation for (at present) about 60 genetic conditions similar to phenylketonuria (PKU). This is called *genetic screening at birth*.

Genetic screening at birth does not result in abortion and may soon become the single greatest reason for widespread, presymptomatic genetic testing. According to the March of Dimes Foundation, at least 9 major congenital disorders easily can be identified at birth, and more than 60 others can be detected, but only 30 percent of American babies are tested for the basic 9 congenital disorders.[34] States vary widely about which tests they require at birth, but almost all require testing at birth for PKU (because the retardation resulting from PKU can be prevented by a special diet). At press, California was considering a law to require tests at birth of 60 hereditary conditions.

Why does it matter? Consider Ben Haygood, born in August 2000 in Mississippi. Ben did fine for two years, then suddenly got sick in day care and died that night. He had a rare but treatable hereditary disease, MCADD (Medium-Chain Acyl-Co-A-Dehydrogenase Deficiency), that prevented metabolism of fats. Ben's death may have been prevented by a slight modification of his diet and by discovery of MCADD which would have been revealed by a $25 test at birth.[35] Similarly, Ysabel Gonzalo had LCHAD (Long-Chain 3-Hydroxyacyl-coenzyme A Dehydrogenase Deficiency), another fatal metabolic disease and suffered extensive brain damage; her injury probably could have been prevented with a low-fat, high-carb diet started immediately after birth.

Tandem mass spectrometers can detect 50 congenital diseases using blood from one heel-stick of a baby. Most states budget little money for expanded genetic screening. As a result, according to the chief of the CDC's newborn screening branch, many American children may die each year of preventable illnesses.[36]

The above expresses the view of passionate advocates for newborn testing for genetic diseases, led by the March of Dimes Foundation. In 2005, an important federal panel recommended that all states test all newborns for 29 different genetic diseases, setting off a national controversy.[37]

Perhaps, however, we should not endorse this push for testing so quickly.

Some critics question whether we know that testing for about 20 of the conditions would do more good than harm.[38] Without good studies to prove benefit of treatments, identifying conditions and then giving unproven treatments might be harmful.

History could repeat itself when all states mandated testing babies for phenylketonuria (PKU). In 1959, Robert Guthrie, a microbiologist at the University of Buffalo, developed a simple blood test for PKU in babies and campaigned passionately to test all babies.[39] If they tested positive, Guthrie argued, PKU babies could be raised on a special diet low on phenylalanine. Without testing, PKU would not be discovered in babies until they were brain-damaged.

Guthrie assumed that a positive result from his test meant that a baby really had phenylketonuria (in statistical terms, he assumed his test was very sensitive), and second, he assumed that the special diet was safe for babies misdiagnosed with PKU. But his assumptions were false.

Some babies testing positive for PKU had a benign mutation and were normal. Worse, the diet low in phenylalanine damaged their normal brains. Shortly after testing started, leaders in pediatrics discovered in alarm that they didn't know what a positive test meant, how to differentiate a true positive from a false positive test, or the right diet for the right kid. Unfortunately, a moral juggernaut had started for testing and it was unstoppable.

Some critics fear that the same thing will happen again, especially for 5 or 6 tests where clinical trials have not yet proven that the current medicines help. In other cases, we really don't know how many false positives the tests will generate (where a baby can test positive, but never have the disease).[40]

Defenders claim that 20 of the conditions are so rare that it would take decades to prove that testing and treatments save lives. In the meantime, they say, babies will die who otherwise could be saved.

In conclusion, what initially looked like an open-and-shut ethical mandate to save babies from death and brain damage, now looks more complex.

7.9 Sending the Wrong Message?

It is interesting that when a couple chooses not to have a child who is blind or deaf for genetic reasons, they are said to be "sending the wrong message" to people living with these genetic diseases. Is this really so?

First, some selective perception may be involved here. There are thousands of other personal choices that people make that, according to the above logic, also send the wrong message. For example, if a couple reflects on having children and chooses to be childless, does that decision send a message to other couples that children are undesirable? If people don't find children in wheelchairs to play on their soccer or baseball teams, doesn't this send a message to children in wheelchairs? Doesn't having a "Special" Olympics send a message? Doesn't it send a message not to mainstream retarded children with gifted children? Not to admit everyone to medical school?

Second, abortion is a private decision. It is not something you announce in the paper like an engagement to be married. As such, one wonders how such private decisions "send a message" to people with disabilities? If you don't know that I've ever had a first-term abortion, how can my abortion send a message to you? This is like saying that a person secretly smoking in his home is sending a message to nonsmokers in favor of smoking.

Last, the new technology allowing abortions to avoid genetic diseases during the first trimester reinforces these points. The earlier the abortion, the more private it is. And the more private and earlier it is, the less realistic it is to claim that it sends any message at all to people with disabilities.

After learning the fetus they were carrying had Down syndrome, the Dryers decided to abort. They conceived again and had their new fetus tested at 12 weeks and it also had Down syndrome. In this case, they decided to bring the fetus to term and have the baby.

Nevertheless, the Dryers felt uncomfortable in their church and neighborhood. About a month after their child was born with Down syndrome, they accepted new jobs on the other side of the country and moved.

CONCLUSIONS

Since the first few couples began testing first-trimester fetuses and since companies began offering a one-time panel for a wide variety of genetic conditions, the practice has quietly been growing. Overall, the rate of births in America of babies with Down syndrome is probably dropping. One hard piece of evidence concerns babies with spina bifida, the number of which dropped between 1991 and 2002 from 887 to 734 per year, and the number of babies with anencephaly dropped in the same period from 655 to 348 births per year.[41] Trends for babies with Down syndrome probably matched this trend.

On learning the information of this chapter, people may feel that science is giving prospective parents too many choices and that these parents lack the wisdom to make good choices. In essence, people fear that prospective parents will make bad choices. Such fears may evaporate as the same tools allow prospective parents to choose for or against conditions they value or disvalue highly.

For the sake of argument and for example, suppose a gene is verified for causing homosexuality. Will the same people who oppose allowing couples to choose against genetic diseases not want the freedom to choose against gay embryos? Suppose a tendency to join a church is gene-based. Won't some want children with such genes?

The topic of this chapter will be important for decades to come in bioethics because it combines many controversial areas: abortion, eugenics, rights of persons with disabilities and discrimination against them, parental choice over children and their future traits, and wise public policy about such matters. These issues will be confronted by not just genetics counselors in medical centers, but by physicians in primary care whom prospective patients increasingly ask for information about their future babies, raising new stakes in the fight against malpractice.

This chapter has argued that parents really are going to have more choices about genetic disease. After decades of false alarms, three new forces are coming to a head: ability to test fetuses in the first trimester rather than the second, ability to do a large number of genetic tests in that first trimester for a reasonable cost, and, finally, families seeking genetic information not from genetic specialists but from primary care physicians. These three developments will result in more fetuses being testing for genetic defects.

None of these together, however, would match the exponential leap of testing that would occur when the first malpractice awards occur for not testing. Once that occurs, ordinary physicians may be forced to offer all parents such testing in the first trimester, and that, indeed, would be a significant change.

Will that occur? An old cartoon strip, "Pogo," once had a strip with the conclusion, "We have met the enemy and it is us!" Widespread testing will not be caused by racism, desires for a Master Race, or even perfect babies. Rather, when the legal system awards compensation for babies with genetic diseases who could have been theoretically prevented by testing, then such testing will be upon us.

Will that be a new "eugenics" or just another false alarm? It could mean thousands fewer babies born in America with genetic diseases. That result would require thousands of abortions specifically to prevent these conditions, as well as testing of millions of normal fetuses. Whether you see those results as good or bad will depend partly on how much you value autonomous choice over children and partly on your worldview.

FURTHER READINGS

Baird, Robert M., and Stuart E. Rosenbaum, eds. *The Ethics of Abortion: Pro-Life vs. Pro-Choice.* Buffalo, NY: Prometheus, 2001.

Feinberg, Joel, ed. *The Problem of Abortion.* Belmont, CA: Wadsworth Publishing, 1984.

Fletcher, Joseph. *The Ethics of Genetic Control: Ending Reproductive Roulette: Artificial Insemination, Surrogate Pregnancy, Nonsexual Reproduction, Genetic Control.* Buffalo, NY: Prometheus, 2001.

Greenwood, Joan. "The New Ethics of Abortion." *Journal of Medical Ethics* 27, Suppl. II (October 2001), pp. ii2–ii34.

Guterman, Lila. "Choosing Genetics." *Chronicle of Higher Education*, May 2, 2003, pp. A22–26.

Kevles, Daniel. *In the Name of Eugenics.* New York: Basic Books, 1985.

Marquis, Don. "Why Abortion Is Immoral." *Journal of Philosophy* 86, no. 4 (April 1989), pp. 183–202.

Robertson, John. *Children of Choice.* Princeton, NJ: Princeton University Press, 1996.

Thomson, Judith Jarvis. "A Defense of Abortion." *Philosophy and Public Affairs* 1, no. 1 (1971), pp. 46–66.

Tooley, Michael. *Abortion and Infanticide.* Oxford, England: Clarendon Press, 1983.

Warren, Mary Anne. "On the Moral and Legal Status of Abortion." *Monist* 57, no. 1 (January 1973), pp. 43–61.

CHAPTER 8

Can Research Be Just on People with Schizophrenia?

This chapter discusses general ethical issues in medical research and particular issues in research on schizophrenia. It discusses the enormous growth in American research over the last 50 years, as well as informed consent, schizophrenia, the Nuremberg Code, the Tuskegee Syphilis Study, and conflicts of interests. The case focuses on the ethics of research on schizophrenia.[1]

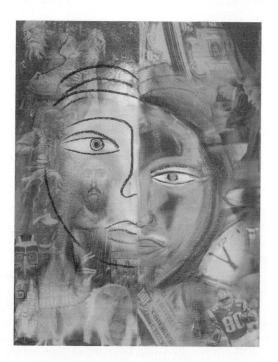

In 1984, Claudia and Joe Friend thought that their 20-year-old son, Greg, would get the best help possible for his schizophrenia if they enrolled him in a research trial. Claudia worked as a high school librarian and Joe Friend was a retired naval lieutenant commander. They enrolled Greg at the Maryland Psychiatric Research Center (MPRC) in Cantonsville, Maryland, run by the University of Maryland. Six months before, Greg had been treated at Wyman Park Medical Center in Baltimore.

At admission, he was disheveled, drooled constantly, and was incontinent. He "sat in a praying position on the floor and said he'd seen God, that others could read his mind, and that his name was being called over the television set."[2]

During the next four months, psychiatrists tried several drugs on Greg and finally discovered that Proloxin helped. At discharge, Greg could dress and shower by himself, and he had gained weight.

Nevertheless, he remained silent most of the time; he tired easily, and suffered bad pain in his knees, a known side effect of Proloxin.

At this point, probably because his insurance would no longer pay for treatment at Wyman, he needed a new facility. With his consent, his parents entered him in MPRC's federally funded study. Researchers hoped to discover whether Greg's schizophrenia or the Proloxin caused his silence and lethargy. At MPRC, his parents hoped Greg would get good care.

8.1 Research to Cure Schizophrenia, Money, and Care for People with Mental Illness

Most medical research on humans carries a tension between two values. On the one hand, patients, their families, and researchers want cures. On the other hand, new experiments may not benefit most patients and may even harm some.

In research on people with schizophrenia, special problems arise because it is difficult to create animal models. Schizophrenia is a disorder of higher-order thinking and no nonhuman animals think just as humans do. Thus the research must be done on people with schizophrenia themselves. To find cures, a population that is itself sick and fragile must be the subjects of experiments.

Why do families allow their sons or daughters with schizophrenia to enroll in experiments at all? The answer to that question is: because by doing so, families can get good, low-cost care.

Many people mistakenly believe that medical insurance policies cover long-term treatment for people with severe mental illness. In fact, virtually none do. Even good policies usually only cover 30 or 90 days of inpatient hospitalization and only reimburse physicians for testing or procedures, not supervision of patients over decades.

According to Senator Peter Domenici (R, NM), medical insurance policies have excluded mental illness from the very beginning, on the premise that such illnesses were not real medical diseases.[3] Even though that thinking changed about schizophrenia, lack of coverage did not.

Faced with a new case of schizophrenia in a young relative, virtually all families lack the financial and emotional resources to help. As a result, such families refer their relative to whatever clinics exist for public psychiatry.

Such public resources vary widely from state to state. Vermont and New Hampshire fund excellent, low-cost systems with good outpatient clinics and group homes run by psychiatric social workers and supervised in a state-run psychiatric system. Most other states or big urban areas do *not* fund outpatient clinics or group homes and thus the only alternative to care within families is warehousing the relative in a large, state facility.

Mental illness, broadly defined, may be more widespread than people think. According to a controversial (and possibly self-serving) 2005 study from the National Institute of Mental Health (NIMH), more than half of Americans will develop a mental illness at some point in their lives (defined by the criteria of the *Diagnostic and Statistical Manual of Mental Disorders (DSM)* of the American Psychiatric Association).[4]

For most families, not just poor ones, getting a mother or son into a research study may be the *only* way to get good inpatient care. As such, the ability to decline to participate in such a study is compromised. Already under a high degree of stress, perhaps over many years, families may be ready to hand off a relative to an inpatient research study where she or he will get better monitoring from research nurses and clinical staff than the relative would get living at home while family members go off to work during the day.

8.2 Nazi and American Research, and the Tuskegee Study

During World War II, the leaders of German medicine joined the Nazi party—most of them voluntarily—and led the Racial Hygiene Movement that idealized Aryan features and despised Jews, Gypsies, gay men, and people with mental or physical disabilities. The Final Solution to eradicate such "inferior" people from Germany was the Holocaust, where 6 million people were killed, mostly where victims were gathered in camps for more effective mass killing (hence, "concentration camps").

Physician-experimenters used people awaiting death in these camps in atrocious medical experiments. Josef Mengele, obsessed with changing non-Aryan peoples into people with Aryan traits, experimented on sets of twins by exchanging blood between pairs, sewing wrists together, and, in one case, sewing a hunchback to a normal child's back.[5] He subjected victims to electric shocks to establish human limits. He studied infertility by sterilizing Polish nuns with radiation. He injected blue dye into the eyes of children to see if he could produce blue eyes.

Another Nazi physician, Sigmund Rascher, developed a "sky ride wagon" to stimulate rapid changes in altitude, strapping victims inside and subjecting them to extreme, rapid changes. He experimented with reviving victims made unconscious by freezing waters. Other German physicians infected victims with typhus and malaria to study these diseases.

After the war, most of these Nazi physicians were convicted and hanged as war criminals (Mengele escaped to Paraguay). Their defense at their trials was always that they were just following orders.

As a result of these crimes, the *Nuremberg Code* came about, which has 10 principles governing research on human subjects. Its principles require informed consent of subjects, absence of coercion, proper scientific design of experiments, and beneficence (therapeutic intentions) toward subjects.

American Medical Research During World War II

Researchers experimented on orphans in America in 1941 at the Ohio Soldiers and Sailors Orphanage, on inmates with retardation at the New Jersey State Colony for the Feeble-Minded, and on patients at a mental institution in Dixon, Illinois.[6] To develop a vaccine against shigella (a bacterial disease causing dysentery), other researchers injected deadened forms of this bacteria into subjects. No one died, but many got very sick.

Some questionable research used military personnel as subjects. Cornelius Rhoads, director of the leading American cancer hospital, Memorial Sloan Kettering in New York City, led the military's secret chemical warfare service. Subjects were "volunteers" who did not know what they were volunteering for: Researchers made no attempt at informed consent.[7] Among other things, researchers tested mustard gas on 4,000 to 5,000 subjects, discovering that it killed white blood cells and could be an anticancer agent.[8]

When subjects of the chemical research later applied for treatment at veterans' hospitals, the Veterans Administration (VA) denied, as part of a cover-up, that they had been exposed to toxic agents, so these subjects couldn't get any special treatments for their conditions. This scenario would be repeated after the Vietnam War and Operation Desert Storm.

The wartime mentality of researchers continued after the war: Disease was the enemy, researchers were the soldiers, and victory could be won—with enough resources and enough will. While World War II was still in progress, considerations of ethics and informed consent carried little weight. As critic David Rothman writes, "Some people were ordered to face bullets and storm a hill; others were told to take an injection and test a vaccine."[9]

Postwar experimentation continued such doubtful practices. During World War II, Americans (like their opponents) sought cures for dysentery, malaria, and venereal diseases, but when the war came to an end, the fight against diseases in the United States did not. In fact, the prospect of winning the war against syphilis and cancer gave researchers in the 1950s and 1960s a sense of urgency that kept alive the wartime spirit of research.

After the war, faith in the inevitability of scientific progress wavered, and with it, faith in medical research. In 1962, Rachel Carson's *Silent Spring* described the ravages of pesticides; the Cuban missile crisis edged us close to nuclear war, and a failure to adequately test thalidomide (used to treat morning sickness) on pregnant animals resulted in births of dozens of children who lacked arms and legs.

The military has a long history of justifying secret, dangerous medical research by appealing to national security. In other words, the end of a safe, secure country justifies using unethical means on subjects. For example, to assess the effects of nuclear radiation, soldiers were made to stand miles away from the blasts and watch explosions, wearing only sunglasses for protection. Supposedly justified by national security, military physicians cannot be sued for abuses from research, and the Department of Defense has a special exemption from Federal Drug Administration scrutiny.

So it was not surprising that soldiers mustered out in 1991 for Operation Desert Storm had to take an experimental anthrax vaccine with a booster containing squalene, an adjuvant stimulating the immune system and making the vaccine effective more quickly. Squalene may have caused autoimmune diseases in soldiers and might explain their Gulf War Syndrome.[10]

Before World War II, randomized clinical trials were not common in medicine. Their introduction to clinical medicine may be one of the most important advances in the last half century, for they supplanted the guesses and subjective biases that informed many medical decisions before their standard usage.

After their introduction, medical research began to be considered more critically. In 1966, in the *New England Journal of Medicine*, Harvard medical professor Henry Beecher criticized 22 medical experiments involving human subjects because none had obtained informed consent from subjects and because several bordered on abuse.[11] Beecher claimed that these studies were not exceptions but the rule. At approximately the same time, British physician Henry Pappworth criticized 500 worldwide medical experiments on similar grounds.[12]

In addition to the Nuremberg Code, the *Declaration of Helsinki* has been adopted by many professional organizations and contains a list of rights of research subjects.[13] The most important requirement is that in any kind of research, every patient must get the best proven diagnostic techniques and drugs. This declaration bans placebos in drug studies when an effective drug already is used in practice.

One study that violated the Declaration of Helsinki was the Tuskegee Syphilis Study. Revelation of it in 1972 changed the way Americans, especially black Americans, viewed medical research.

The Tuskegee Study

The Tuskegee Study was a 40-year, federally run study of untreated syphilis in 400 illiterate black men who were poor Alabama sharecroppers. Started by the United States Public Health Service (USPHS), it ended under the Centers for Disease Control (CDC) in Atlanta. With the exception of a black nurse who stayed in Tuskegee, white men ran the study.

The study began in 1929 when 600 men with latent syphilis were identified in rural Macon County by a charity that planned to treat them with the best treatment then available: heavy metals such as arsenic and mercury, given in a paste on the back.[14] When the Depression began, the charity's plans collapsed and USPHS decided to follow 400 of the men who had not received treatment (200 were treated and not followed) as a *study in nature* to see how syphilis progressed.

Even when penicillin was discovered and made available in the mid-1940s, these men were never told they were in a study of untreated syphilis, nor given penicillin. Local physicians actively conspired with USPHS to prevent them from getting antibiotics or joining the armed services (preventing them from getting penicillin there).

Originally chosen in 1929 because Macon County had the highest percentage of citizens with syphilis in America, the black men were perfect for a long-term study in nature because they were so *vulnerable* (to use a concept now important in the ethics of research). Being illiterate, they were unlikely to read about penicillin; being poor, they were unlikely to see private physicians; being tied to the land as sharecroppers, they were unlikely to leave Macon County; being black and all of the above, they would have had few opportunities to change their career or fate in life and, thus, were stuck in Macon County until they died.

The Tuskegee Study was not a secret. Over a dozen articles about it appeared in medical journals over the decades of the study.

When Jean Heller, a reporter for the Associated Press, broke the story in 1972, it led to cries for reforming American medical research. Congress required that future federally funded research be reviewed by Institutional Review Boards (IRBs), composed of both private citizens and researchers. Congress also mandated informed consent of subjects.

Ethical Relativism and the Holocaust

This chapter has already described some evil events in medical history. Such atrocities call into question the theory of *ethical relativism.* Because a relativist denies the existence of any absolute ethical standards, he denies that any perspective exists from which to condemn the Holocaust or Nazi medical atrocities. Although such events look bad from the standard of our present society, he argues that within Nazi society or Nazi ideals, these events were not wrong.

It is hard to see how the relativist can defend these claims. Certainly Nazi society was not better for its victims, and certainly few people would choose to live in that society rather than our own. Relativists must acknowledge that they cannot give impartial reasons why our society is better than Nazi society or why medicine should abhor such experiments.

Given the continuing kinds of genocide that have occurred in the Congo, Serbia, and around the world, we have learned that, unless protected by strong moral stands defending human rights and justice, ethnic hatred and racism easily flare up and destroy thousands of people. When that occurs, virtually no one in such countries is better off, and the whole society may descend into chaos. Is that the price of believing in ethical relativism?

At the heart of the experiment in Greg Friend's case was a provision in this federally funded study that required a washout period *of four weeks to enable drugs to clear from Greg's blood, liver, and kidneys. Drug companies and psychiatric researchers believe new drugs should be tested on fresh subjects with systems not contaminated by old drugs. Subjects need a period to "wash out" old drugs from their bodies.*

Adults with schizophrenia do not automatically lack capacity to consent to their own treatment. Indeed, Greg was asked to sign, and did sign with his parents, a consent form mentioning such a washout period.

In Greg's study and during its washout period, subjects did not stay at MPRC but saw physicians periodically as outpatients. The consent form warned that their old symptoms could recur during the overall study but did not warn of any specific dangers during the washout period.

After four weeks without Proloxin or any other antischizophrenic medication, Greg experienced nightmarish hallucinations and extreme feelings of self-loathing. He saw a small child, thought, "I could kill him," and to prevent himself from doing so (or to punish himself for the thought) broke his own arm on the metal railing of his parents' Columbia townhouse. Taking a huge amount of aspirin, he then tried to kill himself.

8.3 Schizophrenia

Schizophrenia stems from the Latin *schizo* (split) and *phrenia* (mind). As a psychological disorder, the term signifies a disintegration of personality and a break or split from reality. It is commonly confused with having multiple personalities. According to the National Institute of Mental Health, in any given year, about 1 percent of Americans over age 18, or over 2 million adults, have schizophrenia.[15]

Although schizophrenia is a serious mental disorder (it is responsible for half of long-term patients in mental hospitals), modern drugs allow many people with schizophrenia to lead productive lives and often in halfway homes ("halfway" between a large, state institution and a regular home, a house where a half-dozen adults live independently with help of a live-in case worker).

The rule of fourths predicts long-term prognosis for schizophrenics: One-fourth will get well with drugs and be stable; one-fourth will fare moderately well on drugs and live on their own; another fourth will do well enough to live in a halfway home under supervision; the final fourth will do poorly and will be institutionalized.[16]

A more accurate phrase is "schizophrenic disorders," which reflects the diversity of symptoms that tend to be labeled under "schizophrenia." These disorders have two main divisions in causes and treatment. Type 1 (active) symptom pattern involves thought disorders such as hallucinations and delusions. The

Type 2 (passive) symptom pattern involves extreme social withdrawal and flat affect.

Biochemical imbalances seem to cause Type I patterns, which respond well to antipsychotic medications. Type II patterns seem to be caused by structural deformities in the brain and do not respond well to antipsychotic medications. A diagnosis of Type I schizophrenia disorder has a much better prognosis than a Type II.

The core pathology at the heart of schizophrenia is a very disorganized thought process, followed by hallucinations, where victims see, hear, smell, feel, and taste things or events that do not exist.

Most scientists today believe that schizophrenia stems entirely from biological or genetic causes. Heredity is a major factor. In a large study of identical twins, if one twin became schizophrenic, the other had a 50 percent chance of the same.[17]

Schizophrenia is not the same as schizoaffective disorder, which combines the distortions of thought of schizophrenia with distortions of mood. Schizoaffective disorder is a very severe mental illness with a poor prognosis.

8.4 Informed Consent and Schizophrenia Research

Western medical ethics allows patients to volunteer in nontherapeutic research, but such consent must be free, voluntary, and informed. If it is not, then we regress to the kinds of research performed during World War II.

During the 1960s, informed consent began to be the standard of care for medical research. In the late 1960s, the USPHS began to require it. In 1972, the *Canterbury* v. *Spence* decision in federal court established that informed consent must be obtained for medical procedures. According to this decision, "informed consent" did not mean what the community of medical professionals thought one should know, the *professional standard*, but what a reasonable person would want to know in the subject's position, the *objective standard*. In *Canterbury* v. *Spence*, a singer was not told that one possible complication of a laminectomy (a fusion of vertebraes) was paralysis and the loss of his voice. (The paralyzed singer claimed that, had he known, he would not have risked his livelihood.)

In the early 1970s, many midcareer physicians didn't like the new standard of informed consent. For decades, they had been accustomed to telling patients only what physicians deemed necessary and having patients follow their orders. Physician R.H. Kampmeier once recalled that in the 1940s and 1950s he often marched into a patient's room, announced that he was taking out the gall bladder the next morning, and the patient gratefully thanked him, having no understanding of the risks or possible complications involved.[18]

The patients' rights movement began in the mid-1970s to oppose such paternalism. It demanded that patients be informed in advance of risks and benefits so they could make informed decisions about participation.

In reality, many patients currently sign a multipage consent form without comprehending what they are reading. Residents, nurses, or medical students are often asked to "consent" the patient (i.e., get her to sign the consent form and answer her questions) even though they may not really know answers to her questions. For the most part, many patients rely on whether they trust their physician, and if so, sign without reading.

Franz J. Engelfinger, who edited the *New England Journal of Medicine* for decades, once called this "informed (but uneducated) consent" and argued that most patients have no idea what they're doing when they sign a typical consent form for medical experimentation.[19] For him, only the integrity of virtuous researchers protects patients from abuse. In rebuttal, patients ask how they can know if a researcher has integrity.

All of the above discussion is somewhat bureaucratic in analyzing *procedures* for obtaining informed consent and the history of legal requirements to do so. What it has omitted is the ethical justification for doing so, and that justification centers on *respect for autonomy* of research subjects. Without disclosure of true intentions by researchers, without full understanding by participants, and without full, voluntary consent by subjects, medical research is not justified. Given the force of (what might be called) the research imperative, and given the tendency of patients and researchers to lapse into medical paternalism, respecting autonomy of patient-subjects emerges as a check on these two powerful forces, like checks and balances in a political system. In other words, without real concern for patient autonomy, bad things will occur of the kind associated with dictatorships and abuses of people under dictatorships.

In 1989, Greg Aller, an adult with schizophrenia, lived in California near his parents and functioned well on medication, earning high grades in college and working part-time. His parents, Robert and Gloria Aller, had helped make a documentary at UCLA Medical Center explaining research on autistic children. Impressed with the compassion they filmed, the Allers hoped that psychiatrists would treat their son compassionately when they enrolled him in a study at UCLA.

*The Allers believe that the consent form at UCLA misled them by downplaying dangers of the study's washout period. It misleadingly said that Greg could get better, stay the same, or get worse, implying equal odds of each. In fact, as Robert Aller later said, "The researchers did not reveal to us that in a previous trial, 92 percent of patients got worse."[20] Nor did researchers reveal that the real purpose of the study was, upon withdrawal of medica-*tion, to investigate the signs and symptoms of a psychotic relapse.

After his medication was stopped in 1990, Greg's mental health dramatically declined. He became violent and his family feared him. The new medication did not return him to his previous level of functioning, and worse, neither did resumption of his previous medication. Because he had been in a study requiring a washout period, Greg Aller was worse off than he had been before.

In 1991, the Allers warned UCLA officials that washout periods were dangerous for people with schizophrenia. During that year, Tommy Lamadrid, another adult subject with schizophrenia in the same UCLA study, committed suicide during the washout period by jumping off the engineering building at UCLA.

In 1993, Abigayle McIntyre, an adult with schizophrenia and daughter of physician Judith Vukov, entered a UCLA research study because Vukov believed that it would give her daughter the best treatment.[21] Taken off all her previous medications for three weeks, Abigayle screamed and cried for hours. She was then given Haldol, a standard antipsychotic drug, which gave her terrible headaches and dangerously high blood pressure. A month later on a day pass and while still in the protocol, Abigayle killed herself by swallowing a large number of aspirin pills.

After Greg Aller's experiences, Robert Aller and his wife joined with the parents of Greg Friend, the Lamadrid family, and another family to form a small coalition publicizing the dangers of washout periods in studies on subjects with schizophrenia. In 1997, Robert Aller and other parents testified with Joe and Claudia Friend before the National Bioethics Advisory Commission's hearings on the ethics of psychiatric research.[22]

Confusions and Myths About Schizophrenia

Schizophrenia appears to most people as a mysterious and terrifying disease. As such, it is poorly understood; people who suffer from schizophrenia are often wrongly seen as sicker or more dangerous than they really are.

In fact, a small percentage of people diagnosed with schizophrenia completely "recover." They lose their hallucinations, function normally for decades, and even enjoy professional careers. Take Don Fisher. Diagnosed in his mid-twenties, Fisher had a PhD in biochemistry; two years after earning it, he spent four months in a psychiatric hospital.[23] With a supportive family (his father taught at Johns Hopkins Medical School), he went on to medical school at George Washington University and completed a residency in psychiatry at Harvard. Afterward, he had a long career as a psychiatrist and as an advocate for psychiatric patients.

More common is the situation of mathematician John Nash, portrayed in the Oscar-winning film *A Beautiful Mind*, starring Russell Crowe. By late in his life, and in a scene depicted in the movie, Nash recovers enough to receive a Nobel Prize (admittedly for work done before his schizophrenia started), attend the ceremony, and make a brief speech. (Like many schizophrenics, Nash still hallucinated during the ceremony, but like many functional people with schizophrenia, Nash *knew* he was hallucinating).

Swiss psychiatrist Manfred Bleuler started to change the image of people with schizophrenia in his landmark study in which he interviewed 200 patients who had been diagnosed with schizophrenia 20 years earlier. Manfred's findings contradicted the work of his own father, Eugene Bleuler, who had believed that schizophrenia was an inexorable, incurable mental disease. Manfred discovered that 20 percent were no longer schizophrenic and 30 percent had substantially improved. Rather than slipping inexorably into psychosis or catatonia, half got better.

Other scientists gradually confirmed Manfred Bleuler's discovery. For example, in 1987, Yale University School of Medicine psychologist Courtenay Harding followed 269 former patients from Vermont's state mental hospitals. She found that— by loose criteria—almost two-thirds were judged by researchers to be either fully recovered or functioned well in general, all with the exception of one area where they fared differently (they still needed medication or still heard voices). Contrary to popular beliefs, some of these former mental inmates, even while hearing voices, held down regular jobs. All in all,

> the belief that recovery from schizophrenia occurs only occasionally is belied by at least seven studies of patients who were followed by more than 20 years after their discharge from mental hospitals in the United States, Western Europe, and Japan. In papers published between 1972 and 1995, researchers found that between 46 and 68 percent of patients had either fully recovered—they had no symptoms of mental illness, took no psychiatric medication, worked and had normal relationships—or were, like John Nash, significantly improved in one area of functioning.[24]

In short, most people with schizophrenia live more normal lives than is commonly believed.

Problems of Consent in Schizophrenia Research

Since the Nuremberg Code, ethical research has required the consent of subjects of medical research. Adults with schizophrenia are not necessarily so impaired that they cannot understand an experiment and consent to participate.

On the other hand, such adults do suffer a disorder of thought and judgment. The authors of the influential 1978 *Belmont Report* considered such adults, along with prisoners, children, and patients of mental institutions, to be vulnerable subjects who needed special protections. Their mere consent was not sufficient justification for their participation in research.

Adults with schizophrenia and their families suffer from four major problems involving consent. First, their consent may be coerced because the physician or institution asking for their consent may be their primary caretaker. If they decline to participate, they may fear loss of sympathetic treatment. Second, if the physician or institution is normally the primary caretaker, they may not understand that the researcher may receive substantial payment for recruiting each subject. Third, they may not appreciate the dangers of the washout period or getting a placebo when they are off medications. Finally, as critic and University of Maryland at Baltimore professor Adil Shamoo points out,

> In withdrawal [of drug] studies, there usually is a small likelihood of great personal benefit and a large likelihood of personal harm. This is one of the most difficult research situations for potential subjects to evaluate, unlike high benefit/low risk research that is easy to accept or low benefit/high risk research that is easy to reject.[25]

For all these reasons, several commissions and alliances for persons with mental illness support independent confirmations of the adequacy of consent for adults with schizophrenia. This could be in the form of a psychiatrist independent of the researchers, a consent auditor, or having such adults or members of their families on IRBs that review protocols.

Moreover, consent only *begins*, and does not end, protection of such subjects. Take *challenge studies*, where a drug is introduced under controlled circumstances to research subjects in order to observe a hypothesized result.[26] In such nontherapeutic challenge studies, subjects may be given drugs such as amphetamines, L-dopa, or ketamine to induce psychosis. In such studies, only a very great benefit to future subjects would justify inflicting this harm on subjects.

In the UCLA study with Greg Aller and others, Yale law professor Jay Katz accused researchers of misleading subjects about the intentional creation of psychotic episodes with placebos and washout periods and argues that "the subject-patients' consent was manipulated."[27] Katz believes the consent form should have emphasized in bold letters that the study "WILL

NOT HELP YOUR CONDITION." The form also stated that "all medications will be stopped" and that "they would continue to receive regular care," which is contradictory. Katz concluded, "What transpired in this study is not unique to UCLA: It is symptomatic of the flawed nature of current regulations and current practices protecting the human rights of subjects." To use different terms, this study violated both the autonomy of subjects and the requirement not to harm them.

Lastly, given how poorly medical insurance covers care for schizophrenia, and how meager the resources are of most states for public psychiatry, we know that most families desperately seek to admit their relative into, and give consent for, any kind of public facility where normal care can be obtained at low cost. If the price of admission is participation in research, many families are willing to pay.

With reproductive ethics, critics worry that large sums of money offered to young women for their eggs, or to be surrogate mothers, coerce them into foolish decisions, paternalistically implying that young, competent women cannot make such choices. On the other hand, everyone seems to have overlooked the structural problems of a system, lacking in resources for persons who are mentally ill, that may force bad decisions on families.

Family Dilemmas

Caring for a relative with schizophrenia is no easy job and often traumatizes families. Indeed, some psychiatrists think of schizophrenia not as a disease of one person but as a *family illness*. It certainly creates a crisis in many families.

Because some adults with schizophrenia can function normally on drugs or be returned to normal, families constantly seek better drugs when traditional drugs fail to work or no longer work.

Support for families with a schizophrenic relative is less extensive than many believe. Over 40 million Americans lack good medical insurance, and only superb insurance policies provide full care for schizophrenia. When drugs or care, or both, are offered for free, families may enroll their relative in the program both to save money and in hopes of obtaining better medications.

The media and medical marketers so create the impression of great pharmacological success that families may find it hard to believe that schizophrenia cannot be cured. This may especially be true when the relative is in his 20s, with his whole life ahead of him.

Families may also have unrealistic expectations of researchers. Already, 1 in 10 adults with schizophrenia will commit suicide. Can researchers really monitor subjects 24 hours a day to prevent suicide? It would seem they can do so only if subjects are locked up and monitored as inpatients, an expensive endeavor for which few researchers are funded. Realistically, new protocols for drugs may need to take chances with outpatient subjects to save money and also to maximize freedom and autonomy of subjects.

When a subject commits suicide, everyone may accuse researchers of having evil motives or of not caring. When a 25-year-old son or daughter commits suicide, few parents will see it as an unavoidable, natural consequence of schizophrenia but in some cases, that is just what it is.

Critics rebut this argument by saying that, on medication and under supervision, the rate of suicide is much lower than 1 in 10. Moreover, as for monitoring subjects, fragile people with schizophrenia do in fact need special monitoring, and if they are going to be guinea pigs in a research study, why shouldn't they be carefully monitored? Thus, critics question whether such studies should *ever* be done on an outpatient basis.

8.5 Virtue Ethics, Integrity, and Conflicts of Interest

The primordial role of a physician to a patient is one of healer to one who is sick, the *healer/comforter role*. Even if a physician has reached the limits of healing, he or she must still act as a comforter to the patient who suffers.

A physician may make money by recommending a treatment to a patient, but the patient may not need it. What protects the patient is the moral integrity of the physician. It is her character that keeps in check the impulse to make extra money by doing procedures of no benefit to patients.

The same character must also protect patients from conflicts of interest experienced by physicians from financial gain and conflicting roles. As medicine evolved in the 19th and 20th centuries, roles of physicians became more complex as some became *medical experimenters*. Whereas the healer/comforter role derived from Kantian and Christian ethics, the new role derived from utilitarian ethics.

For this reason, a physician engaging in medical research has dual loyalties—both to her individual patient-subject and to her future patients. Such physician-experimenters have conflicting demands that ideally are balanced in a satisfactory way. A crucial requirement of informed consent is that the patient-subject understands the research doctors' predicament and understands that the balance may tilt against him.

One could argue here, and critics do, that structural changes in American research over the last decades have undermined the ability of virtuous researchers to resist abuses. If the *institutional culture* has become corrupted, what hope is there for individual virtue?

In America over the last 20 years, this conflict has intensified. In the early 1970s, the majority of research was funded by the federal government and, as such, was funded through "RO-1" grants with national review by respected peers. Previously, drug companies funded some research, but they pocketed all the money. With the goal of encouraging transfer of biomedical technology, the Bayh–Dole Act of 1980 erased an ethical bright line between academic and corporate medicine and allowed universities and their researchers to patent and reap royalties together.

Twenty years later, pharmaceutical companies fund most research into drugs and devices at universities; they do not fund independent peer review of their new drugs and do not publicize bad results. By indirectly paying physicians to test new drugs (through funds to university departments) and by financially encouraging physicians to recruit patients for experiments, drug companies may influence physicians to ignore the best interests of their patients.

In 1998, a study by the Department of Health and Human Services concluded that IRBs could no longer handle the job of protecting subjects from abuses in medical experimentation.[28] It found that IRBs were underfunded, overworked, and that the volume of work expected of volunteers could not be accurately and conscientiously performed. Another study in 2002 by the Institute of Medicine reached similar conclusions.[29]

Several scandals erupted in the 1990s wherein a few physicians and their associates appeared to have taken millions of dollars from drug companies for dubious research.[30] Some doctors in Georgia allegedly made at least $4 million over seven years from aggressively soliciting people with schizophrenia for drug trials; they made another $6 million over the same period from testing other drugs.[31]

In 1994, Susan Endersbe, a 41-year-old woman with schizophrenia and suicidal impulses, after a two-week washout period, was put on the experimental drug Sertindole, despite contraindications for suicidal impulses. Abbott Laboratories, which paid a psychiatrist to test Sertindole on patients with schizophrenia, enrolled her in the study.[32] As nurses' notes attest, Endersbe repeatedly told staff that she would kill herself, and after three days on Sertindole, she did just that by leaping to her death off a bridge into the Mississippi River.

Clearly, not every psychiatrist has had the moral integrity to withstand the siren call of increased financial gain. Where such powerful conflicts oppose a patient's interests, one wonders how many psychiatrist-researchers have the character to resist the lures of increased fame, status, and money in achieving successful research. Indeed, in any fee-for-service area of medicine, one wonders where physicians obtain the integrity to resist any treatment not in patients' interests but that financially furthers their own.

In the early 1990s, researchers at MPRC searched for a chemical cause of schizophrenia. Creating a reproducible medical problem, such as a head injury, is often the most important first step in developing a cure for the problem. They hit upon ketamine, a chemical cousin of the street drug PCP, an anesthetic used on large mammals by veterinarians. On the streets, it is also called "Special K" and a "date rape" or "predator" drug. Humans who were anesthetized with ketamine often awakened temporarily psychotic and sometimes reported terrible nightmares. Ketamine also causes hallucinations, short-term amnesia, and dissociation, a feeling of the mind's separation from the body.[33]

Researchers hypothesized that ketamine might reliably produce schizophrenic psychosis and become a benchmark for studying such psychosis. If it could be shown that ketamine played a role in producing schizophrenia-like states, the next step would be to discover how to eliminate the body's ketamine-like compounds.

Nevertheless, giving ketamine to a normal person to produce schizophrenia, or giving ketamine to a person with schizophrenia who was doing fine, unquestionably harms that person; subjects would be worse off after taking ketamine than before taking it. In the language of medical research, giving patients such drugs is a nontherapeutic experiment.

At MPRC, several psychiatrists received substantial amounts of money from the federal government to study schizophrenia. Institutions employing Drs. Adrienne Lahti and Carol Tamminga received over half a million dollars to see if injecting schizophrenics with ketamine worsened their schizophrenia.[34] In the study of Proloxin in which Greg Friend was enrolled, MPRC received $600,000.

It is also true that researchers tend to see the glass as half full (i.e., ambiguous results are seen to favor their own research). In the ketamine study, Dr. Tamminga downplayed harm to subjects. When asked by Alto Charo, a member of President Clinton's Bioethics Commission, "Why does anybody *say yes to enrolling in your [ketamine] research?" Tamminga looked startled and replied, "I've never really thought about it."[35] Charo's fellow commissioners did think about it and concluded that inducing psychosis in mentally fragile schizophrenic patients was not something to be done without great moral justification.*

Researchers Defend Themselves

Many psychiatric researchers believe that placebo studies of new drugs to fight mental disorders are necessary and appropriate. They defend themselves on utilitarian grounds. From a Kantian viewpoint, each patient may not get the best drug, but on the whole, randomized clinical trials with washout periods and placebos best prove which new drugs work. For example, we now have drugs for schizophrenia that do not cause tardive dyskenesia (uncontrollable spasms, often irreversible) because researchers used placebo-controlled studies on past patients.

Paul Appelbaum, a professor of psychiatry at the University of Massachusetts Medical School, offers a modest defense of continuing to research new drugs for schizophrenia.[36] First, the main lobby for persons with mental disorders, the National Alliance for the Mentally Ill, does not favor cessation of all research. Second, almost all patients on medication will at some time experience a relapse, showing the need for better drugs. Third, "it has been known for many years that some schizophrenic patients can have their medication discontinued without experiencing relapse for a substantial period of time." Fourth, washout periods provide all subjects in drug trials with the same baseline and minimize adverse drug interactions with maintenance drugs.

He also argues that compromise is possible: Patients with a high risk of severe relapse can be screened out, and evidence suggests that tapering off drugs, rather than abrupt withdrawal, minimizes severe episodes. Furthermore, subjects can be closely monitored for relapse by having such studies only done as inpatients. Finally, consent can be required only not of the subject but of the "person who is responsible for the health care of the subject."

On a more serious topic, although inducing psychosis with ketamine in persons with schizophrenia would seem to most people to harm such subjects, some researchers defend the practice. Trey Sunderland, a Yale University psychiatrist who was chief of geriatric psychiatry at the National Institute of Mental Health (NIMH) and chair of its IRB, said he believes that use of ketamine in such so-called "challenge studies" could "yield answers for some of the most devastating mental illnesses."[37]

Critics of such research speculate that each time a subject with schizophrenia has a psychotic episode, he or she gets worse, almost as if toxic chemicals build up in the brain, causing structural damage. This so-called *kindling theory of psychosis* sees neural pathways as getting hotter and hotter until "combustion" occurs.

Dr. Sunderland disputes the kindling theory, saying there is no evidence that ketamine causes flashbacks in patients undergoing surgery and that no subjects at the NIMH have complained of any damage from such studies.[38] He continues, "This is a medicine which is given under close scrutiny for a short-term basis. There is no repeat long-term exposure." Moreover, ketamine's street use is "not an issue in these studies" and not mentioned in forms providing informed consent.

Finally, Dr, Sunderland defended the form providing informed consent in these studies. "It does mention you might get an altered mood, hallucinations. . . . The main side effects of the medication are listed in black and white."[39]

8.6 Harm to Subjects and the Kantian Ideal of Patient Care

The unusual aspect of the two main studies discussed in this chapter (washout and ketamine studies) is that researchers understood that bad things would happen to subjects, intended for this to happen, and did not really inform subjects or their families about such consequences. Psychiatrist Appelbaum says that while only 16 percent of patients maintained on medication will relapse, when medication is withdrawn, nearly 55 percent will.[40] Moreover, "abrupt discontinuation of medication induces a threefold greater risk of relapse than gradual discontinuation over a period of weeks to months."

Such protocols violate the Declaration of Helsinki. When an effective drug exists, a new drug must be compared to the old drug, not a placebo.

The study inducing psychosis with ketamine is unusual in the recent history of American medicine. Even the Tuskegee Study did not *inflict* a disease on its patients, but just *observed* a disease that could have been treated.

The protocol violates the ideal of patient care in Kantian ethics of treating each patient as a member of the "Kingdom of Ends." It also violates the traditional rule of medical ethics, "First, do no harm," also known as the principle of nonmaleficence.

In animal research, researchers injure primates to create a baseline of injury for further study. At the University of Pennsylvania, Thomas Genneralli inflicted tremendous head injuries on chimpanzees in attempts to simulate the effects on humans in automobile crashes. Edward Taub, at the University of Alabama at Birmingham, severed the nerves on one side of primates to simulate injury from stroke in humans.[41] But it is unusual for medical researchers to intentionally harm human subjects.

Indeed, it appears that psychiatric researchers took liberties with adults with schizophrenia that other medical researchers would consider unethical. Oncologists do not *induce* cancer in human subjects to study cancer, nor do they try to *reintroduce* cancer in patients who've been treated and who are in remission. Cardiologists do not try to *create* heart attacks to study cardiomyopathy, nor do they *induce* arrhythmias in patients who once had heart attacks.

Washout periods and placebos also don't necessarily guarantee that a previous drug is completely gone from a patient's system. That depends on whether the drug enters the patient's blood directly or indirectly via metabolites. If the latter, researchers may not really know the decay curve for metabolites or how long, if ever, it would take to create a perfectly drug-free state.

8.7 Vulnerable Subjects and Social Justice

During the 20th century, the worst abuses in medical research occurred with *vulnerable* subjects, people who have little power to decline participation in experiments. Besides prisoners and illiterate sharecroppers, children, the elderly, people under the influence of drugs, and people suffering from mental illnesses can be vulnerable subjects in medical research.

Greg Friend later said that he was vulnerable at the time he consented to participate in the MPRC study and that he could not have given real, informed consent. Friend's case illustrates another problem about vulnerability: If the only way to get free or good care is in a medical experiment, then people without superb medical insurance will always be the subjects of medical research. In Friend's case, his parents may have exhausted their medical insurance (why he left the first facility is not explained) and may have been seeking not only good treatment at MPRC but free treatment.

Friend's case and that of others illustrate the problem of *social justice* in medical research. In America, poor people overwhelmingly are the subjects of medical research. With the exception of research on cancer, rich people, as well as middle-class people with good medical coverage, unless they have no other medical options, do not participate in medical research. Is this just?

> *Claudia and Joe Friend were shocked to learn about what had happened to other patients with mental disorders during their washout periods and began a crusade to have all such washout periods banned. Over the next two decades, from 1984 to 2004, they lobbied for an end to washout periods in psychiatric research.*
>
> *Fourteen to 15 years after Greg Friend's attempted suicide (which Greg survived, going on to live many more years), in 1997–1998, several significant events occurred: First, Robert Whitaker's series in the* Boston Globe *exposed abuses of subjects in psychiatric research. Second, the Institute of Medicine issued a report critical of the regulation of research in America.[42] Finally, President Clinton's National Bioethics Commission held hearings on both washout periods in psychiatric research and the deliberate induction of psychosis by giving ketamine.[43] Comments by individual commissioners were critical of both kinds of research, but especially the latter.*

8.8 Structural Critiques of Modern Psychiatric Research

Several critics, such as the Alliance for Human Research Protection (AHRP) and Public Citizen, have battled for the rights of patient-subjects in modern psychiatric research, focusing on problems caused by (1) research that seeks profits for stock-financed drug companies, (2) conflicts of interest in those who receive payments for research and in those who regulate such research, and (3) lack of protection for vulnerable schizophrenic subjects on whom the research is done.[44]

In some drug studies, according to the *Wall Street Journal,* psychiatrists who recruited patients to studies where drugs were tested for schizophrenia and Alzheimer's received as much as $30,000 per patient.[45] Former deputy editor of the *New England Journal of Medicine,* Marcia Angell, charged (in her last editorial before leaving that periodical) that corporate influence in academic medicine now determines what research is done, by what methods, by whom, and which results were reported or suppressed.[46]

One of the chief complaints of critics is that new drugs are commonly tested on younger, healthier subjects than those likely to be prescribed the drug, thus minimizing known side effects. In other words, older, sicker people who eventually are prescribed the new drugs will likely experience *worse symptoms*, especially in combination with other drugs they're taking.

During the decade from 1995 to 2005, the NIH budget (which funds most research in America) doubled from its previous high. During this period, three important new drugs were brought to market to help people with schizophrenia: Zyprexa (olanzapine), Risperdal (risperidone), and Seroquel (quetiapine).

Perhaps this explains how the drug Vioxx could have been given to so many millions of elderly patients for arthritis without it being known previously that it caused heart attacks. For critics, Vioxx is a perfect example of how finances lead companies to suppress bad results and how the Federal Drug Administration (FDA) has allowed pharmaceutical companies to rush new drugs to market without adequate testing. For example, of the 32 members of the FDA advisory panel screening new drugs, 10 members had received money from Merck or Pfizer, manufacturers of Vioxx and Celebrex.[47] Critics raised similar concerns about Bextra, as well as using antipsychotic drugs such as Zyprexa and Risperdal for dementia (elderly patients who took these drugs were 1.7 times more likely to die prematurely than similar patients given placebos).[48]

Of relevance to Greg Friend's case, critics such as Vera Sharav of AHRP claim that washout periods have a hidden effect desired by drug companies: *Washout periods make people with schizophrenia sicker and thus exaggerate the benefit of any new drug begun later.* Remember that in clinical practice, patients do not undergo washout periods in switching from one drug to another, so the benefit is unlikely to be matched with real patients.[49]

In a 1998 ground-breaking series of articles on the ethics of research on people with schizophrenia and under the Freedom of Information Act, the *Boston Globe* obtained results of clinical trials submitted to the Federal Drug Administration. It found that three main drugs for schizophrenia were tested during the 1990s: Zyprexa (olanzapine), Risperdal (risperidone) and Seroquel (quetiapine). Serlect (sertindole) was also tested but withdrawn after questions arose about its safety in a meeting of an FDA advisory committee. The *Globe* discovered that 12,176 patients from the United States and abroad were tested in trials for all four drugs. There were 88 deaths, including 38 suicides, for an overall death rate of 1 of every 138 volunteers.

Psychiatric researchers rebut that some percentage of people with schizophrenia will commit suicide regardless of whether they are in a drug study. They emphasize that patients in such clinical trials for schizophrenia will likely be sicker than patients not in such trials.

Critics concede these points, but note that the rate of suicide of patients with schizophrenia in clinical trials is two to five times higher than the norm for people with schizophrenia, which is 2 to 5 deaths per 1,000. Moreover, they say, people with very severe cases of schizophrenia are almost certainly too sick to participate in such trials without being inpatients and under close monitoring.

Finally, it is startling that no objective standard exists of when a new drug achieves a benefit that exceeds that of a placebo to classify it officially as therapeutic. Researchers and regulatory agencies have a wide latitude in judging exactly what improvement counts as a benefit to patients.

Drug researchers paid to find new and better drugs will obviously interpret their results to show benefits. Surprisingly, Thomas Laughren, MD, the head of the FDA's Psychiatric Drug Division in 2000, conceded that "there is a certain amount of myth" in the claim that new psychiatric drugs have any benefit above placebo. In other words, all we know is that the new drug had some minimal effect beyond placebo, but "there isn't any standard for what *effect size* is required to get a psychotropic drug on the market. We have never, in my experience, not approved a drug because of finding that the effect size is too marginal."[50]

8.9 NBAC's Report on Psychiatric Research

In mid-1997, the National Bioethics Advisory Commission, appointed under President Clinton, began 18 months of hearings about research on individuals who are mentally challenged. Realizing that such research had been neglected by previous commissions, NBAC wanted to proactively improve regulations. It issued its report in 1998.[51]

Unfortunately, the NBAC did not recommend the elimination of washout studies in research on people with schizophrenia, nor did it call such studies unethical. Instead, it merely urged the Institute of Medicine (IOM), the intellectual wing of the American Medical Association, to evaluate challenge, washout, and placebo-controlled studies in psychiatric research.

The NBAC did make some suggestions, but rather than making specific suggestions about *content*, most involved setting up *processes* where *other people* would make the specific judgments about content. It is the nature of committees not to be radical, even when confronting something that needs condemnation, and many people on such committees want *someone else* to be the ones who tell researchers they can no longer do their experiments. Thus the NBAC suggested independent auditors of consent in subjects with mental impairments, as well as special panels at NIH. The NBAC did not say it was unethical for researchers to induce psychosis in subjects, but urged IRBs to "exercise heightened scrutiny."

Conclusions

The crusade of the Friends has failed. Greg Friend's parents strove to eliminate washout studies in psychiatric research, but at the end of 2005, such studies are still being used. Although not as common as they once were (perhaps because IRBs and drug companies have become more sensitive to this issue), there is no federal ban on this kind of psychiatric experiment. Nor are challenge studies banned.

In 1997, the NBAC anticipated that drug companies would throw billions into finding new drugs for mental disorders. That did not occur. Over the last decade, drug companies have maximized profits by successfully lobbying to change the law to give them longer patents on their old drugs, focusing on "lifestyle drugs" such as Viagra, and changing their focus from inventing new drugs to directly marketing existing drugs to consumers.[52]

In the late 1990s, it appeared that real change might occur in the regulation of research on people with schizophrenia. The NBAC held hearings and made its report, Robert Whitaker's investigative reports in the *Boston Globe* were syndicated nationally, and groups emerged to champion the rights of patients with mental illness. But soon the media's attention shifted elsewhere.

Psychiatric researchers have aggressively defended washout periods and placebo-controlled studies of new drugs for mental illness.[53] Despite three decades of sporadic investigation, medical research on people with schizophrenia has changed little over this time, and, despite the existence of IRBs and a branch of the federal government charged with preventing abuses in experimentation, abuses in research may have even gotten worse. Many medical schools let drug companies draft and edit research on results in their schools from drug company–sponsored research.[54] Robert Whitaker's 2003 book, *Mad in America*, which won a Polk journalism award and a nomination for a Pulitzer Prize, documented a shocking increase in abuses by the pharmacological industry and psychiatric researchers over the last 20 years. Whitaker then concluded that adults with schizophrenia were much better protected 25 years ago in the United States and are better protected in India and Nigeria.[55]

In 2004, the *Los Angles Times* revealed that Trey Sunderland, chief of geriatric psychiatry at the National Institute of Mental Health, had not reported $517,000 of consulting fees over a five-year period from Pfizer pharmaceuticals, presumably for consulting about drugs for research on people with schizophrenia, a violation of federal ethics rules.[56] It appeared that the fox was guarding the henhouse.[57]

The year before, *The New York Times* reported that an Emory psychiatry professor published favorable reviews of drugs manufactured by companies where he was given, or already had, large stock options.[58] These options represented a net gain of over a million dollars. Several physicians publicly rebuked him for failing to disclose his conflicts of interest.

In February 2005, the NIH announced new ethics rules that prohibited its scientists from consulting privately at pharmaceutical companies. The new rules took effect immediately and banned scientists from owning stock in such companies. Angered by the new rules, NIH scientists huffed and predicted that without such compensation, good people wouldn't work at NIH.[59]

Let us end this chapter on a topic mentioned at the beginning. Much of the questionable research described in this chapter results from the desperation of patients and their families to get adequate care for schizophrenia. We have not really raised the question of finance and distributive justice, but we raise it here: Why should a just, compassionate society single out this biological disease? Why should the federal government pay for kidney dialysis and/or kidney transplants, but not care for people with schizophrenia? Why do companies pay for dental and optical care, but not care for mental illness?

Alone among the developed countries of the world, America lacks a comprehensive national medical plan to help our sickest patients. Our patchwork system, loosely based on employment, poverty, old age, or disability, increasingly falls apart as more and more companies are choosing not to provide good medical coverage to employees. Among the victims of this continuing national tragedy are people with schizophrenia and their families.

As this book went to press, important news broke: Some, new, expensive drugs for schizophrenia described in this chapter (Zyprexa, Seroquel, Risperdal, and Geodon) gained FDA approval based on short-term studies financed by drug companies comparing the new drug to a placebo. A new study financed by the U.S. Government discovered that these new drugs were no more effective or no safer than perphenazine, an older generic drug.[60] None of the new drugs had been systematically compared to one another in a long-term trial designed to decide which to try first. The Clinical Antipsychotic Trial of Intervention Effectiveness (CATIE) study followed 1,493 patients with schizophrenia randomly assigned to take one of the four drugs; in CATIE, neither doctor nor patient knew which drug was being tested.

Zyprexa, with sales of $2.4 billion in America in 2004, costs about $12 a day, whereas perphenazine, about $1. Switching patients on Medicaid back to perphenazine might save states and the federal government millions of dollars.

FURTHER READINGS

Declaration of Helsinki. See World Medical Association Web site: http://www.wma.net/e/policy/b3.htm

DuVal, Gordon. "Ethics in Psychiatric Research: Study Design Issues." *Canadian Journal of Psychiatry* 49, no. 1 (January 2004), pp. 55–59.

Research Involving Persons with Mental Disorders That May Affect Decision-Making Capacity. Rockville, MD: National Bioethics Advisory Commission, 1998. http://www.georgetown.edu/research/nrcbl/nbac/capacity/TOC.htm

Shamoo, Adil E. *Ethics in Neurobiological Research with Human Subjects: The Baltimore Conference on Ethics.* Amsterdam, Holland: Gordon & Breach Publishers, 1997.

Weijer, Charles. "Thinking Clearly About Research Risks: Implications of the Work of Benjamin Freedman." *IRB: A Review of Human Subjects Research* 21, no. 6 (November–December 1999).

Whitaker, Robert. *Mad in America.* New York: Perseus, 2003.

Zipursky, Robert. "Ethical Issues in Schizophrenia Research. *Current Psychiatry Reports* 1 (October 1, 1999), pp. 13–19.

CHAPTER 9

Is There a Duty to Die?

This chapter explores cases in medical ethics that combine end-of-life issues with those of scarce medical resources. One of the premier subjects of bioethics, death and dying, has been a topic of intense public discussion for over 30 years; it includes topics such as brain death, requests to die by competent adults, physician-assisted dying, and when to cease treatment for incompetent patients in irreversible comas (discussed in Chapter 6 about Terri Schiavo). Discussion about scarce medical resources has existed since Shana Alexander's 1962 article in *LIFE* describing the God Committee in Seattle (discussed in Chapter 3 about Ernie Crowfeather).

What is unique to this chapter is discussion about the end of life in the context of great amounts of money and effort expended on creating extra years or months of life with a limited quality of life for those affected. Could such efforts be futile or even unjust? What is the opportunity cost of extraordinary care at the end of life?

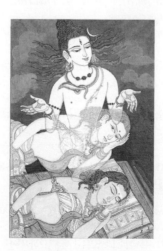

Virginia Newcomb forgot her grandchildren's names when she was 78 years old. Since her husband, a Lutheran minister, died of a heart attack 20 years before, she had been living alone in her San Francisco area home. Both of her children were in their 50s and had families of their own. Virginia Newcomb and her daughter, Jessica, also a widow, both lived south of San Francisco.

Jessica and Virginia talked at least once a week. At first, Jessica was only mildly alarmed that Virginia had to be reminded of her grandchildren's names. People in her mother's family had always been absent-minded and often forgot birthdays and anniversaries, so it was natural for Jessica to downplay Virginia's lapses.

Over the next several months, the character of Virginia's forgetfulness changed. At first, she forgot how to work the remote on the television, to which she adjusted by always leaving the TV on the same channel. Then she forgot how to get home from the corner convenience store, to which she adjusted by refusing to go out anymore. Then she forgot Jessica's phone number, to which she adjusted by insisting that Jessica call her every morning.

One day in June, a day Jessica will always remember, the San Francisco fire department called her to say that Virginia had been picked up, wet and disheveled, underneath the Golden Gate Bridge. When asked how she got there or why she was wet, Virginia told an incoherent, rambling story about seeing a lost relative from her childhood and pursuing him as he tried to get away.

Jessica arrived and took Virginia home with her. The next week, down at Stanford Medical Center, a blood flow scan of the brain and MRI revealed that large portions of Virginia's brain were white, not gray, and had degenerated. The diagnosis came back as Alzheimer's disease. The neurologist said that, at this point, Virginia had probably had the disease for "several years."[1]

9.1 Gov. Lamm's Famous Remarks and His Historical Predecessors

In 1984, Richard Lamm, the governor of Colorado, ignited an ethical firestorm while addressing the Colorado Health Lawyers Association at St. Joseph's Hospital. He suggested that elderly patients with terminal diseases should not cling to each month of life (which consequently costs society hundreds of thousands of dollars in each case), but instead had a *"duty to die."*[2] People who die without having life artificially extended are like "leaves falling off a tree and forming humus for the other plants to grow up. . . . You've got a duty to die and get out of the way. Let the other society, our kids, build a reasonable life."

In an article published later, Governor Lamm criticized the costs of dying in our modern medical system: "For 10 generations, American mothers and fathers left a richer and more productive country to their children, but my generation broke the link of trust . . . we have improved and are improving our standard of living at the expense of our children."[3]

At the time of the governor's remarks, debate about death and dying focused on whether competent individuals with terminal illnesses had a *right* to die, not on a *duty* to die. Critics jumped on Governor Lamm's statement, claiming it was evidence of how granting a right to die could quickly turn into a duty to die.

For such critics, it was unthinkable that any patient would have a duty to die to help others save resources. To them, the transfer of resources should flow from well-off young people to elderly persons. The old do not have any obligations to live fewer years or to forgo medical treatment for the benefit of the young.

Lamm championed a duty to die based on intergenerational justice. Even in 1984, he did not think it fair that the elderly were costing so much to die in a way that transferred wealth from younger workers to them.

We often hear that America has the best medical system in the world. Governor Lamm did not think that claim could remain true.[4] The present system's inability to limit or stop care is driving it to bankruptcy. Dying today is too costly.

Spending exorbitant amounts of money on the elderly is unfair in several ways. First, the young will never experience the same kind of medical care because the system will become bankrupt. Second, today's financing of medical care for the elderly is an involuntary transfer from the young to the old and thus unjustifiable. A special injustice falls on working people without medical insurance: Society unfairly taxes them to support coddling elderly patients with extravagant, unnecessary treatments, for example, $300,000 liver transplants for 85-year-old patients.

Other medical systems around the world do better because they focus more on prevention and get better value from each dollar spent on health. American society would get a better marginal return on its medical dollars by redirecting monies spent on the end of life to preventive care for younger people.

Governor Lamm believes we cannot go on buying extravagant care for the insured while giving only minimal emergency care to the uninsured. Medical care is not an *individual* but a *social* good. "Once we admit that we cannot pay for everything, we must ask ourselves not only what does a patient need, but how do we spend our resources to buy the maximum health for the largest number of citizens."[5]

Spending a half-million dollars on each elderly patient as he or she dies may in effect deny minimal care for the uninsured:

> We are spending millions of dollars on esoteric improvements at the margins in American medicine while spending pennies on the access problem where we could buy far more health. We give some people too much health care and others too little. We have money for ECMO [Extra Corporeal Membrane Oxygenation] machines but not prenatal care. We spend incredible amounts of money on kidney dialysis, but practically nothing on educating people to stop smoking and abusing alcohol. We have far too many MRI machines, but 30 percent of the women in America give birth without adequate prenatal care in their first trimester.[6]

So for Lamm, a duty to die is cast in terms of a battle for resources between young and old, an issue of intergenerational justice, almost as if the greedy medical needs of the elderly make young working people into taxed slaves.

Lamm's Historical Predecessors

Governor Lamm was not the first to argue that an individual life was not of supreme value, not a value that should trump all others. In the fifth century BCE, the philosopher Socrates drank hemlock, a poison, to kill himself, partly as a duty to his Athenian society. As his student, Plato, tells us, the real study of philosophy for Socrates was to find wisdom, and part of wisdom is finding a way to calmly and courageously face one's own death.[7]

Ancient Athens deeply imbued its citizens with the view that people existed for the good of the city-state, not vice versa. Given the constant invasions of Athens and Greece by other city-states and by Persian leaders such as Darius and Xerxes, ancient Greeks had to be ready at a moment's notice to fight and lay down their lives for their country. Death was common and the average expected life span at birth was only 35 years. Many young men died in battle at a much earlier age.

As such, when one was dying, it was considered base or ignoble to cling to an extra few months of life, if doing so placed a heavy burden on one's fellow citizens or family. (Socrates was 70 years old when he drank his hemlock.) If the ancient Greeks had possessed the means to extend dying the way modern medicine can, doing so would have been seen as selfish in many cases.

In the two millennia since, a long line of philosophers and thinkers have agreed with Socrates. Roman emperor Marcus Aurelius and Roman slave Epictetus both were Stoics and championed suicide in the face of undignified suffering. In the 18th century, Scottish philosopher David Hume argued that taking one's own life after diagnosis of terminal illness had very little negative effect on others and, at most, represented a withdrawal of good works from society, nothing more.[8] As such, not fighting death when terminally ill was morally permissible, even admirable.

Problems of Defining a Right to Die

Obviously, a "duty to die" implies different things. It certainly differs from a "right to die." A right to die is an option that may or may not be exercised, and one is neither moral nor immoral for either exercising it or not. On the other hand, if there is a duty to die, good people should obey it because it would be wrong to go on living when one should die. But what then does "a duty to die" mean?

It could mean that, when the time comes where it could be offered, one forgoes expensive medical attempts to prolong life.

For example, if there is a duty to die and if one is dying of coronary artery disease, one could refuse a heart transplant, citing this duty.

That seems too broad a definition because it would include premature babies and children, who certainly have no duty to die and forgo such resources (in part, because they cannot make voluntary choices). Characteristically, a duty to die is asserted for elderly people who have lived rich, full lives.

Rather than merely forgoing extra treatments, a duty to die may imply more active methods, such as killing oneself. In this case, the old maxim "ought implies can" becomes relevant (i.e., one must have both the kind of disease and the resources where killing oneself is a real option). For example, this would not be a real option in the latter stages of dementia, when one will be in a locked unit in a nursing facility, where all sharp objects and weapons will have been removed, and where only a nurse has access to drugs in a locked cabinet. Similarly, if one is suddenly rendered paralyzed from the neck down by an accident, one will not easily be able to kill oneself without a friend's help (in most states, making the friend guilty of a crime). Indeed, and despite the brave talk of some people that "I'd kill myself before I'd live like that," most people sink into disability, dementia, and dysfunction slowly and by degrees. They may not recognize their own descent until it is too late to do anything about it.

Philosopher Jan Narveson argues that duties are always *to* a particular person and presuppose a rough agreement in the background about what they are.[9] In other words, new duties can't just be asserted by some people out of nowhere and to society in general, and then be used to make people feel they must comply. Narveson also distinguishes between a weak and strong sense of a duty to die. Narveson thinks a strong sense of a duty to die would be "enforceable" in some sense. He cites our nearly universal condemnation that we have a duty not to kill innocent strangers. His weak sense of a duty to die implies much less, merely that patients should not insist that caregivers ruin their own lives to allow them to live extra years.

In the past, critics picked up on the combination of championing dignified death for the dying with efforts to contain costs and predicted that the two together would lead to exactly what this chapter discusses: a duty to die.[10] Disability activists and antieuthanasia champions fear that a focus on the great expense of maintaining people with disabilities, people with schizophrenia, and the nondying but infirm elderly will, combined with glorification of dignified dying such as that presented by the Hemlock Society, make these patients and their relatives turn to direct and indirect suicide as a quick, cheap solution. Indeed, for some of these activists, a right to die and a duty to die are two extremes, and although different, they are on the same spectrum of ethical possibility, linked by a concern over wasting medical and familial resources.

But a right to die and a duty to die really do differ conceptually. A right to die is what political philosophers call a right of noninterference, a right to be left alone, and, in this case, a right not to be forced to live against one's will. In contrast, a duty to die is an obligation to do something one may not want to do but which one does either because it's the right thing to do or to benefit other people. In the first case, one is likely to want to die and will need to take action to implement that desire. In the latter case, one may not want to die but may do so for some other good.

Medical Coverage and Lack of Coverage in America

Unlike Canada and England, America lacks a national, single-payer, unified system of medical care. Most Americans who have medical coverage have it in one of four ways: employment-based coverage, age-based through Medicare, poverty-based through Medicaid, or through CHAMPUS (the system of medical care for people in the armed services).

That leaves about 40 to 44 million Americans who lack any medical coverage at all or who are grossly underinsured. Contrary to stereotypes, most of these Americans are not unemployed, but work (most likely they work in service industries such as restaurants or hotels, or work for employers with fewer than six employees). FICA taxes, as well as state and city taxes, are deducted from these workers' paychecks to pay for medical services for patients in Medicaid and Medicare programs. Part of some sales taxes are also used. Thus, workers whose employers don't provide medical coverage subsidize medical treatment of patients covered by Medicaid, Medicare, and CHAMPUS.

Starting in 2005, Medicare will cover expenses for some drugs after patients have spent $800. Medicare does not cover a room in a long-term-care facility or aides for invalids cared for at home. State Medicaid policies vary greatly in what they cover and how much one can make and be eligible for them, with California the most generous and Alabama the least.

At first, Jessica enthusiastically took Virginia into her home, making a bedroom for Virginia in the guest bedroom above the garage. For a year, this arrangement worked. Drugs such as donepezil (brand name: Aricept) seemed to arrest further loss of memory. Virginia also took drugs for arthritis and for other ailments. All in all, her medications cost $1,000 a month; none were covered by Medicare.

One night, Virginia woke up screaming, broke a window, and jumped from her second-story bedroom, breaking her leg in the fall. She returned home in a cast and, two months later, broke her foot again trying to chase a cat in the yard.

At this point, Jessica reluctantly decided that Virginia would be better off in a senior care facility designed to prevent falls, where assistance would be available to her 24 hours a day. (Jessica unfortunately had to be gone during the day to work.) So Virginia entered the Garden Acres Retirement Community, at a cost of $4,000 per month.

To pay for her care, Jessica sold Virginia's modest home south of San Francisco for a million dollars. Like many of her generation, Virginia had always told her children and grandchildren that money from sale of the house would send them to college and would pay for downpayments on their own houses.

Virginia also had surgery for a gallstone, but developed a postoperative infection that put her in the hospital for three days, during which she experienced transient psychosis. When she returned to Green Acres, she was very disoriented for the first few days.

9.2 John Hardwig: Defending a Duty to Die

In 1997, philosopher John Hardwig revived Governor Lamm's cause and championed the duty to die.[11] However, Hardwig argued in a very different way from Lamm, avoiding claims about intergenerational justice and focusing instead on the much more realistic and common plight of an overly stressed family trying to help a dying elderly relative. Hence, Professor Hardwig presented and justified a duty to die *as an obligation to one's family.*

Hardwig criticizes what he says dominates bioethics: "the individualistic fantasy." This paradigm sees the individual in isolation from family, friends, and co-workers. Within that fantasy, the only real value is personal autonomy or, legalistically, informed consent. Suicide and assisted dying for terminal patients are often discussed as if individuals had no families or relationships (e.g., the cases of Larry McAfee, Dax Cowart, and Elizabeth Bouvia).[12]

One theory in contemporary ethics is called *communitarian ethics* and emphasizes that ethical issues and their resolution typically occur not among unrelated, equal individuals but among a nexus of relationships. Families, both nuclear and partial, old and blended, form the central core of this nexus, which also includes neighbors, friends, church members, and co-workers.

Although he doesn't put it this way, Hardwig's defense of a duty to die stems from this tradition. For Hardwig, what generates a duty to die for someone terminally ill *is consideration for the interests of others whom one cares about.* Put simply, there comes a point for Hardwig where he thinks it is immoral to burden those one loves. "Ending my life if my duty required might be difficult. But for me, a far greater horror would be dying all alone or stealing the futures of my loved ones in order to buy a little more time for myself."

Professor Hardwig inserts a perspective missing from many discussions in bioethics that feature trade-offs between individual rights and the greater good of society. Hardwig attacks this "bald dichotomy" as a false dilemma: first, because more than two sides exist here; and second, because this is not the lived experience of most patients. They feel no guilt in taking resources away from an anonymous, amorphous society. What rings true for patients is the trade-off between their own self-interest and that of those in their circle of caregivers.

It is easy to dismiss Hardwig's views, or reduce them to an absurd position, but they need a fair hearing. His ideal case is one where an elderly person (call him John) has had a rich, long life and has been befriended by younger relatives. Now, at age 85, with the usual multitude of problems (say, diabetes, coronary artery disease, and kidney failure), caring for John takes all the time of his single 63-year-old daughter, Joan (John's wife of many years died the year before). Not having the money for a long-term-care facility (not covered by Medicare) and owning his own home (unable to qualify for Medicaid), John can only be taken care of at home by Joan. This means helping him with his insulin shots, driving him to his dialysis appointments three times a week, waiting three hours until the dialysis is complete, driving John home, and helping him with routine chores around the house that his heart condition prevents him from doing.

At this juncture, suppose John is offered a kidney transplant. As an elderly patient, he will have a long downtime to recover from the surgery, but a new kidney might help him live another decade of life. Another decade, that is, if Joan goes all out and essentially dedicates her life to taking care of her aged father.

But Hardwig asks, what about Joan's life? Did she sign on for this? We unthinkingly believe that children owe their parents care in their old age, but that intuition came from long ago, when parents died before 65 and when no one age 70 faced the next decade being a nurse to a father who was 90.

In such a situation, for the good of his daughter, Hardwig argues that John should forgo the transplant. Hardwig hesitates to say that John should actually kill himself, but with our proposed choice, Hardwig would have no hesitation in arguing that John should forgo the transplant and that he has a *duty* to do so. "The fact of deeply interwoven lives debars us from making exclusively self-regarding decisions, as the decisions of one member of a family may dramatically affect the lives of all the rest."[13]

Hardwig argues that we are tempted to see the father's impending death as the greater evil because it is a bad event that is coming soon, whereas Joan's life is open-ended and can recover after her father's death. But Hardwig thinks that judgment gives too little weight to the crushing burden on Joan of caring for her father. As for her father's coming death: "Death—or ending your own life—is simply not the greatest evil or the greatest burden."[14] Even if it were the greatest burden, a simple utilitarian calculation covering only the extended family shows that such a death does not outweigh all other values: "The fact that I suffer greater burdens than others in my family does not license me simply to choose what I want for myself, nor does it necessarily release me from a responsibility to try to protect the quality of their lives."

Hardwig agrees with Elisabeth Kübler-Ross, a Swiss psychiatrist who pioneered a new openness about death and dying in American hospitals, that we fear death too much. "Our fear of death has led to a massive assault on it," he writes.[15] By conquering that fear and by seizing control of our own death, he says we can affirm our own agency and self-worth. In so doing, we can also plan our deaths and draw meaning from greater connections to our family and loved ones.

In adopting the perspective of a family, rather than of an individual (or of a physician treating an individual patient), Hardwig reframes the typical discussion and emphasizes how a serious illness is not just an individual misfortune but a *family* misfortune. As such, how the patient responds affects not only him but his entire family. If we think of virtues and vices, then such misfortunes show true character, with some people acting courageously and unselfishly for the sake of their grandchildren or spouses, and others acting childishly and selfishly. Hardwig concludes, "Those of us with families and loved ones always have a duty not to make selfish or self-centered decisions about our lives."[16]

Whether a particular patient has a weak or strong duty to die depends on all the particular details about the medical condition, the course of his life, and the resources of the family. In general for Hardwig, the more the burdens imposed on the family—financial, emotional, destruction of marriages, postponement of retirement—the greater the obligation to die. The older we get, the less we give up by not fighting for every extra year of life: "As we age, we will be giving up less and less by giving up our lives, if only because we will sacrifice fewer remaining years of life and smaller portion of our life plans." The quality of our life usually declines dramatically in our final years, and as we approach death, what we give up is of less and less value.

For all these reasons, and as a professor of philosophy, Hardwig agrees with Socrates that if we have lived to age 75 and are not at peace with the idea of our own dying, we lack moral character and wisdom. We are "out of touch with life's basic realities."

Suppose, at age 80 with a diagnosis of pancreatic cancer, one says, "I have lived a good and full life. I have no complaints and could not have wished for a better career, spouse, or children." In that case, Hardwig echoes the common sentiment that one has a stronger duty to die over another, different person who never got a break in life, never had one good relationship, and always struggled to pay the bills. The latter can hope that his extended dying may bring him that one great friendship, or even love, but the former person should be ready to go—at least, according to Socrates and Hardwig.

Today, many of us fear progressive neurological diseases such as Parkinson's, Alzheimer's, ALS, and cascading strokes. In such cases, and when the part of you "that is capable of giving love" will be gone, Hardwig thinks we have a duty to die and not bequeath the bodily shell to our families for a decade of incremental dying.

Finally, Hardwig believes that the duty to die builds somewhat on how responsible or irresponsible one has been with one's health and life. If Jim has saved nothing for retirement— has no pension, long-term-care insurance, or any other assets— can Jim rightfully expect his brother or son to transfer all their savings to his doctors for the care that Jim failed to prepare for? No, he cannot.

To conclude, in some ways Hardwig uses "duty" in a rhetorical sense. His real point is closer to the central idea in ancient Greek virtue ethics of a nobility of style, a desire for personal honor and dignity, and an honorable refusal to cling to each scrap of life, as one gradually loses all control and self-possession as life ebbs away in long-term-care facilities and with more and more debilitating operations.

When offered an arranged escape, Socrates chided his friend Crito and asked what quality of life he would have as one banished from Athens and condemned to beg and to wander from port to port. Rejecting such a low quality of life, Socrates nobly chose death at a time and manner of his own choosing, preserving his dignity and contributing to the good of his city-state. In some ways, Professor Hardwig is our new medical Socrates, asking us to at least consider drinking the hemlock as an unselfish alternative to an expensive, lingering death plagued with CPR, chemotherapy, artificial hearts, and ending in the ICU.

9.3 Alzheimer's and Dementia

Dementia is not, as frequently conceptualized, a benign condition of old age characterized by lots of sleep and loss of memory. Although it has these characteristics, as Alzheimer's or Lewy body disease (the second most common form of dementia in elderly patients), it is a terminal disease. Instead of the body's being killed by cancer or a dying heart, in this case, the brain itself is slowly dying.

The average elderly dementia patient takes 8.6 years to die, from first diagnosis to final days.[17] Donepezil (brand name: Aricept) is thought to slow the disease for at least six months, but not cure it; patients on this drug take nine years to die. Aggressive control of diet, blood pressure, and infections may give such patients another three to four years of life.

Family support is also a good predictor of how long patients with dementia will live. Those with attentive family members will live years longer than those with no family at all.

Supporting a dementia patient also requires dental care. For some patients, aggressive dental care is the difference between life and early death. However, such care can be expensive, especially because most dentists don't like to work on dementia patients and heavy sedation can cause such patients to have even greater, immediate, irreversible loss of more memory.

Alzheimer's patients like Virginia Newcomb can expect to live at least 10 years, maybe 20, although the last few will be in a nursing facility for dementia patients that is much more costly than a retirement home for independent seniors. Taking donepezil may slow down progression of mild Alzheimer's for a few years, but after 3 years, it probably has no effect.[18]

After Virginia's two years at Garden Acres Retirement Home, the administrators were fed up with her. Virginia had been wandering the halls of the facility and couldn't then remember which unit was hers. Once, she entered the kitchen at mealtime, sat down, and started making mashed potatoes with the staff. Another time, she locked herself in a walk-in ice box and almost froze to death.

Faced with Virginia's deteriorating situation, Jessica found a Lutheran long-term-care facility, EverBright, that was near her home and specially designed for dementia patients. It cost $6,000 per month. Unfortunately, and despite the fact that Virginia's husband had been a Lutheran minister, EverBright had no vacancies. It should be noted that no medical coverage—Medicare, Medicaid, BlueCross BlueShield— covers living in such a unit. Only if a patient has purchased long-term-care insurance can such bills be paid and, even then, such policies have many loopholes, deductibles, and qualifications.

Luckily for Jessica and Virginia, eventually a spot opened up. Because she can pay for it and because she is Lutheran, Virginia is admitted.

As a survivor on her husband's policy, Virginia gets social security of $1,000 a month. With this income and money from the sale of Virginia's house, Jessica will pay Virginia's bills.

Besides costs of her long-term-care facility, Virginia also must pay for city, state, and federal taxes, Medicare co-payments and deductibles, premiums for medigap private insurance, parts of doctor and hospital bills not covered by Medicare or other insurance, eye and dental care, diapers, shampoos and hair care, and miscellaneous expenses. All in all, her monthly bill expenses come to nearly $8,000.

If Virginia lasts 10 years, she will exhaust her resources and leave nothing to her children and grandchildren. Virginia's children may themselves have to pay for the last 2 years of her care. During these last years, Virginia will not recognize any of her children, know her own name, or be able to understand shows on television.

9.4 Rawls and Callahan on Justice and Natural Limits

As discussed in Chapter 4 about Paul Farmer, the late philosopher John Rawls conceived a theory of justice that favors, if not a duty to die, then at least a shift of medical resources towards helping the young and uninsured. Rawls asks us to imagine the kind of society we would choose in a hypothetical social contract where we know nothing about our personal characteristics (i.e., we choose from [what he calls] the *original position*, where we choose under a *veil of ignorance*, knowing nothing about social position, income, race, and so forth). In such a position, Rawls argues that we would choose two principles: first, maximal, equal liberty for all, and second, inequalities or differences that are just only if they benefit everyone, including the poorest, sickest citizens.

From such a strategy of choice, Rawls thinks we would choose a society that provides a minimal level of medical care for everyone. That is, providing minimal medical care to everyone is required for Rawls as a matter of *justice*.

Each state heavily subsidizes medical students' education in public universities. Physicians in specialties make $250,000 to $300,000 a year, in primary care, around $150,000. Physicians acquire knowledge and rights (e.g., to write prescriptions for drugs) that other citizens lack. All these benefits stem from a medical system that gives physicians unequal rights. Is this system just?

Only if this way of organizing medicine primarily benefits the poorest, sickest people. Does it? Would a system of more primary care physicians benefit more? Or a system where nurses functioned as primary care physicians, treating colds and writing common prescriptions? What about a nationalized system such as Canada's, where every citizen has medical coverage (versus 44 million people who don't in America)? In many ways, and just viewed domestically, American medicine is not just.

If we ask a grander question of justice, "Is American medicine producing the physicians who will cure the ills of the world's sick?" then the answer is "No." Paul Farmer's career is so abnormal that he seems like a saint, not a predictable product of the system.[19]

A follower of Rawls, Tufts professor Norman Daniels, elaborates on what a Rawlsian view of medical care requires. He believes that each of us in the original position would see that each dollar of health care could be spent to guarantee a rough equality of opportunity of health. Rather than spending 75 percent of such dollars on last-ditch efforts when citizens are very old and have aging bodies, redistributing such dollars could keep younger people healthier for longer periods of time.

Under the veil of ignorance, if people imagined how money should be spent over their lives for medical care, Daniels believes they would opt for spending more money earlier to maximize their chances of reaching retirement and not opt to extending the last year of their life at age 90. Daniels agrees that just Rawlsian medical care requires more dollars be shifted to earlier years of life and to uninsured people, rather than spending such dollars on overinsured people at the end of life.

Daniel Callahan and Natural Limits

As Norman Daniels tied his conception of fair allocation of medical resources to the biologically fixed concept of species-normal functioning, in turn bioethicist Daniel Callahan ties his to natural limits in aging. Although Callahan rejects a duty to die, he is sympathetic to the tone of Hardwig's remarks and the idea that it is selfish to squander resources at the end of life, especially when such great inequities exist for the working young.

Callahan's enemy is the myth of medical progress and trying to keep people forever young. For him, the quest for bodily immortality is a quixotic quest.

Callahan thinks American medicine unnaturally extends human life past its natural boundaries with expensive technology: "We will not indefinitely continue to have the ability to pay for an expanding healthcare system, or for those endlessly emerging marvels of technology that promise to extend life."[20] In *What Kind of Life? The Limits of Medical Progress*, he writes, "The very nature of medical progress is to pull to itself many more resources than can be of genuine benefit to many individuals, and much, much more than can be socially justifiable for the common good."[21]

Instead of this false, future-looking conception of medical progress, Callahan likes a medicine that accepts the built-in limits of our bodies, our minds, and our society's capacity to provide cures:

> I have before my mind's eye a future healthcare system that seeks not to constantly conquer all disease and extend all life, but which seeks instead to enhance the quality of life; which seeks not always to overcome the failings and decline of the body, but helps people better accept and cope with them; which tries to keep in view that health is a

means to a decent life, not a value in its own right; which works to help society curb its appetite for ever higher quality and constant improvements in health care. It is a system that aims to intensify inward, seeking not the endless conquests of all frontiers, but only those that promise a more coherent individual life within a more coherent societal life.[22]

In 1990, Callahan wrote that "Whether it is intensive care for the premature newborn, low birth weight baby, bypass surgery for the very old, or AZT therapy for AIDS patients, the eventual outcome will not likely be good; and when those problems are solved, there will be others to take their place."[23] For Callahan, medicine should not focus on the "curative" function here, but its "caring" function (for example, like a hospice, when natural limits are accepted).

Critics reply that it is good that medical research didn't heed his view and didn't accept HIV disease as a "natural limit" for HIV-infected people. Protease inhibitors have now transformed HIV infection to a chronic condition, one that is no longer inexorably terminal.

Yet for Callahan, medicine can do little in the face of disease and death:

Now, if we agree that there is evil in the pain and suffering brought on by biological causes, what kind of evil is it? Even if some of the evil is avoidable, much of it is not and never will be. It is simply part of the way things are. In that case, medicine would do well to understand that its task must be to help people live with that evil, not fool themselves into thinking that it can someday be utterly eliminated.[24]

Despite his denial that elderly patients have any duty to die, Callahan certainly thinks that society is not obligated to fund more and more expensive drugs, devices, and research to help them live longer.

Callahan takes a pessimistic view of what medical research can accomplish. One could argue that the evidence justifies a more optimistic view. One who expressed such a view was octogenarian comedian Art Linkletter, whose interview in a 2002 article in *Parade* magazine credited medical research "with allowing my generation to have another 20 years of good, high-quality life.[25] In the past, it was common for my father and grandfathers to be cut down in their mid-60s with heart attacks, stroke, or cancer, but thanks to modern medicine, these conditions are either prevented or turned into manageable chronic conditions where people can live happy lives."

Surely there is something correct in this view. Part of what has made life better for the elderly is also Medicare, which covers most medical expenses for those over age 65, and Social Security, which is a system of payments for elderly people (starting as early as age 62) and disabled people that is financed by FICA taxes from the paychecks of persons in the active workforce.

> *After Virginia Newcomb had lived in EverBright for six years, a crisis occurred. Even when Jessica decided that aggressive care was not necessary, the long-term-care facility made sure that Virginia had weekly visits from a physician and all her drugs, even those that slowed down the last stages of deterioration of her dementia. They had no choice. As one geriatrics professor said, "The long-term care facility industry in America is more tightly regulated than the nuclear power industry. Their hands are tied."[26]*

> *When Virginia's condition declined to where she could no longer swallow—a sign of imminent death and gross physical deterioration—Jessica signed the form to forgo a feeding tube. However, Jessica's older sister, Jenny, who had hitherto contributed nothing to Virginia's care and who had been absent, suddenly came on the scene and insisted that "I don't want mother to starve to death like Terri Schiavo." Jenny called the facility's top administrator and threatened to sue him if her mother wasn't fed.*

> *Afraid of a suit, EverBright and its physician went ahead and had a surgeon put a feeding tube in Virginia. Now there would be a big deal one day about how and when to remove it.*

Feeding Tubes, Starvation, and End-of-Life Care

It is a common perception that terminal patients suffer by not being fed. This issue came up in the Schiavo case, where critics said it was cruel to remove her feeding tube and let her "starve."

Physicians in palliative care, the branch of medicine charged with making dying comfortable, claim that dying patients rarely suffer when food is withdrawn. Patients near death often voluntarily stop eating on their own.

Dying patients who are fed normally through a feeding tube often show signs of fluid overload, and such forced feeding may even be painful to them. Dry mouths and lips are not the same as hunger and thirst, and may be relieved with ice chips or misters.

Dehydration in dying patients may also ease the dying process, as it results in less swelling of extremities, passing of fluids as waste, lung secretions, and vomiting.[27]

Finally, one little known fact is that competent adults with a terminal illness may control the manner and timing of their death simply by refusing to eat. Since this is not painful, this gives them some measure of control over their last days and reduces technological interventions associated with feeding and hydration.

9.5　Global Reallocation? Dying Simply So Others Can Simply Live

When bioethicist John Hardwig revived Richard Lamm's defense of a duty to die, University of Utah philosopher Margaret Battin similarly defended such a duty, only on very different grounds.

Margaret Battin argues for a duty to die for those in developed countries in order to transfer resources to improve the longevity and quality of life of those in developing countries. As we read in Chapter 5, life expectancy of Botswanans has declined from 61 years in 1993 to 39 years in 2001.[28] Where a newborn Japanese baby can expect to live 81.5 years, a Zambian baby can expect to live only 32.5 years, a difference of nearly half a century.[29] And we know that AIDS and tuberculosis (TB) kill far too many people in developing countries.

In different parameters, people in developed countries have only about 15 percent of the world's population but consume nearly 90 percent of the world's health resources.[30] As Battin says, "People in rich countries live far longer, far healthier lives, and die much, much later than people in poor countries."[31]

But does the fact that a baby in North America can reasonably expect to live to 80 good years of life, while a baby in Zambia will be lucky to live to 30, impose any duties on the North Americans? And specifically, how could it impose on them, at the end of their lives, a duty to die early and not to consume expensive medical resources?

Margaret Battin builds on Hardwig's arguments, while noting the limitations of his position. In particular, Hardwig's duty to die concerns only an obligation arising from the needs of a family. As such, it has no implications for the resources of America, much less the medical needs of people in developing countries.

Although Rawls originally conceived his theory of justice to apply to one country, Professor Battin extends Rawls's theory to covering the globe. So she asks, if we brought all the people of the world together to choose under the veil of ignorance in the original position, what kind of society would we choose? What kind of world?

The answer is that we would not choose a world where rich North Americans consume 90 percent of the world's medical resources, while two-thirds of the people on the planet have their life expectancy halved because of lack of the most basic health care. As a matter of justice, it is wrong that North Americans and Europeans spend so much medical money on themselves while those in developing countries have so little.

In *Living High and Letting Die,* philosopher Peter Unger slams this point home, arguing, "As I write these words in 1995, it's true that in each of the past 30 years, well over 10 million children died from readily preventable causes. And, except for a lack of money aimed at doing the job, most of the deaths could have been prevented by using any one of many means."[32] For example, he argues that each year millions of children die from malnutrition, bad drinking water, and diseases associated with these two causes (e.g., dehydrating diarrhea). A packet of oral rehydration salts from UNICEF, which costs about 15 cents, can save the life of a child.

Unger, like Battin, thinks that people in developed countries live unjust lifestyles in consuming so many resources (medical care, food, gas, and so on) and ignoring hundreds of millions of others who languish for lack of the most minimal resources. Just as we look back and condemn Jefferson and Washington for seeing the evil of slavery but not freeing their own slaves, so Unger thinks people will one day look back on our own time and condemn us for living such lavish lifestyles while so many died in unjust poverty.

In sum, for Battin and Unger we have a weak duty to die in the sense that we should not pursue drugs, technology, and advances in longevity that allow us to eke out a few more marginal years of life. Instead, we should take that money—from our own budgets and from NIH research—and spend it on helping others live longer in developing countries.

Critics object that we did not start with Rawls's original position and then design a global medical system.[33] Because the assumptions of Rawls's system are not met, we cannot draw conclusions about behaviors that deviate from those that Rawls's theory dictates if those conditions were met.

But Rawls never intended his theory to describe what actually happened or what actually could happen in a social contract under a veil of ignorance. Instead, he has given us an *ideal* of world justice, to use to see whether our world is moving toward or away from that state.

The Transfer Problem

We may think of basic medical treatment as a simple thing perhaps because the minimal treatment that people need to live (a bag of rice a month, clean water) can be obtained for such a small percentage of our average income. Moreover, because basic medical care is indisputably necessary for the continued satisfaction of all other needs, it is easy to jump to the conclusion that getting such care is a right that can be demanded against those who have more treatment. On first glance, such a right would seem to justify redistribution of resources.

The big problem here is the assumption that medical treatment is a simple thing. More often than not in the world, it is not. In the many developing countries of the world where starvation is everywhere, medical treatment and food are not just simple needs, but rather amount to *all* needs. For complex reasons, as we shall see, neither food nor medical treatment can be simply transferred from well-off Americans to starving Ethiopians.

The writings of Nobel Prize–winning economist Amaryta Sen emphasize that famine and diseases of malnutrition take place within a locus of legalized power relationships that allow it to occur. As he writes,

> Market forces can be seen as operating through a system of legal relations (ownership rights, contractual obligations, legal exchanges, etc.). The law stands between food availability and food entitlement. Starvation deaths can reflect legality with a vengeance.[34]

What Sen is saying is that in much of the undeveloped world, having power over food and medical treatment is like citizens of developed countries having power over their savings, house, land, and inheritance. Therefore, just as developers or environmentalists can't go into an existing suburb and raze it for their own ends, so well-intentioned philanthropists can't go into a poor country and *change its laws about property to end the power of dominant groups over food and medical care.*

Egalitarians such as Peter Unger think starvation (and the diseases associated with it) are the result of too few people owning too much, so they would take away property from the well-off, either forcibly or through external incentives. But political systems that try to forcibly redistribute property almost always do more harm than good. Attempts failed in Russia, China, Cuba, and Nicaragua to redistribute farmland by force. Such redistribution did not stop subsequent famines in Russia and China, and ultimately these planned, centralized, overcontrolled economies failed because they could not provide food and goods as efficiently as market capitalism. Any great revolution in land rights will be accompanied by chaos, deaths, and instability for decades. Only the most cold-hearted utopians can feel confident that such revolutions ultimately create the greatest good for the greatest number.

Certainly on the national and international levels, one person's forgoing expensive medical care will not translate into any help for someone else: There are too many steps in between, too many legal barriers, too many others claiming the property. Even if a thousand people chose to forgo kidney transplants, saving Social Security millions, Congress would not necessarily allocate that money toward prenatal care or medical care for poor, young people. Other costs may have increased and offset this savings or Congress might redistribute the money to a more pressing need, such as national defense.

Even in the family, forgoing treatment certainly might not translate into more or better medical treatment for younger relatives. Lack of a will and tax planning might mean that the government gets half of the savings. Children might get the money and spend it on nonmedical goods. Adult children might suddenly get the money and now be able to purchase medical insurance, but still be unable to quit smoking and drinking, leading to a similar bad early death. All in all, the assumption that one person's savings from forgoing expensive medical care can be transferred to benefit the health of another needy person is one that needs more justification than it normally receives.

9.6 Mary Warnock vs. Felicia Ackerman on a Duty to Die

Whether one is sympathetic to a duty to die seems partly a matter of culture and economic class. Some poor people insist on maximal expenditure of resources for their family member, especially if they suspect the medical establishment of wanting to save money by limiting care.

At the end of 2004, Dame Mary Warnock, described by the media as "Britain's leading medical ethicist," suggested that elderly patients should consider suicide rather than being a financial burden on their families and on society.[35] Her own husband, Geoffrey, a famous moral philosopher, was a case of physician-assisted dying when a general physician prescribed increasing morphine for him.

Again, the sentiment expressed by Warnock was more affirmation of the virtue of unselfishness than advocacy of a new, real, social duty to die. "I know I'm not allowed to say it," she said at age 80, "but one of the things that would motivate me [to die] is [that] I couldn't bear hanging on and being such a burden on people."

She dreaded entering a long-term care facility: "If I went into a long-term care facility, it would be a terrible waste of money that my family could use far better." In the same interview, she suggested that parents who insist their brain-damaged babies be kept on ventilators be charged for this expense, rather than maintaining such vegetative babies at public expense.

Philosopher Felicia Ackerman argues that Hardwig's position "reflects our society's devaluation of the old and ill, a devaluation that some old people accept uncritically, just as many women used to accept the idea that women should be subordinate to men."[36] She thinks that "Hardwig's conception of what can constitute an unacceptable family burden seems astonishingly weak." She cites two examples: first, where mental disease renders a spouse "distant, uncommunicative, unresponsive, foreign, and unreachable," and second, where money saved for college for children must instead be spent on medical costs, necessitating borrowing for college tuition by children.

So is Hardwig defending selfishness among younger, healthier children? Ackerman thinks so: "we fear too much . . . having our lives and plans disrupted by the medical needs of our loved ones. This fear may cause us to magnify such disruptions out of proportion to the point where having to work and borrow one's way through college or live with a distant and uncommunicative spouse seems so terrible that the sick person's death seems preferable and even obligatory."

9.7 Within the Family: Our Parents' Keepers

Many people might find that there is something deeply wrong with this whole discussion. Isn't it just *obvious* that children should take care of their parents in old age as they die, *no matter what the cost?* After all, if a child is born dying or with a terrible disability, parents are obligated to care for the child, *no matter what the cost.*

The late philosopher Joel Feinberg once wrote, "My benefactor once freely offered me his services when I needed them. . . . But now circumstances have arisen in which he needs help, and I am in a position to help him. Surely I *owe* him my services now, and he would be entitled to resent my failure to come through."[37]

Yes, it is true that some medical expenses at the end of life may be wasteful and unnecessary, and as Jan Narveson has pointed out, the elderly may feel this as intensely as their children.[38] After all, it is *their* lives that are deteriorating and they are the subjects of all the needless, expensive procedures.

But to shift from emphasizing the permission to forgo expensive medical procedures to the obligation, however weak, is a step in the wrong direction. Too easily, we forget about past wrongs to marginalized groups of people and how easy it was to abuse or kill people in such groups. Moreover, medicine in the decades after World War II has been largely untested: We have not lived through a Great Depression or world war in quite some time, and when we do again, scarcity will pressure whatever ethical bulwarks we have erected against sacrificing people who are elderly and mentally ill for the greater good.

Taking Care: Ethical Caregiving in Our Aging Society, the last report of the President's Council on Bioethics under Leon Kass, attacked both the economic "ownership" individualism of Republicans and the social individualism of Democrats.[39] It also attacked adulation of autonomy in bioethics, as symbolized by living wills. Instead, it advocated the primacy of the family and concluded that senior citizens should acknowledge their dependency by signing over a durable power of attorney to a relative. Contrary to Hardwig, Kass and his Council assume that a family will do everything possible to keep a relative alive with Alzheimer's, no matter what the cost to them in money, time, or effort.

Stephen Post hypothesizes in *The Moral Challenge of Alzheimer Disease* that public policy cannot both imply that persons with Alzheimer's disease lack value and also "invest in home care assistance, caregiver respite services, assisted living facilities, improved nursing homes, and hospice services for persons with severe dementia?"[40] More globally, Post argues that "the value of a human being is not diminished by even profound cognitive decline; we must assume equal moral seating and awaken a new beneficence toward those who can no longer remember."[41]

9.8 Dworkin's Defense of Advance Directives and Autonomy

Virginia Newcomb, like most members of her generation—one that Tom Brokaw called "the Greatest Generation"—saved all her life, so much so that her grandchildren thought of her as tight-fisted. One of these grandchildren brings up this trait one day and says, "Grandmother would have been horrified if she knew that so much money was being spent on her. She would have never wanted this."

Assume this is an accurate statement. Assume that Virginia Newcomb had written down general instructions stating that she did not want her money spent this way or to exist this way. Even assuming both things, what weight should we give this advance directive in deciding her care?

Ronald Dworkin, one of America's most distinguished law professors, argues in *Life's Dominion* that such advance directives should be honored, even if the person who wrote it has vanished and a new, diminished person wants to live.[42] Dworkin admits that the new, different person, perhaps a shell of the former, robust self, presently has an acceptable quality of life and wants to live. It's just that the quality of life of the new slimmed-down Virginia Newcomb would horrify the former, real Virginia Newcomb.

Dworkin puts this point this way:

> But what about a patient's *precedent autonomy?* Suppose a patient is incompetent in the general, overall sense but that years ago, when perfectly competent, he executed a living will providing for what he plainly does not want now. Suppose, for example, that years ago, when fully competent, Margo had executed a formal document directing that if she should develop Alzheimer Disease, all her property should be given to a designated charity so that none of it could be spent on her own care. Or that in that event she should not receive treatment for any other serious, life-threatening disease she might contract. Or even that in that event she should be killed as soon and as painlessly as possible? If Margo had expressed any of those wishes when she was competent, would autonomy then require that they be respected now by those in charge of her care, even though she seems perfectly happy with her dog-eared mysteries, the single painting she repaints, and her peanut-butter-and-jelly sandwiches?[43]

Dworkin distinguishes between a person's present, *experiential interests* and her overall, higher *critical interests.* The latter constitutes our full, rich selves, which ground our conception of ourselves as autonomous persons and the satisfaction of which decides whether our life has been successful or not. Someone who considers her true self to be as a painter and mother might be experientially happy in the later stages of Alzheimer's but, because she was unable to paint or recognize her daughter, consider her real self dead.

What are we to make of Dworkin's argument? For one thing, it recognizes the phenomenon in rehabilitation medicine known as the *adaptation effect,* where a person who is suddenly a quadriplegic announces that he'd rather die than continue to live this way but then, six months later, has adapted and come to find his quality of life acceptable.

Dworkin argues that when disease has weakened our bodies and minds so much that we are merely shallow versions of our former, full selves, judges and physicians should honor the principle of patient autonomy and respect our advanced directive, not putting us on a respirator or, in Virginia Newcomb's case, not spending so much money on her care when her mind has gone.

Indeed, Dworkin argues that we *disvalue* the former person and her life by continuing to spend money on her in ways she forbade. Such treatment "compromises the life as a whole" and violates its dignity. "Value cannot be poured into a life from outside; it must be generated by the person whose life it is, and this is no longer possible for him."[44] To treat a person in contradiction to her advanced directive is like ignoring her will and giving her money not to her children but to a charity.

Dworkin's argument becomes most powerful: In the last stages of Alzheimer's, when nothing remains, even a being with some experiential pleasures. "In many respects, the demented person is in the same position as an unconscious, permanently vegetative patient."

He also writes,

A doctor is no more justified in contradicting a competent adult's judgment about dementia than in contradicting his judgment about permanent unconsciousness.[45]

In other words, how can judges honor a competent person's advance directive not to be maintained in PVS but ignore a similar directive not to be maintained in Alzheimer's?

We should honor the formerly competent person's advance directive, Dworkin concludes, for three reasons: to respect her precedent autonomy, because it is compassionate, and because it respects her dignity. "We cannot say that we would be showing compassion for Margo if we refused to do what she wanted when she was competent, because that would not be compassionate toward the whole person, the person who tragically became demented."[46] Moreover, "Why is indignity a special kind of harm, whether self-inflicted or inflicted by others, and why does it seem worse when the indignity is not recognized by its victim?"[47]

Dworkin argues that the answer is that treating us later, when we are demented, in ways we forbade, violates our critical interests, and it is these critical interests that give us "intrinsic value—the sanctity or inviolability—of our own lives."[48] Dworkin surprisingly then argues that continuing to maximally treat a vegetative, demented patient against her advance directives *violates society's value of the dignity and sanctity of life.* This is a remarkable conclusion because all other advocates of the sanctity of life come to exactly the opposite conclusion, namely, that life must be maintained no matter what its quality and no matter what the former person's advance directive dictated.

In making this argument, Dworkin has fleshed out the value of autonomy for medicine at the end of life. A tendency exists, both in medicine and in society, to let autonomy slide as cognitive abilities slide at the end of life. But the previously robust, autonomous person may have anticipated this slide and made plans accordingly. If such plans have been made, then Dworkin says we disvalue our core ethics if we ignore those plans.

One problem with Dworkin's argument stems from the fact that even competent people incorrectly predict their future wishes. The famous SUPPORT study (Study to Understand Prognoses and Preferences for Outcomes and Risks of Treatments) on advance directives and end-of-life care discovered that people do not accurately predict what they will later find acceptable or unacceptable as quality of life.[49] For example, people who predicted that they would rather die than go on a ventilator most often did *not* choose to die but instead went on a ventilator. It's one thing to say abstractly that one would "rather be dead than live like that," but when actually faced with death, most people decide to live, even with bad quality of life.

Given the fallibility of predictions of competent people about their actual wishes at the end of their lives, if we have a person with Alzheimer's whose life seems to have some pleasure and not too much pain, then letting her die cannot be justified solely by appealing to her former wishes. Chances are too high that she incorrectly forecast her future preferences.

Where Dworkin's argument is persuasive is when she has become vegetative and nothing at all remains, no sentient being of any kind. In such a situation, an explicit advance directive covering such a situation should be honored. Although it is illegal in all states to kill such a human by not feeding her, because of Dworkin's argument and because the person has left, it can be ethical to do so.

9.9 Medical Professionals and Medical Futility

So far we have analyzed a duty to die through the eyes of the patient affected, the family, the country, and peoples in developing countries, but what about the medical team that must actually treat the elderly person? What about the effects of all this on them?

Certainly some physicians in primary care must feel a great sense of injustice in their daily lives. In one morning, they may see a 55-year-old overweight man who has irregular heartbeats, diabetes, and high blood pressure, and who, without medical coverage, cannot pay for a pacemaker, insulin, or the medicine to control his blood pressure that costs $100 a month. The next patient, brought in using a walker by her 70-year-old-daughter, is an 89-year-old woman who fell and broke her hip. Already this woman has had a quadruple heart bypass, a previous hip replacement, and gallstone surgery. She is now considering a second hip replacement, at a cost of several thousand dollars and, because of her age and ill health, probably a week in intensive care for several thousand dollars more. During this surgery, she could easily spiral downward, necessitating a series of expensive, last-resort treatments to keep her alive. She could even end up in a coma and on a feeding tube.

After being put on a feeding tube, Virginia Newcomb defied expectations that she would only live another 11 months. Because of Jenny's insistence, she was aggressively treated for two bouts of pneumonia and a fall that left her with a broken ankle. She died five years later at age 93.

For the first few years, Virginia could at times recognize Jessica when she came to visit. (Jenny never visited her mother or came to EverBright again.) "When you come around, she perks up," the nurses told Jessica (making her feel guilty for not visiting every day). "Otherwise, she just sleeps all the time."

At Virginia's funeral, Jessica and Jenny were not speaking to each other.

CONCLUSIONS

Asserting that the old and infirm have a duty to die is one of the most controversial claims in bioethics. The two basic ways that a duty is justified is as beneficence to one's family and as a saintly unselfishness toward the world's resources. If done in the name of poor people in developing countries or younger people in North America, a duty to die rests on shaky ground because of the transfer problem. On the other hand, if asserted in a weak sense, a duty to die certainly resonates in some families. Some high-minded elderly people, who have lived good lives, may take it seriously.

FURTHER READINGS

Battin, Margaret Pabst. *The Least Worst Death: Essays in Bioethics on the End of Life*. New York: Oxford University Press, 1994.

Callahan, Daniel. *What Kind of Life? The Limits of Medical Progress*. New York: Simon and Shuster, 1990.

Chatterjee, Deen. *The Ethics of Assistance: Morality and the Distant Needy*. New York: Cambridge University Press, 2004.

Clements, Jonathan. "The Flawed, Expensive Insurance Policy That You Really Ought to Consider." *Wall Street Journal*, October 13, 2003.

Daniels, Norman. *Am I My Parents' Keeper? An Essay on Justice Between the Young and the Old*. New York: Oxford University Press, 1988.

English, Jane. "What Do Grown Children Owe Their Parents?" In *Having Children*, ed. Onora O'Neill. New York: Oxford University Press, 1979.

Fagerlin, Angela, and Carl E. Schneider. "Enough: The Failure of the Living Will." *Hastings Center Report* (March–April 2004), pp. 30–38.

Gunderson, Martin. "Being a Burden: Reflections on Refusing Medical Care." *Hastings Center Report* 34, no. 5 (September–October 2004).

Hardwig, John. *Is There a Duty to Die and Other Essays in Medical Ethics*. New York: Routledge, 2000.

Humber, James, and Robert Almeder. *Is There a Duty to Die?* Totawa, NJ: Humana Press, 2000.

Lamm, Richard D. "St. Martin of Tours in a New World of Medical Ethics." *Cambridge Quarterly of Healthcare Ethics* 3 (1994), pp. 159–67 (reprinted in Gregory Pence, *Classic Works in Medical Ethics*, McGraw-Hill, 2000).

Post, Stephen. *The Moral Challenge of Alzheimer Disease: Ethical Issues from Diagnosis to Dying*, 2nd ed. Baltimore: Johns Hopkins University Press, 2000.

President's Council on Bioethics. *Taking Care: Ethical Caregiving in Our Aging Society*, September 2005, www.bioethics.gov

Stone, Deborah. "Shopping for Long-Term Care." *Health Affairs* 23, no. 4 (July–August 2004), pp. 191–96.

CHAPTER 10

*T*reating Jehovah's Witnesses Professionally

This chapter explores issues about how medicine deals with members of minority religions who refuse ordinary medical treatment in life-threatening situations. It focuses on the views of Jehovah's Witnesses. Other similar religious minorities in North America include Seventh-day Adventists, Christian Scientists, and Latter Day Saints.[1]

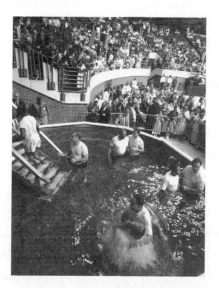

At 2 AM on a Saturday, a distraught couple in their 50s, Samuel and Mary Hepnah, come to the emergency room at St. Claire's Hospital with their 17-year-old daughter, Sara. They are Jehovah's Witnesses.

*Out of nowhere, Sara has had blurred vision and
difficulty saying words. Consulting neurosurgeon Heath
Throckmorton admits her to the hospital.*

*The family carries BlueCross BlueShield medical insur-
ance. Financing any possible medical treatment is not a
problem for them.*

*An MRI the next morning reveals a meningioma, a
nonmalignant brain tumor. Pressure inside the skull from
the growing tumor makes it life-threatening, thus it must be
immediately removed.*

*Dr. Throckmorton may need to give Sara blood during
the surgery, but encouraged by her parents, Sara refuses
the surgery. Dr. Throckmorton shows the family Sara's
MRI and exclaims, "She will have more and more
seizures. When the next one comes, she could be driving.
The next time she could hemorrhage. She could die on
the spot."*

*Dr. Throckmorton belongs to a local Church of Christ.
The Hepnahs' refusal angers him. He has thought a lot about
cults and Christianity. Nothing angers him more than false
religion posing as true Christianity, much less cults that force
their believers to die needlessly.*

*"If you follow your cult's beliefs, your daughter will die,"
Throckmorton testily informs Samuel. "If you want to be
treated in this hospital, you'd better let us give her blood.
It's our way or the highway."*

*Upon hearing this, Samuel and Mary Hepnah become
agitated and call their local Witness coordinator, who tells
them he is on his way. Despite her refusal to permit surgery,
Dr. Throckmorton lets Sara stay another night in the hospital
"for observation." He secretly hopes she will consent to surgery
after she thinks it over.*

10.1 Jehovah's Witnesses and Medicine

Charles Taze Russell founded Jehovah's Witnesses in 1870 when
he rejected his Presbyterian roots and started a Bible Study
group. A decade later, he started the Watchtower Bible & Tract
Society, a nonprofit Christian corporation that publishes magazines and tracts to promote its ideas.

Russell prophesied that the Second Coming of Jesus would occur in 1914. When that did not happen, the Watchtower Society fell on hard times until it was rejuvenated in 1931 by new president Joseph Rutherford, who called its members "Witnesses" (after Isaiah 43:10, "Ye are my witnesses, saith Jehovah").[2]

Jehovah's Witnesses meet in Kingdom Halls. Its members must spend time each week spreading the word of Jehovah's kingdom; in this activity, they resemble Latter Day Saints, who as young adults spend two years as missionaries. Such proselytizing caused Jehovah's Witnesses to soar from a few members in 1870 to 6 million in 2002.

Headquartered in a tall building overshadowing the Brooklyn Bridge, the Watchtower Society prints 15 million copies of its magazines each week. From this Brooklyn skyscraper, it sends out its message in 120 languages to 230 countries.

Nathan Knorr became president of the Watchtower Society in 1942. Like some Orthodox Jews and Southern Baptists, Jehovah's Witnesses view scriptures as inerrant and literally true. As such, they believe in the Second Coming, where God's Chosen will rule on Earth; their writings emphasize the imminent Apocalypse and Final Judgment. However, they reject the Incarnation, the doctrine that Jesus is literally God-in-the-flesh, holding instead that Jesus was God's son and first creation.[3]

They do not pledge allegiance to nations of this Earth, nor do they sing national anthems. They do not smoke, drink alcohol, or use illegal drugs. Their doctrines forbid abortion and mercy killing.

Because of the imminent end of the world, Witnesses believe that most Christians focus too much on the affairs of this world and not enough on gaining admission to the next. Witnesses emulate early Christians in emphasizing that there is only one real value in life—gaining personal salvation.[4] Because all nation states are temporary and because all human progress is illusory, they believe nothing in this world really matters except gaining eternal life for themselves and their families. Because no wars are worth fighting, Witnesses are pacifists.

Nathan Knorr also gave Witnesses their most characteristic medical belief: Giving or receiving blood transfusions is forbidden.[5] Witnesses base their beliefs on the Bible, and specifically on these passages:

> Every moving animal that liveth shall be meat for you; even as the green herb have I given you things. But flesh with the life thereof, which is the blood thereof, shall ye not eat. (Genesis 9:3–4)

> And whatsoever man there be of the house of Israel, or of the strangers that sojourn among you, that eateth any manner of blood; I will set my face against that soul that eateth blood, and will cut him off from among his people. (Leviticus 17:10)

> But that we write unto them, that they abstain from pollutions of idols, and from fornication, and from things strangled, and from blood. (Acts 15:28)[6]

Jehovah's Witnesses believe the above passages and others in the Bible forbid the transferring of blood from one person to another. They see blood transfusions as "feeding" the body, just like nourishment. Because the Bible expressly forbids such eating of blood, they see blood transfusions as explicitly forbidden. Jehovah's Witnesses who violate this commandment are damned and expelled from Kingdom Halls.

Provided that technicians completely drain organs and tissues of blood before transplantation, Witnesses allow donating or receiving organs. Although organ donation is discouraged, it is left up to individuals.

Witness theology forbids Witnesses from accepting whole blood and some of its components, namely, red cells, white cells, platelets, and plasma. However, it allows some components to be received (e.g., hemoglobin).

Witness theology makes an analogy with a truck: if a vehicle has been dismantled in a salvage yard, the original truck differs from the dismantled battery, tires, scrap metal, and bumpers. Statements true of the whole do not necessarily apply to the parts. In sum, Witnesses can receive some parts of blood, just not the whole.

Witness theology also permits acceptance of artificial blood, but forbids donation to the blood supply. Witnesses are also not allowed to store their own blood for future surgery because this constitutes blood being out of the body (in contrast, blood in the closed system of hemodialysis is considered inside the body).

10.2 Professionalism, Religious Minorities, and Tolerance

The Massachusetts Citizens for Children is an organization dedicated to preventing the suffering of children in religious groups. It lists at least 20 groups in the United States that practice denial of medical care to children, including:

> Faith Assembly Christian Science, The Believers Fellowship, Faith Tabernacle, Church of the First Born, Church of God of the Union Assembly, Church of God Chapel, Faith Temple Doctoral Church of Christ in God, Jesus through John and Judy, Christ Miracle Healing Center, NE Kingdom Community Church, Christ Assembly, The Source, True Followers of Christ, "No Name" Fellowship, End Time Ministries, Faith Cathedral Fellowship, Living Word Assembly of God, and Traveling Ministries Everyday Church.[7]

From outside, the views of the above groups and Jehovah's Witnesses seem to be those of cults. But what is a *cult?* In essence, a cult is a nontraditional religion that mainstream religions regard as crazy, deviant, founded on falsehood, or one that harms its members. Ordinary people see members of cults as either irrational religious fanatics or as people who have been brainwashed.

If one views it from far enough away, almost any religion can be seen by someone as a cult. Hindus may ask if Christians really believe in Transubstantiation during Communion (i.e., do Christians really believe that during this ceremony, the wine becomes the blood of Jesus Christ and the wafer, Christ's body)? If so, Hindus ask, when Christians eat and drink such substances, are they cannibals?

How strange a religion seems from afar depends on what part of that religion critics emphasize. If they focus on Shi'ite fundamentalism, Islam seems like a rigid, sexist, fatalistic religion. But if one looks at Indonesia, a country with the world's largest Muslim population and one rich in banking and international trade, one sees a sophisticated, flexible Sunni Islam that hardly resembles Shi'ia Islam. In the same way, the Christianity of urban Episcopalians in Oxford, England, hardly resembles the Christianity of Appalachian snake handlers.

Thus, it is important to de-cult Jehovah's Witnesses and try to understand why they refuse blood and blood products. Consider an analogous stand for a Christian: What if Dr. Throckmorton, as a condition of surgery, made Christian patients renounce Christ?[8] Renouncing Jesus would certainly create a problem for Christians in gaining salvation ("Jesus saith unto him, 'I am the way, the truth, and the life: no man cometh unto the Father, but by me.'" John 14:6).[9] In any case, if a patient did so and then died during surgery, would he enter Heaven? As the price of getting surgery, even life-saving surgery, surely no Christian would give up salvation ("For what is a man profited, if he shall gain the whole world, and lose his own soul?" Matthew 16:26). So why should Dr. Throckmorton ask Jehovah's Witnesses to do the same?

Remember that Witnesses believe that Jesus will return soon, that Armageddon is coming, and that the teachings of Jesus must be respected about how to be "born again." In the oldest Gospel, Mark, the Pharisees repeatedly ask Jesus for practical guidelines to pressing moral problems of their day, but Jesus refuses to give answers. Despite the fact that a third of the world existed under that most evil institution, slavery, and that most people suffered under that other evil, dictatorship, Jesus makes no comment against either, other than to advocate resignation and nonresistance.

The Pharisees wanted a better code of moral principles to govern relations with others and criticized Jesus for failing to give them one. For Witnesses, an honest reading of Mark reveals that the message of Jesus contradicts giving such principles or, indeed, discussing *any* bioethical, political, or social problem of his day. For the dominant message of Jesus there is that the Kingdom of God is at hand, that only those who repent and ask forgiveness of God for sin can gain everlasting life, and that such salvation is not gained by doing good works or by following moral principles but by establishing a personal, one-on-one relationship with God, the Father.

Given this theme, no wonder Jesus did not denounce slavery or dictatorship. Given the coming End of Days, why bother? Soon everything will be ashes and only the Elect will sit with Jesus in Heaven.

Of course, most Christian churches today reject this controversial interpretation. Over 1,600 years, organized Christianity has interpreted these teachings and reinterpreted them again.[10] Be that as it may, our concern here is not with biblical interpretation or the history of Christianity. Instead, we seek to understand Witnesses and their views.

In doing so, a new perspective may emerge. If one believes that the world is ending soon, that our only task on Earth is to enter into a personal relationship with God and be saved, that the manual for doing so is revealed teachings in Scripture, and if one believes that having a blood transfusion condemns one to Hell, shouldn't one reject blood transfusions?

But what about Jehovah's Witnesses from the point of view of medical professionals? Forgoing treatment by Jehovah's Witnesses sparks controversy in medicine because most physicians do not believe that Witnesses have the correct theology. Moreover, these physicians correctly believe that some Jehovah's Witnesses do not wish to die by refusing blood products, but are forced to do so by their theology.

As such, physicians differ about what constitutes *professional* behavior in treating such patients. Some physicians immediately honor the wishes of such patients and refer them to a more accommodating physician. (Such "honoring" is seen by some physicians as getting rid of problematic patients.) Other physicians try to work with these patients, seeking compromises that will allow them to maximize their chances of living.

Almost everyone would agree that Dr. Throckmorton's behavior is *unprofessional.* Why is that? First, his actions seem more about his own ego and beliefs than about the care of his patient. Second, by presenting his ultimatum, Dr. Throckmorton has backed his patients into a corner; he has challenged the Hepnahs to act on their foundational religious beliefs, beliefs that place a high value on heroic sacrifice in medical situations. (The literature of Jehovah's Witnesses recounts examples of other people being converted after seeing a Witness die for her beliefs, just as seeing the deaths of early Christian martyrs caused non-Christians to convert.)

If we ask, "Did Throckmorton's actions contribute to the problem or to its solution?" the answer is the former. He not only contributed to the problem, he also *caused* an adversarial relationship between the patient, her family, and him.

> *Dr. Alvin Kleinberg, another neurosurgeon who has had 40 years of experience with all kinds of cases, gets Sara Hepnah to confess that she fears death and that if her parents weren't so adamant against it, she might allow the surgery. Sara also reveals that, if she does have the surgery, she fears the wrath of her parents and fears that if she dies during surgery, she will go directly to Hell.*
>
> *Dr. Kleinberg spends many hours with the Hepnahs. He does not call them members of a cult. He indicates, by his actions, tone, and concern, that he respects their beliefs and respects their decision to let their daughter risk death for these beliefs. After several days, the Hepnahs feel good about their relationship with Dr. Kleinberg.*

10.3 Parental Owners vs. Parental Stewards of Children

Our views of what parents owe their children stem from two contrasting sources of parental authority. University of Hawaii bioethicist Kenneth Kipnis contrasts parental *dominion* over children with parental *custody*.[11] Dominion of children stems from a model of family law that sees children as *property* of their parents. To do surgery on children without the consent of parents violates rights not only of the child but also dominion rights of parents over their children.

According to Kipnis, in 1874 a different view began which saw parents merely as temporary stewards of children, not as owners. Custody implies that the governing relationship of parents over children is like marriage: legalized, regulated, and revocable by the state. On the ownership model, the state has virtually no legitimate justification for interfering with parental decisions over children, but on the custodial model, the state can intervene in cases of abuse and neglect.

Kipnis thinks these conflicts about parental roles enter medicine when cases arise concerning male and female circumcision, surgical assignment of sex, and "flogging" dying children with experimental treatments because parents can't bear to see them die. In such cases, physicians may be acting as custodians of the child's best interests while parents are asserting ownership.

10.4 Virtue Ethics, Treatment Refusal, and Religious Minorities

Although some people may mock Jehovah's Witnesses for risk ing death, they should not be too quick to scorn such actions. As mentioned in previous chapters, autonomy is one of the values that has been most emphasized in bioethics over the last half century. It represents the idea that the patient, not the physician, best knows how to rank benefits and burdens in a worldview. Especially when it comes to views of God and what it's worth dying for, personal autonomy becomes crucial in ethics and politics.

To think of this issue from a different perspective, many physicians lament that patients do not take more responsibility for decisions about their health. Recall here the alcoholics discussed in Chapter 2 whom the disease model saw as passive victims of a disease. The Hepnahs are taking *all* the responsibility for their decision, even fighting physicians over it. In a strong sense, in refusing normal medical treatment, the Hepnahs are taking control over their lives.

From the perspective of virtue ethics, who can dispute the courage shown by a Jehovah's Witness who is willing to risk death for her beliefs? Jehovah's Witnesses in developing countries frequently get punished for their beliefs, as in the case of a Witness child in Zambia who was expelled from public school for refusing to sing the national anthem or salute the national flag.[12]

Some other religious people, faced with such a choice, might elect to change their beliefs. Jehovah's Witnesses show real courage in refusing to take blood and in following other unpopular teachings.

To return to the role of Dr. Throckmorton in our case in producing problems, consider his complete contempt for the heroism of this family. He certainly exhibits neither understanding nor compassion for a Christian Witness about to undergo martyrdom. Surely he would not condemn the deaths of the early Christian martyrs.

Let us consider another issue. An old debate in virtue ethics concerns whether one can be courageous in the wrong cause. Is the thief courageous in his dangerous feats, or merely daring and cunning? Were Nazi soldiers courageous in fighting, just like Allied soldiers, even though they fought for Hitler?

In the same way, one can ask whether Jehovah's Witnesses show bravery in risking their lives for their beliefs about personal salvation. Socrates believed that one can only be courageous in a just cause.[13] If so, then for those of different faiths, Jehovah's Witnesses who sacrifice their lives for their beliefs are not brave and, if their theology is false, fools.

But how far can this logic be taken? Such thinking implies that if Hinduism is true and not Christianity, then Christian martyrs are fools. Or if there is no God or Heaven, and atheists are correct, are all people who die for their religious beliefs fools?

Better to hold that one can be courageous for many different ends. On this view, Nazi soldiers can be as brave as their Allied counterparts. Anyone risking death for their religious beliefs is brave. On this view, fundamentalist in southern Utah, Seventh-day Adventists, Christian Scientists, and Jehovah's Witnesses can be brave in refusing medical care.

10.5 Legal Issues

According to the 1990 *Cruzan* decision by the U.S. Supreme Court, a competent adult has the right to refuse life-saving medical procedures. American courts have also recognized the right of adult Jehovah's Witnesses to refuse blood transfusions, even when such transfusions might save their lives.

In a landmark 1944 decision, the U.S. Supreme Court in *Prince* v. *Commonwealth of Massachusetts* declared that although adult Jehovah's Witnesses have the right to sacrifice their lives for religious reasons, they do *not* have the legal right *to sacrifice the lives of their children.*[14]

> The right to practice religion freely does not include the liberty to expose the community or the child to communicable disease or the latter to ill health or death. . . . Parents may be free to become martyrs themselves. But it does not follow they are free, in identical circumstances, to make

martyrs of their children before they have reached the full
and legal discretion when they can make that choice for
themselves.

Subsequent legal decisions affirmed and reinforced this
precedent-setting decision, which has held for over 60 years.

10.6 Medicine and the Good of the Child/Adolescent

In cases such as this one, adolescents in medicine—in other
words, those between ages 13 and 18—pose unique problems.
Neither children nor full-adults, they often have adult-sized
problems concerning sexuality, consent, and drugs.

As Kipnis notes, pre-20th-century law conceptualized
children—including adolescents—merely as property of their
parents. The 20th century saw progress in moving toward
the custodial model, and thus more protection for interests of
adolescents.

According to law professor Angela Holder, an authority
in pediatric-adolescent law, the 1960s posed a unique crisis
because "adolescents were contributing to an epidemic of
venereal disease in this country."[15] Because adolescents feared
physicians would inform on them to their parents, they
avoided medical clinics and treatment for venereal diseases,
and so:

> By the end of the 1960s, all states had enacted statutes
> permitting treatment of minors for venereal diseases with-
> out parental consent. . . . and many states enacted statutes
> providing that minors might consent generally to medical
> or surgical care.[16]

Courts gradually accepted the view that older adolescents
can understand as much as adults and consent like adults. This
is known in pediatrics as the *mature minor rule*. Its application
balances the severity of the problem, public health considerations, and adolescent autonomy. For example, without the
required consent of their parents, adolescents may get contraception at Planned Parenthood, drug or alcohol treatment, or
free medical care in public clinics. The more severe the action,
the more physicians want to involve parents or courts. An
adolescent would not be allowed to refuse treatment for skin

cancer without contacting his or her parents. Similarly, if an adolescent seeks an abortion, states may pass laws requiring notification or consent of a parent before the abortion is performed, and indeed most states have passed such laws.

In reality, because most adolescents get medical insurance under their parents' policies, parents must be involved for physicians to get reimbursed. Exceptions involve publicly funded services that explicitly target adolescents, for example, treatment for HIV infection under a veil of complete confidentiality.

Emancipated minors may make decisions without notification of their parents. These are defined legally as adolescents who marry, join the armed services, run away, or are financially independent of their parents. Also, "In almost all states unmarried minor mothers, as young as eleven or twelve, are emancipated even if they are living with their parents."[17]

Society vacillates in how it sees such adolescents: it allows them to serve in the Armed Forces but won't allow them to buy alcohol. In some states, they can have an abortion at age 14 but cannot vote.

American courts ruled in 1990 in *In the Interests of E. G.* that a Jehovah's Witness adolescent could refuse the life-saving blood transfusions needed to cure her leukemia.

> The trial judge decided that [she] understood her situation, understood that she would die without treatment, and that her refusal was based on her religious convictions and not on parental coercion or fear of abuse if she consented. . . . The decision was upheld on appeal.[18]

A Canadian court of appeals ruled that a 15-year-old Jehovah's Witness could refuse a transfusion in a similar case because he was competent as a mature minor and could understand the consequences.[19]

But later American courts mostly ruled that adolescents may *not* refuse life-saving medical care. They ruled that a 16-year-old Witness, after being severely injured by the impact of a train, could not refuse a blood transfusion and appointed a guardian for him, who allowed transfusions.[20]

Adolescent autonomy figures prominently in this chapter's case because Sara desires surgery, even with blood, whereas her parents oppose it. In this sense, Sara is in limbo, neither child nor adult, torn between her own desires and those of her faith and parents. And courts have made contradictory decisions in cases of adolescents with life-or-death issues.

From the point of view of Kantian ethics, it would seem that the good of the child requires the surgery, even if it involves a blood transfusion. In the same way, a virtuous parent or a compassionate one would do what is medically best for the child and agree to surgery. In secular culture, or modern Christian culture, there is no doubt that the surgery is for the good of the child. To keep her alive, we must operate and give her blood to save her life.

However, such interpretations assume a certain metaphysics or eschatology (views of the end of the world). If you accept the premises of Jehovah's Witnesses, then the good of the child is foremost to obtain salvation, so virtuous parents would want their child saved, not condemned to eternal hell.

Like interpretations of the Golden Rule, even deciding what is best for the child is not transparent. Only when we agree on a worldview can we judge unequivocally what is best for Sara Hepnah.

10.7 Bloodless Surgery and Jehovah's Witnesses

Because of requests of Jehovah's Witnesses, bloodless surgery has skyrocketed in North America and some surgery centers advertise that they can do all minor surgery without blood transfusions. Because Jehovah's Witnesses value choice of physicians and medical centers, they often enroll in plans for medical insurance, such as BlueCross BlueShield, that give them maximal choices. In that way, they can refer themselves and their members to hospitals and physicians who minimize the use of blood during surgery or promise not to transfer any blood at all.

With 6 million members worldwide, Jehovah's Witnesses command attention in medical centers as new sources of revenue. They allow centers with poor profits to reposition themselves as specialty surgery centers. This ever-growing population has prompted programs such as the Center for Bloodless Medicine and Surgery at the Hackensack University Medical Center in New Jersey and the Bloodless Medicine and Surgery Program at DCH Regional Medical Center in Tuscaloosa, Alabama. Prior to surgery, patients receive hematopoietic agents (iron supplements and other medication) to produce red blood cells. Microsampling is used for laboratory tests, which uses fewer samples and less blood.

During the operation, surgeons use different methods to conserve blood. One of these methods is hemodilution, which dilutes patients' circulatory systems to minimize blood loss. They use volume expanders (nonblood fluids) to enhance circulation. Surgeons use blood salvaging to recover spilled blood in the chest or abdominal cavity. To stop bleeding, a machine filters blood and returns it to the patient. Surgeons use surgical lasers, electrocautery, and argon beam coagulators. Through tiny holes in the skin, interventional radiologists close off bleeding vessels. Through refining these techniques, surgeons develop safer surgeries for all patients.

Harking to the adage in bioethics, "Follow the money trail," we see that the rise of bloodless surgery has toned down the indignation in medicine against Jehovah's Witnesses. Now that some physicians make good money with Witness patients, other physicians in other centers have taken notice and have begun to learn bloodless techniques.

Nevertheless, almost all surgeons consider it unprofessional to promise a Jehovah's Witness that blood will never be used during surgery or to swear that bloodless surgery is safe and fine. In unforeseen cases of anatomical anomalies discovered only after surgery begins, or with idiosyncratic reactions to anesthesia, or combinations of drugs, blood transfusions will be necessary to stabilize the patient. Witnesses should understand that their chances of dying during bloodless surgery exceed those of normal patients (assuming the surgeon honors their prior wishes and does not give them blood during a surgical emergency).

After many days, including a day of discussion with a local Jehovah's Witness counselor, the Hepnahs decide to let a local judge order their daughter to be allowed to get blood during surgery. They specified that they wanted Dr. Kleinberg to do the surgery, not Dr. Throckmorton.

Sara donated two units of blood to be used in case she needed the blood during surgery. The surgery was scheduled

*for the next week and proceeded uneventfully. No blood
transfusion was needed and the operation was successful.
Sara expects to live many more years.*

10.8 Consistency in Handling Cases of Minority Views in Medicine

Some people see immigrant, ethnic, religious minorities differently than domestic, religious minorities. The same people
who would agree that American Jehovah's Witness adolescents
should not be allowed to die for their beliefs might be quite
willing to let a Hmong adolescent girl refuse surgery for her
beliefs. In the latter case, they might argue, a thousand-year-old
cultural history supports a worldview that illness is caused by
"loss of the soul" or possession of the soul by evil *dab* (spirit).[21]
The fashion among some physicians is to cut more latitude for
such immigrant minorities than domestic ones.

But is the asymmetry justified? Jehovah's Witnesses have
just as much a worldview as the Hmong and both are certainly
tied to a different metaphysics than the biophysical model of
Western medicine. Indeed, there seems to be no reason for
treating religious minorities who recently arrived from a foreign country differently than our indigenous religious minorities. Both may endanger their children with strange beliefs, and
whatever standards apply to one should apply to the other.

When either group comes to American hospitals, the frustration of American physicians such as Dr. Throckmorton is
understandable. It's like such minorities both do, and do not,
want physicians to treat them by American standards.

Legal Update

Because courts have consistently refused to let adult Jehovah's
Witnesses make martyrs of their children, the leadership of
Jehovah's Witnesses has realized that it cannot win this particular legal battle. Thus, they have adopted the compromise seen
in this case where parents themselves do not consent to surgery
for their children and thus do not themselves risk eternal
damnation.

In this compromise, Witness coordinators often know a
specific local judge who will work with them and respect their

beliefs. As in this case, they often specify which surgeon will operate. They may also specify a center that minimizes use of blood. They usually add a stipulation revoking their consent after the surgery or after a period of time.

Thus, practices of contemporary Jehovah's Witnesses distinguishes between a *willingness to allow* blood transfusions in children and a *willingness to consent* to such transfusions. So long as the parent or parents do not *themselves* consent verbally or consent in writing to the transfusion of blood for their child, they are not damned and are not accomplices in any possible damnation of their child. The thinking here may involve the acting–omitting distinction, where by not consenting, the parents are not acting and are merely omitting active resistance to the transfusion. The status of the adolescent in the afterlife is unclear.

CONCLUSIONS

The case in this chapter would unambiguously be characterized as "a medical ethics case" inside hospitals and would automatically be sent to a hospital ethics committee. It is also a case that legally has an open-and-shut answer within modern medicine because courts have held for 60 years that parents "cannot make martyrs of their children."

On the other hand, much of the extant literature in medicine about Jehovah's Witnesses demonizes them, making them into a cult with unfathomable beliefs. In contrast, if we adopt a sympathetic view of their beliefs—one which does not mock their acceptance of a worldview—then risking death by forgoing surgery emerges in a new light, one to be described not in terms of superstition but in terms of courage.

All of which is to say that, both in this chapter and in all the cases in this book, good answers in bioethics are usually more complicated than they seem at first.

FURTHER READINGS

Davis, Dena S. "Does 'No' Mean 'Yes'?: The Continuing Problem of Jehovah's Witnesses and Refusal of Blood Products." *19 Second Opinion* 34 (January 1994).

Dixon, J. Lowell. "Blood: Whose Choice and Whose Conscience?" *New York State Journal of Medicine* 88, no. 9 (September 1988), pp. 463–64.

Fadiman, Ann. *The Spirit Catches You and You Fall Down: A Hmong Child, Her American Doctors, and the Collision of Two Cultures.* New York: Farrar, Straus and Giroux, 1997.

"Jehovah's Witnesses: The Surgical/Ethical Challenge." *Journal of the American Medical Association* 246, no. 21 (November 27, 1981), pp. 2471–72.

Sheldon, Mark. "Ethical Issues in the Forced Transfusion of Jehovah's Witness Children." *Journal of Emergency Medicine* 14, no. 2 (1996).

Smith, Martin L. "Jehovah's Witness Refusal of Blood Products." *Encyclopedia of Bioethics.* New York: Macmillan, 2004.

Endnotes

Chapter 1

[1] This case is a collage of many cases over decades that occurred in American hospitals. No names in the case are real.

[2] Joseph Collin, "Should Doctors Tell the Truth?" *Harper's Monthly Magazine* 5, no. 155, (1927), pp. 320–26.

[3] Onora Nell (former name of Onora O'Neill), *Acting on Principle* (New York: Columbia University Press, 1975), p. 3.

[4] Immanuel Kant, "On a Supposed Right to Lie from Altruistic Motives," in *Critique of Practical Reason and Other Writings in Moral Philosophy*, ed. Lewis White Beck (Chicago: University of Chicago Press, 1949), p. 348.

[5] Sissela Bok, "Kant's Argument in Support of the Maxim 'Do What Is Right Though the World Should Perish'," in *Applied Ethics and Ethical Theory*, eds. D.M. Rosenthal and F. Shedadi (Salt Lake City, UT: University of Utah Press, 1988), p. 192.

[6] Lindsey Tanner, "More Physicians Giving Apologies to Avoid Lawsuits," *Birmingham News*, November 12, 2004, p. A10.

[7] Sandra M. Gilbert, *Wrongful Death: A Memoir* (New York: W.W. Norton, 1997).

[8] John Lantos, *Do We Still Need Doctors?* (New York: Routledge, 1997).

[9] Committee on Quality of Health Care in America, Institute of Medicine, *To Err Is Human: Building a Safer Health System*, eds. Linda T. Kohn, Janet M. Corrigan, and Molla S. Donaldson (Washington, D.C.: National Academies Press, 1999). See: http://www.nap.edu/catalog/9728.html

[10] Robert Pear, "Panel Seeks Better Disciplining of Doctors," *The New York Times*, January 5, 2005, p. A19.

[11] Sandra Boodman, "Medical Errors Come Home: Mistakes Grow After Release from Hospital," *Washington Post*, 18 February 2003, p. H1.

[12] Danielle Ofri, "They Sent Me Here," *New England Journal of Medicine* 352 (April 28, 2005), pp. 1746–48.

[13] Sir Walter Scott, *Marmion*, Canto 6, Stanza 17 (1808).

Chapter 2

[1] I am grateful to Ben Hippen, MD, a kidney transplant surgeon now practicing in Charlotte, NC, who carefully critiqued this chapter when he was a fellow at UAB in 2005.

[2] "Guidance for authors on the policy of the Journal of Studies on Alcohol regarding the appropriate use of the term 'binge,'" *Journal of Studies on Alcohol,* http://www.rci.rutgers.edu/~cas2/journal/Binge.html

[3] Rene Fox and Judith Swazey, *The Courage to Fail: A Social History of Organ Transplants and Dialysis,* rev. ed. (Chicago: University of Chicago Press, 1978).

[4] http://kidney.niddk.nih.gov/kudiseases/pubs/peritoneal/

[5] http://kidney.niddk.nih.gov/kudiseases/pubs/hemodialysis/

[6] Martha Knisely Huggins, Mika Haritos-Fatouros, and Philip Zimbardo, *Violence Workers: Police Torturers and Murderers Reconstruct Brazilian Atrocities* (Berkeley: University of California Press, 2002).

[7] Thomas Szasz, *The Myth of Mental Illness: Foundations of a Theory of Personal Conduct,* rev. ed. (New York: Perennial Currents, 1984).

[8] Ivan Ilych, *Limits to Medicine: Medical Nemesis, the Expropriation of Health* (New York: Penguin, 1976).

[9] Norton Hadler, *The Last Well Person: How to Stay Well Despite the Health-Care System* (Montreal: McGill-Queen's University Press, 2004).

[10] See Al Jonsen, *The New Medicine and the Old Ethics* (Cambridge, MA: Harvard University Press, 1992).

[11] R. Fox and J. Swazey, *The Courage to Fail,* pp. 278–79.

[12] R. Fox and J. Swazey, *The Courage to Fail,* p. 300.

[13] Shana Alexander, "They Decide Who Lives, Who Dies: Medical Miracle Puts Moral Burden on a Small Committee," *LIFE,* November 1962.

[14] R. Fox and J. Swazey, *The Courage to Fail,* p. 291.

[15] R. Fox and J. Swazey, *The Courage to Fail,* p. 300.

[16] Immanuel Kant, *Foundations of the Metaphysics of Morals* (1785), trans. Lewis White Beck (Indianapolis, IN: Bobbs-Merrill, 1959), p. 39.

[17] Walter Robinson, *Medical Ethics: Lahey Clinic Medical Ethics Newsletter* 11, no. 2 (Spring 2004), p. 8.

[18] *Medical Ethics: Lahey Clinic Medical Ethics Newsletter* 11, no. 2, p. 1.

[19] *Medical Ethics: Lahey Clinic Medical Ethics Newsletter* 11, no. 2, p. 6.

[20] Alcoholics Anonymous World Services, Inc. Accessed 6/29/04. Web site http://www.Alcoholics-anonymous.org/default/en_about_aa_sub.cfm? subpageid=56&pageid=9

[21] R. Fox and J. Swazey, *The Courage to Fail*, p. 267.

[22] R. Fox and J. Swazey, *The Courage to Fail*, p. 268.

[23] E. Quertemont, "Genetic Polymorphism in Ethanol Metabolism: Acetaldehyde Contribution to Alcohol Abuse and Alcoholism," *Molecular Psychiatry* 9, no. 6 (June 2004), pp. 570–81.

[24] D. W. Crabb, M. Matsumoto, D. Chang, M. You, "Overview of the Role of Alcohol Dehydrogenase and Aldehyde Dehydrogenase and Their Variants in the Genesis of Alcohol-related Pathology," *Proceedings of the Nutritional Society* 63, no. 1 (February 2004), pp. 49–63.

[25] Connie Mulligan et al., "Allelic Variation at Alcohol Metabolism Genes (ADH1B, ADH1C, ALDH2) and Alcohol Dependence in an American Indian Population," *Human Genetics* 113 (July 12, 2003), pp. 325–36.

[26] I owe this point to a conversation with my colleague Harold Kincaid.

[27] Personal accounts of overcoming heavy drinking often say the same. See Dennis Wholey, *The Courage to Change: Personal Conversation About Alcoholism* (New York: Houghton Mifflin, 1984).

[28] Herbert Fingarette, *Heavy Drinking* (Berkeley: University of California Press, 1988).

[29] C. Mulligan et al., "Allelic Variation," p. 329.

[30] The Harm Reduction Coalition's Web site is: http://www.harmreduction.org/ prince.html

[31] See Ludwig Fleck, *The Genesis of a Scientific Fact*, eds. Thaddeus J. Trenn and Robert K. Merton, trans. Frederick Bradley (Chicago: University of Chicago Press, 1981). (Originally published in German in 1935.)

[32] Stanton Peele, *The Diseasing of America: Addiction Treatment Out of Control* (Lexington, MA: Lexington Books, 1989).

[33] Stanton Peele, "Herbert Fingarette: Radical Revisionist: Why Are People So Upset with This Retiring Philosopher?" in *Rules, Rituals, and Responsibility: Essays Dedicated to Herbert Fingarette*, ed. Mary I. Bockover (La Salle, IL: Open Court Press, 1991), pp. 37–53.

[34] Dr. DeLuca's professional Web site is: http://www.doctordeluca.com/

[35]Brad Rodu, *For Smokers Only* (Los Angeles, CA: Sumner Press, 1998); see the "For Smokers Only" Web site at: http://main.uab.edu/smokersonly/show.asp?durki=63612

[36]Alvin Moss and Mark Seigler, "Should Alcoholics Compete Equally for Liver Transplantation?" *Journal of the American Medical Association* 265, no. 10 (March 13, 1992), p. 1295.

[37]C. Cohen and M. Benjamin, "Alcoholics and Liver Transplantation," *Journal of the American Medical Association* 265, no. 10 (March 13, 1992), pp. 1295–1301.

[38]Lawrence K. Altman, "Artificial Kidney Use Poses Awesome Questions," *New York Times,* October 23, 1971. Quoted from R. Fox and J. Swazey, *The Courage to Fail,* p. 266.

Chapter 3

[1]The case of Laura Giese, and the recipient of her donated kidney, Willie Boyd, were described in a three-part story by Deborah L. I. Shelton in the *St. Louis Post-Dispatch,* December 1, 2, and 3, 2002. "Man's Second Chance Hasn't Turned Out Like He Expected," "Donor Has Physical Pain, but Peace About Decision," "Good Samaritan Donors Need Independent Advocates, Some Say; Donors Say Their Care Often Falls Through the Cracks." See endnote 13 for follow-up story on December 21, 2003. I am grateful to Laura Giese and Willie Boyd for consenting to have their stories told in this chapter and their pictures used.

[2]James Rachels, *The Elements of Moral Philosophy* (New York; McGraw-Hill, 2003), p. 118, paraphrasing Elizabeth Anscombe in G. E. M. Anscombe, *Ethics, Religion, and Politics: Collected Philosophical Papers,* vol. III (Minneapolis: University of Minnesota Press, 1981). See pages 34, 64–65.

[3]Immanuel Kant, *The Metaphysical Principles of Virtue,* trans. James Ellington (Indianapolis, IN: Bobbs-Merrill, 1964), p. 84.

[4]Immanuel Kant, *Foundations of the Metaphysics of Morals,* trans. Lewis White Beck (Indianapolis, IN: Bobbs-Merrill, 1959), p. 47.

[5]Jeffrey Kahn and Susan Parry, "Organ and Tissue Procurement," *Encyclopedia of Bioethics,* 3rd ed. (New York: Macmillan, 2004), p. 1936; see also "A Science Odyssey: People and Discoveries: First Successful Kidney Transplant Performed," http://www.pbs.org/wgbh/aso/databank.entries/dm54ki.html

[6]I distinguish here between donors and organs. More organs still come from cadavers (brain-dead patients). Cadavers yield 1.7 kidneys on average, but live donors of course can only give one kidney. Each year, about 8,500 kidneys come from cadavers and about 5,500 from live donors. See http://www.unos.org.

[7]A. Bass, "New Liver Transplants; Pressure on Parents," *Boston Globe,* December 17, 1989, 1, 75; quoted in Rene Fox and Judith Swazey, *Spare Parts: Organ Replacement in American Society* (Oxford, UK: Oxford University Press, 1992).

[8]Norman Fost, "Conception for Donation," *Journal of the American Medical Association* 291, no. 17 (May 5, 2004), p. 2126.

[9]Charles B. Huddleston et al., "Lung Transplantation in Children," *Annals of Surgery* 236, no. 3 (September 2002), pp. 270–76.

[10]S. Quattrucci et al., "Lung transplantation for cystic fibrosis: 6-year follow-up," *Journal of Cystic Fibrosis* 4, no. 2 (May 2005), pp. 107–14.

[11]V. Fourbister, "Living Donors Dramatize Risk vs. Need," *American Medical News,* September 20, 1999, p. 1.

[12]The death was confirmed by Dr. Jean Edmond in V. Fourbister, "Living Donors Dramatize Risk vs. Need."

[13]Debra Shelton's update is "Donor Has Physical Pain, but Peace About Decision," and "Man's Second Chance Hasn't Turned Out Like He Expected," *St. Louis Post-Dispatch,* December 21, 2003.

[14]Mary Ellison et al., "Living Kidney Donors in Need of Kidney Transplants," *Transplantation,* November 15, 2002, pp. 1349–51. These 56 patients were out of 140,00 patients. Also, UNOS elevates to the top of the list for receiving a kidney anyone who previously donated one and who now needs one.

[15]Carole Tarrant, "For Family, Selfless Act Goes Awry," *The New York Times,* March 12, 2002.

[16]http://www.findarticles.com/p/articles/mi_m0BFU/is_4_86/ai_66882092

[17]http://news.bbc.co.uk/1/hi/education/1150260.stm

[18]http://www.pkdcure.org/aboutPkdArtic10.htm

[19] http://www.cnn.com/2003/US/Midwest/02/08/teacher.kidney.ap/index.html

[20]Stephanie Strom, "Extreme Philanthropy: Giving of Yourself, Literally, to People You've Never Met," *The New York Times,* July 27, 2003 (Week in Review Section).

[21]http://www.wtkr.com/Global/story.asp?S=1946249&nav=0oa7NzJI (Story describes how in 2004 she won a half-million-dollar lottery in Virginia.)

[22]David Lyons, *The Forms and Limits of Utilitarianism* (Oxford, UK: Oxford University Press, 1965).

[23]Denise Grady, "Taking Risks to Save a Friend, Healthy Give Up Their Organs" *The New York Times,* June 21, 2001, p. A11.

[24]D. Grady, "Taking Risks to Save a Friend," p. A11.

[25]D. Grady, "Taking Risks to Save a Friend."

[26]Debra Shelton, "Lives on the Line: Organ Donors," *St. Louis Post-Dispatch,* May 6, 2005, pp. A1ff.

[27]*Transplantation* 69 (2000), pp. 372–76.

[28]D. Shelton, "Lives on the Line," p. A12.

[29]I. Kant, *Foundations of the Metaphysics of Morals,* p. 47. The first version is on p. 39.

[30]James Rachels, *The Elements of Moral Philosophy,* 4th ed. (New York: McGraw-Hill, 2003), p. 131.

[31]This statistic is from the Web site of the United Network for Organ Sharing in 1984, www.unos.org/resources/

[32]C.R. Eisendrath, "Used Body Parts: Buy, Sell, or Swap?" *Transplantation Proceedings* 24, no. 5, p. 2212.

[33]Actually, the raw numbers from UNOS say almost 5,000 Americans, but because hearts and lungs can be transferred from cadavers, and because, even if the organs were available, not all kidney and liver patients could be matched, I have used the conservative number of 3,000 Americans.

[34]Lloyd Cohen, *Increasing the Supply of Transplant Organs: The Virtues of an Options Market* (Austin, TX: Springer/R. G. Landes Company, 1995), p. 5.

[35]Kant, of course, might not agree. But I also think that rewarded cadaveric donation is something that reasonable people could adopt as a universal maxim, for reasons to be sketched in the rest of this chapter.

[36]Judith Jarvis Thomson, "The Trolley Problem," in *Rights, Restitution and Risks: Essays in Moral Theory* (Chapter 2), ed. Willie Parent (Cambridge, MA: Harvard University Press, 1986).

[37]"Bargain Kidneys," *New Scientist* 2188 (May 29, 1999), p. 5, referring to a study by Eugene Schweitzer at the University of Maryland Medical Center in Baltimore. This assumes a transplanted kidney lasts more than three years, a reasonable assumption.

[38]Stephanie Strom, "An Organ Donor's Generosity Raises the Question of How Much Is Too Much," *The New York Times,* August 17, 2003.

[39]Laurie Siminoff and C.M. Saunders Sturm, "African American Reluctance to Donate: Beliefs and Attitudes about Organ Donation and Implications for Policy," *Kennedy Institute of Ethics Journal* 10, no. 1 (2000), pp. 59–74.

[40]A.R. Sehgal, "The Net Transfer of Transplant Organs Across Race, Sex, Age, and Income," *American Journal of Medicine* 117, no. 9 (2004), pp. 670–5.

[41]Author's personal communication with Laura Giese, June 5, 2005.

[42]Author's personal communication with Willie Boyd, June 10, 2005.

Chapter 4

[1]William Cockerham, *Medical Sociology*, 9th ed. (Upper Saddle River, NJ: Pearson Publishing, 2004), p. 34.

[2] http://unstats.un.org/unsd/demographic/ww2000/table3a.htm

[3] http://ucatlas.ucsc.edu/cause.php

[4]W. Cockerham, *Medical Sociology*, p. 68.

[5]John Stuart Mill, *Utilitarianism*, Book II, quoted in *Mill: Utilitarianism—Text and Critical Essays*, ed. S. Gorovitz (Indianapolis, IN: Bobbs-Merrill, 1971), p. 23.

[6]J.S. Mill, *Utilitarianism*, Book I, p. 25.

[7]Tracy Kidder, *Mountains Beyond Mountains: The Quest of Dr. Paul Farmer—A Man Who Would Cure the World* (New York: Random House, 2003).

[8]Laura Landro, "'Disaster Medicine' Becomes a Specialty," *Wall Street Journal*, August 12, 2004, p. D1.

[9]Garrett Hardin, "Lifeboat Ethics: The Case Against Helping the Poor," in *Lifeboat Ethics: The Moral Dilemmas of World Hunger*, eds. George R. Lucas and Thomas W. Ogletree (Nashville, TN: Vanderbilt University Press and Society for Values in Higher Education, Harper-Collins), 1976.

[10]http://library2.barton.edu/libraryinformation/fysmountains.asp#overview

[11]J.S. Mill, *Utilitarianism*, Book I, p. 15.

[12]Lawrence K. Altman, "U.N. Report Shows Concern Over Rise of H.I.V. in Asia," *The New York Times*, July 7, 2004, p. A5.

[13]Bubonic Plague, or the Black Death, was bad, yes, started in Italy in 1347 and lasted for over 300 years, killing at least 25 million people before it disappeared in 1670, but AIDS has the potential to be much worse. Some experts estimate that between 1981 and 2005, HIV has already killed 30 million people worldwide. See: http://www.avert.org/worldstats.htm

[14]Paul Farmer and Nicole Gastineau Campos, "Rethinking Medical Ethics: A View from Below," *Developing World Bioethics* 4, no. 1 (May 2004), p. 25.

[15]E. Marseille, P. Hofmann, and J. Kahn, "HIV Prevention Before HAART in sub-Saharan Africa," *The Lancet* 359 (May 25, 2002).

[16]Nicoli Nattrass, *The Moral Economy of AIDS in South Africa* (Cambridge, England: Cambridge University Press, 2003), p. 104.

[17]Declaration of Helsinki, item #29. See World Medical Association Web site: http://www.wma.net/e/policy/b3.htm

[18]Baruch Brody, "When Are Placebo-Controlled Trials No Longer Appropriate?" *Controlled Clinical Trials* 18 (1997), pp. 602–612.

[19]Benjamin Freedman, "Equipoise and the Ethics of Clinical Research," *New England Journal of Medicine* 317 (1987), pp. 141–145.

[20]Charles Weijer, "Placebo-Controlled Trials in Schizophrenia: Are They Ethical? Are they Necessary?" *Schizophrenia Research* 35 (1999), pp. 211–218.

[21]Marcia Angell, "The Ethics of Clinical Research in the Third World," *New England Journal of Medicine* 337, no. 12 (September 18, 1997), pp. 847–49.

[22]Marcia Angell, "Tuskegee Revisited," *Wall Street Journal*, October 28, 1997.

[23]Public Citizen, News Release, April 22, 1997.

[24]For a copy of this Code at the National Institutes of Health, see: http://ohsr.od.nih.gov/guidelines/nuremberg.html

For a copy of the Declaration of Helsinki at the Food and Drug Administration, see: http://www.fda.gov/oc/health/helsinki89.html

[25]Ronald Bayer, "AIDS: Public Health Issues," in *Encyclopedia of Bioethics*, 3rd ed., ed. S.G. Post (New York: Thomson-Gale, 2004), p. 126.

[26]D. Bagenda and P. Musoke-Mudido, "We're Trying to Help Our Sickest People, Not Exploit Them," *Washington Post*, September 28, 1997, p. C3.

[27]Ruth Macklin, "Ethics and International Collaborative Research, Part I," *American Society for Bioethics and Humanities Exchange* 1, no. 2 (Spring 1997), p. 1.

[28]M. Angell, "Tuskegee Revisited."

[29]Sheryl Gay Stolberg, "U.S. Ends Overseas H.I.V. Studies Involving Placebos," *The New York Times*, February 19, 1998.

[30]Marilyn Chase and Guatam Naik, "Key AIDS Study in Cambodia Now in Jeopardy," *Wall Street Journal*, August 12, 2004, p. B1.

[31]Alexandra Zavis, "South African Leaders Attack U.S. Over Key AIDS Drug," Associated Press, December 18, 2004 (*Birmingham News*, p. A9).

[32]Michael Saag, MD, quoted from his son's video/CD about UAB's efforts fighting AIDS in Zambia, "The Plague That Thunders" (2004).

[33]Peter Singer, "Famine, Affluence, and Morality," *Philosophy & Public Affairs* 1, no. 3 (Spring 1972), pp. 229–43; and *One World: The Ethics of Globalization*, 2nd ed. (New Haven, CT: Yale University Press, 2004).

[34]I owe this point to Charles Cardwell, a reviewer of this text and philosophy professor in Tennessee.

[35]Michael Kamber, "Haiti's Wounds Overwhelm a Suffering Public Hospital," *The New York Times*, November 29, 2004, p. A4.

[36]Tracy Kidder, "Because We Can, We Do," *PARADE Magazine*, April 3, 2005, pp. 4–6.

[37]Sabin Russell, "AIDS Doctor Heads to Rwanda," *San Francisco Chronicle* and *Birmingham Post-Herald*, May 20, 2005, p. A4.

[38]J. S. Mill, *Utilitarianism*, Book II, p. 23.

Chapter 5

[1]Aleta St. James, quoted in an interview with Diane Sawyer, *Good Morning America*, November 15, 2004. See also http://www.abscnews.go.com/GMA/prnt?id=24937

[2]Jeremy Gray, "Great Grandmother, 57, Gives Births to Twins at UAB," *Birmingham News*, May 21, 2005, pp. A10–12.

[3]For J. Marion Sims, see Seale Harris, *Woman's Surgeon: The Life Story of J. Marion Sims* (New York: Macmillan, 1950); also, J. Marion Sims, *Clinical Notes on Uterine Surgery* (New York: J. H. Vail, 1886). On Dickenson, see Elaine Tyler, *Barren in the Promised Land: Childless Americans and the Pursuit of Happiness* (Cambridge, MA: Harvard University Press, 1995), pp. 65–69.

[4]Harry Fisch, *The Male Biological Clock* (New York: Free Press, 2005).

[5]Daniel Callahan, "Bioethics and Fatherhood," *Utah Law Review* 735, no. 3 (1992).

[6]Jeremy Rifkin and Ted Howard, *Who Shall Play God?* (New York: Dell, 1977), p. 115; Daniel Callahan, *The New York Times*, July 27, 1978, p. A16; Leon Kass, "The New Biology: What Price Relieving Man's Estate?" *Journal of the American Medical Association* 174 (November 19, 1971), pp. 779–88.

[7]"Text of Vatican's Statement on Human Reproduction," *The New York Times,* March 11, 1987, pp. 10ff.

[8]M. Hansen et al., "The Risk of Major Birth Defects After Intracytoplasmic Sperm Injection and in Vitro Fertilization," *New England Journal of Medicine* 346 (March 7, 2002), pp. 725–30.

[9]M. Hansen et al., "The Risk."

[10]Leon Kass, "'Making Babies' Revisited," *Public Interest* 54 (Winter 1979), p. 94. Reprinted in *Classic Works in Medical Ethics,* ed. Gregory Pence (New York: McGraw-Hill, 1990), p. 94.

[11]L. Kass, "'Making Babies'," p. 104.

[12]L. Kass, "'Making Babies'," p. 107.

[13]Leon Kass, "The Wisdom of Repugnance," *New Republic,* June 2, 1997; reprinted in *Flesh of My Flesh: The Ethics of Human Cloning,* ed. Gregory Pence, (Lanham, MD: Littlefield), pp. 20–21.

[14]David Benatar, "Why It Is Better Never to Come into Existence," *American Philosophical Quarterly* 34, no. 3 (July 1997), pp. 345–55.

[15]A. Wilcox et al., "Incidence of Early Loss of Pregnancy," *New England Journal of Medicine* 319, no. 4 (July 28, 1988), pp. 189–94. See also J. Grudzinskas and A. Nysenbaum, "Failure of Human Pregnancy After Implantation," *Annals of New York Academy of Sciences* 442 (1985), pp. 39–44; J. Muller et al., "Fetal Loss After Implantation," *Lancet* 2 (1980), pp. 554–56.

[16]Daniel Callahan, *What Kind of Life? The Limits of Medical Progress* (New York: Simon & Schuster, 1990).

[17]John Stuart Mill, *On Liberty* (Indianapolis, IN: Bobbs-Merrill, 1969), p. 39.

[18]American Society for Reproductive Medicine, Patient Fact Sheets, 2005, http://www.asrm.org/

[19]Jane Simeone quoted by Andrew Walsh, "The McCaughey Babies: Covering Miracles," in *Religion in the News* 1, no. 1 (June 1998). (Published by the Greenberg Center for the Study of Religion in Public Life, Trinity College, Hartford CT.) http://www.trincoll.edu/depts/csrpl/RIN%20Vol.1No.1/McCaughey.htm

[20]"McCaughey Septuplets Turn Four," *Dateline NBC,* November 20, 2001, reproduced at: http://www.msnbc.com/news/660542.asp

[21]"McCaughey Septuplets Turn Four."

[22]*Des Moines Register,* December 22, 2004.

[23]Rob Stein, "A Boy for You, A Girl for Me: Technology Allows Choice," *Washington Post,* December 14, 2004, p. A14.

[24]Juliet Tizzard, "Regulating sperm sorting," BioNews, October 22, 2002, Progress Educational Trust, http://www.progress.org.uk/News

[25]Henry Chu, "China: Too many men, too few women," *Birmingham News*, February 12, 2001, p. 23.

[26]R. Stein, "A Boy for You."

[27]R. Stein, "A Boy for You."

[28]R. Stein, "A Boy for You."

[29]R. Stein, "A Boy for You."

[30]R. Stein, "A Boy for You."

[31]Most of the quotations from Professor Iliescu come from an interview with her on *Good Morning America*, April 14, 2005.

[32]Press release, Romanian Professional Association of Medical Doctors, February 3, 2005.

[33]Centers for Disease Control and Prevention, National Center for Health Statistics.

[34]UK National Statistics, "Age Specific Birth Rates," http://www.statistics. gov.uk/STATBASE/ssdataset.asp?vlnk=7672

[35]Harry Fisch, *The Male Biological Clock* (New York: Free Press, 2005).

[36]Martha Nussbaum, *Upheavals of Thought: The Intelligence of Emotions* (New York: Cambridge University Press, 2001).

[37]Gina Bellafante, "Surrogate Mothers' New Niche: Bearing Babies for Gay Couples," *The New York Times*, May 27, 2005, p. A1.

[38]G. Bellafante, "Surrogate Mothers' New Niche."

[39]"Egg Donation," *60 Minutes*, October 2, 1994.

[40]Roberta B. Ness et al., "Infertility, Fertility Drugs, and Ovarian Cancer: A Pooled Analysis of Case-Control Studies," *American Journal of Epidemiology* 155, no. 3 (March 5, 2002), pp. 217–24; Michelle D. Althuis, "Uterine Cancer After Use of Clomiphene Citrate to Induce Ovulation," *American Journal of Epidemiology* 161, no. 7 (2005), pp. 607–15.

[41]Gina Kolata, "Soaring Price of Donor Eggs Sets Off Debate," *The New York Times*, February 25, 1998, p. A1; Adrienne Knox, "Brokers and Fertility Clinics in Bidding War for Women Willing to Sell Eggs from Ovaries," *Birmingham News*, March 15, 1998, p. A3.

[42]Bill McKibben, *Enough: Staying Human in an Engineered Age* (New York: Times Books, 2003).

[43]Charles L. Stevenson, *Ethics and Language* (New Haven, CT: Yale University Press, 1944).

[44]This discussion of emotivism is indebted to James Rachels's *The Elements of Moral Philosophy,* 4th ed. (New York: McGraw-Hill, 2003).

[45]Leon Kass, "The Wisdom of Repugnance," *New Republic,* June 2, 1997.

[46]Quoted from Robert Lacey, *Ford: The Man and the Machine* (New York: Little Brown, 1987).

[47]See Gregory E. Pence, *Who's Afraid of Human Cloning?* (Lanham, MD: Rowman & Littlefield, 1998) or *Cloning After Dolly: Who's Still Afraid?* (Lanham, MD: Rowman & Littlefield, 2005).

[48]Lori Andrews, CourtTV Online transcripts, 1999, http://www.courttv.com/talk/chat_transcripts/andrews.html. Professor Andrews said similar things to Diane Sawyer on *Good Morning America,* April 14, 2005.

[49]Dean Koontz, *Velocity* (New York: Bantam, 2005).

[50]John Paul II, *Memory and Identity: Conversations at the Dawn of a Millennium* (New York: Rizzoli Press, 2005).

Chapter 6

[1]I am indebted to Kenneth Goodman, MD, director, Bioethics Programs, University of Miami, co-director, Florida Bioethics Network, for critiquing a version of this chapter.

[2]Anna Badkhen, "Schiavo Shied Away from the Spotlight," *San Francisco Chronicle,* March 26, 2005, p. A1.

[3]Mark Fuhrman, *Silent Witness: The Untold Story of Terri Schiavo's Death* (New York: William Morrow, 2005), p. 20.

[4]Arian Campo-Flores, "The Legacy of Terri Schiavo," *Newsweek,* April 4, 2005, pp. 22–28.

[5]Scott Schiavo, quoted in "Between Life and Death: The Terri Schiavo Story," A&E Network, April 16, 2005.

[6]Mark Fuhrman, *Silent Witness,* p. 22.

[7]St. Petersburg Police Department Incident 90-024846, Appendix B, Mark Fuhrman, *Silent Witness,* p. 238.

[8]Mark Fuhrman, *Silent Witness,* p. 28.

[9]A. Campo-Flores, "The Legacy," p. 25.

[10]James Rachels, *The End of Life* (New York: Oxford University Press, 1986).

[11]P. Mollaret and M. Goulon, "Le Coma Depasse," *Revue Neurologie* 101, no. 3 (1959). See Gregory E. Pence, "Heart Replacement," *Classic Cases in Medical Ethics*, 4th ed. (McGraw-Hill, 2004), pp. 301–30.

[12]Ad Hoc Committee of the Harvard Medical School to Examine the Definition of Brain Death, "A Definition of Brain Death, A Definition of Irreversible Coma," *Journal of the American Medical Association* 205, no. 337 (1968).

[13]Timothy Dwyer, "A Futile Fight over Virginia Man," *Washington Post*, March 23, 2005, pp. B1–9.

[14]According to Kenneth Goodman, MD, of the Department of Bioethics at the University of Miami. Personal communication, November 14, 2004.

[15]Mark Fuhrman, *Silent Witness*, p. 135.

[16]A downloadable videotape of Terri with her mother is available at http://www.cnsnews.com/rm/2003/schindler101503/ TerriSchindlerschivo08112001.ram

[17]Jonathan Storm and Alfred Lubrano, "Cable Got a Boost, but TV Saturation Had Its Low Points," *Philadelphia Inquirer*, April 1, 2005, p. 18.

[18]Lee Wilkins, quoted in J. Storm and A. Lubrano, "Cable Got a Boost."

[19]Mark Fuhrman, *Silent Witness*, p. 139.

[20]Timothy Quill, "Terri Schiavo," p. 1631.

[21]C. J. Crystal, quoted in " Brothers among those supporting reclusive Michael Schiavo," ABC (Tampa) News story, March 31, 2005. http://www.tampabaylive .com/stories/2005/03/050331brothers.html

[22]A. Campo-Flores, "The Legacy," p. 26.

[23]Jane Brody, "Preserving a Delicate Balance of Potassium," *The New York Times*, June 22, 2004, p. 12. Low-carbohydrate high-protein diets do not create the right kind and amount of potassium for the body, nor do sports drinks replenish potassium lost in exercising nearly as well as fresh fruits and vegetables.

[24]Jeff Johnson, "Doctor Says Terri Schiavo Likely Victim of 'Some Kind of Trauma'," October 29, 2003, CNSNWS.com.

[25]Multi-Society Task Force on PVS, "Medical Aspects of the Persistent Vegetative State," *New England Journal of Medicine* 330, no. 21 (May 26, 1994), pp. 1499–1508 (part 1) and no. 22 (June 2, 1994), pp. 1572–79 (part 2).

[26]I. Dubroja et al., "Outcome of Post-traumatic Unawareness Persisting for More than a Month," *Journal of Neurological Neurosurgery Psychiatry* 58, no. 4

(1995), pp. 465–66. R. Chen et al., "Prediction of Outcome in Patients with Anoxic Coma: A Clinical and Electrophysiologic Study," *Critical Care Medicine* 24, no. 4 (April, 1996), pp. 672–78; Associated Press, "Policeman Who Briefly Emerged from Coma-like State in '96 Dies," *Birmingham News*, April 16, 1997, p. 7A.

[27]Her CT scan is on the Web site of University of Miami Department of Bioethics at: http://www.miami.edu/ethics2/schiavo/CT%20scan.png

[28]Benedict Carey, "Inside the Injured Brain, Many Kinds of Awareness," *The New York Times*, April 5, 2005.

[29]David Hammer, "Different Cases Cast Light on US Right-to-die Cases," Associated Press, *Birmingham Post-Herald*, November 10, 2003, p. C5; Associated Press, "Arkansas Man Wakes After 19 Years in Coma," July 9, 2003.

[30]AP, "Policeman Who Briefly Emerged," p. 7A.

[31]B. Carey, "Inside the Injured Brain"; Hana Hegeman, "Kansas Woman Regains Ability to Talk After 20 Years," *Washington Post*, February 13, 2005.

[32]A. Campo-Flores, "The Legacy," p. 26.

[33]Malcolm Ritter, "Degree of Schiavo's Awareness a Point of Contention Among Doctors," *Birmingham News*, March 25, 2005.

[34]Manuel Roig-Franzia, "Justices Decline Schiavo Case," *Washington Post*, March 25, 2005, p. A1.

[35]Quoted from William Colby, *The Long Goodbye: The Deaths of Nancy Cruzan* (London: Hay House Publishing, 2002).

[36]Carl Zimmer, "What If There's Something Going On in There?" *The New York Times Magazine*, September 29, 2003.

[37]C. Zimmer, "What If There's Something Going On in There?"

[38]Rita Rubin, "Doctors work to understand vegetative states," *USA Today*, March 21, 2005, p. 3A.

[39]Cathy Lynn Grossman, "Pope declares feeding tubes a 'moral obligation,'" *USA Today*, April 2, 2004, p. 1A.

[40]John Paris, quoted by Lisa Greere, "At Pope's Word, New Schiavo Cases?" *St. Petersburg/Tampa Bay Times*, May 1, 2004. http://www.sptimes.com/2004/05/01/Tampabay/At_pope_s_word__new_S.shtml

[41]Mike Allen, "Conservative Groups' Support Steady," *Washington Post*, March 24, 2005, p. A1.

[42]M. Allen, "Conservative Groups'."

[43]Manuel Roig-Franzia, "Catholic Stance on Tube-Feeding Is Evolving," *Washington Post,* March 27, 2005, p. A7.

[44]Frank Savage, quoted in the *Birmingham Post-Herald,* March 28, 2005, p. D1.

[45]Harriet McBryde Johnson, "Overlooked in the Shadows," *Washington Post,* March 25, 2005.

[46]Jonathan Alter, *Newsweek,* April 14, 2005.

[47]Ron Pollack of Families USA, in Jonathan Weisman and Ceci Connolly, "Schiavo Case Puts Face on Rising Medical Costs," *Washington Post,* March 23, 2005, p. A13.

[48]Mark Fuhrman, *Silent Witness,* p. xiv.

[49]Manuel Roig-Franzia, "Florida High Court Overrules Governor in Schiavo Case," *Washington Post,* September 24, 2004, p. A3.

[50]Manuel Roig-Franzia, "Court Lets Right-to-Die Ruling Stand," *Washington Post,* January 24, 2005, p. A12.

[51]Manuel Roig-Franzia, "Court Lets."

[52]Charles Babington and Mike Allen, "Congress Passes Schiavo Measure," *Washington Post,* March 2, 2005, p. A1.

[53]Democrat Jim Jordan, quoted by Charles Babington, "Viewing Videotape, Frist Disputes Fla. Doctors' Diagnosis of Schiavo," *Washington Post,* March 20, 2005, p. A3.

[54]Tamara Lipper, "Between Life and Death," *Newsweek,* March 28, 2005, p. 30.

[55]Manuel Roig-Franzia, "Schiavo's Parents Take 'Final Shot' to Keep Her Alive," *Washington Post,* March 26, 2005, p. A4.

[56]Nancy Weaver Teichert, "Experts: Lack of Food, Water, Does Not Cause Pain for Dying," *Sacramento Bee,* March 28, 2005; *Birmingham News,* March 29, 2005, p. A6.

[57]Associated Press, "Florida Closes Its Inquiry into Collapse of Schiavo," *The New York Times,* July 8, 2005, p. A20.

[58]Autopsy report, p. 5.

[59]Autopsy report, p. 7.

[60]Autopsy report, p. 8.

Chapter 7

[1]Although this a fictional case, we should expect some like it in the near future, and indeed, something like it may have already occurred. See F. Malone, "First-Trimester or Second-Trimester Screening, or Both, for Down's Syndrome," *New England Journal of Medicine*, 353, no. 19 (November 10, 2005), pp. 2001–2011.

[2]Janet Carr, "The Development of Intelligence," in *Current Approaches to Down Syndrome*, eds. David Lane and Brian Stafford (New York: Praeger, 1985), pp. 167–86.

[3]Tom Regan, *The Case for Animal Rights* (Berkeley: University of California Press, 1985).

[4]*Roe* v. *Wade*, District Attorney of Dallas County, 410 U.S. 113 Texas, Supreme Court of the United States, January 22, 1973.

[5]John Fletcher made this distinction several times in his talks, on the bioethics listserv of the Medical College of Wisconsin, and also in personal communications to the author.

[6]Mary Anne Warren, "On the Moral and Legal Status of the Fetus," *The Monist* 57 (1973), pp. 43–61.

[7]Peter Singer, *Re-Thinking Life and Death: The Collapse of Our Traditional Ethics* (New York: St. Martin's Griffin, 1996).

[8]Carl Zimmer, "Michael Gazzaniga: Scientist at Work," *The New York Times*, May 12, 2005, p. D3.

[9]Jane Brody, "Prenatal Tests Now Cheaper, Less Risky," *The New York Times*, August 1, 2004.

[10]Amy Harmon, "In New Tests for Fetal Defects, Agonizing Choices for Parents," *The New York Times Magazine*, June 20, 2004, p. 2.

[11]"American College of Obstetricians and Gynecologists Opinion #296, First Trimester Screening for Fetal Aneuploidy," *Obstetrics and Gynecology* 104, no. 1 (July 2004), pp. 215–17.

[12]Natalie Marie Nyquist, "The Slippery Slope from Prenatal Science to Eugenics," *Ladies Against Feminism*, July 28, 2004.

[13]Daniel Kevles, *In the Name of Eugenics: Genetics and the Uses of Human Heredity* (Boston: Harvard University Press); reprint edition (September 1, 1995), p. 116.

[14]D. Kevles, *In the Name of Eugenics*, p. 133.

[15]Hermann Muller, *Out of the Night: A Biologist's View of the Future* (New York: Vanguard, 1935). Quoted in Daniel Kevles, *In the Name of Eugenics*, p. 164.

[16]J.B.S. Haldane, "Toward a Perfected Posterity," *The World Today* 45 (December 1924). Quoted in Daniel Kevles, *In the Name of Eugenics*, p. 122. See also Ronald W. Clark, *The Life and Work of J. B. S. Haldane* (New York: Coward-McCann, 1968), p. 70.

[17]Gunnar Broberg and Nils Roll-Hansen, *Eugenics and the Welfare State: Sterilization Policy in Norway, Sweden, Denmark, and Finland* (Lansing: Michigan State University Press, 1997); revised edition (2005).

[18]Gary Sigley, "'Peasants into Chinamen': Population, Reproduction and Eugenics in Contemporary China," *Asian Studies Review*, no. 3 (1998), pp. 309–38; Frank Dikotter, *Imperfect Conceptions: Medical Knowledge, Birth Defects, and Eugenics in China* (New York: Columbia University Press, 1998); Stephen Garton, "Sound Minds and Healthy Bodies: Re-Considering Eugenics in Australia, 1914–1940," *Australian Historical Studies* 26 (1994), pp. 163–81.

[19]Julie Robotham, "Young Women Seeking Prenatal Tests," *Sydney Morning Herald*, August 30, 2004.

[20]A. Harmon, "In New Tests for Fetal Defects."

[21]Mathew Rarey, "Wrongful-Birth Lawsuits Put Doctors in Ethical Dilemma," *Washington Times*, August 5, 1999, p. A20.

[22]"High Court Rules 'Wrongful Birth' Suits Invalid," *Atlanta Journal-Constitution*, July 7, 1999, p. E1.

[23]Suzanne Daley, "France Bans Damages for 'Wrongful Births'," *The New York Times*, January 11, 2002, p. A8.

[24]Amy Harmon, "As Gene Test Menu Grows, Who Gets to Choose?" *The New York Times*, July 21, 2004, pp. A1, A15.

[25]Also, some data indicate that early diagnosis of cystic fibrosis will lead to decreased morbidity (illness) in people affected, but this is not so with fragile X syndrome. Also, the genetic test for cystic fibrosis can be done on newborns.

[26]A. Harmon, "As Gene Test Menu Grows," p. A15.

[27]S.E. McCandless et al., "The burden of genetic disease on inpatient care in a children's hospital," *American Journal of Human Genetics* 74, No. 4 (April 2004).

[28]Stephen Isaacs and Steven Schroeder, "Class—The Ignored Determinant of the Nation's Health," *New England Journal of Medicine* 351, no. 11 (September 9, 2004), pp. 1137–41.

[29]A. Harmon, "As Gene Test Menu Grows," p. A15.

[30]Neela Banerjee, "Church Groups Turn to Sonogram to Turn Women from Abortion," *New York Times,* February 2, 2005, pp. A1–A5.

[31]N. Banerjee, "Church Groups."

[32]Figure is up to December 2003 for the Genetics & IVF Institute of Fairfax, Virginia. See: http://www.givf.com/pgt_sepv.cfm

[33]National Center for Health Statistics. See: http://www.cdc.gov/nchs/pressroom/04facts/pregestimates.htm

[34]Gina Kolata, "Panel to Advise Tests on Babies for 29 Diseases," *The New York Times,* February 21, 2005, pp. A1, A15.

[35]"A Simple Test Could Have Saved Ben's Life," *People* (August 2, 2004), pp. 107–108.

[36]"A Simple Test Could Have Saved Ben's Life," p. 108.

[37]G. Kolata, "Panel to Advise Tests on Babies for 29 Diseases."

[38]G. Kolata, "Panel to Advise Tests on Babies for 29 Diseases."

[39]G. Kolata, "Panel to Advise Tests on Babies for 29 Diseases."

[40]G. Kolata, "Panel to Advise Tests on Babies for 29 Diseases."

[41]T. J. Mathews, "Trends in Spina Bifida and Anencephalus in the United States, 1991–2002." National Center for Health Statistics, http://www.cdc.gov/nchs/products/pubs/pubd/hestats/spine_anen.htm

Chapter 8

[1]I am grateful to Adil Shamoo, PhD, professor, Department of Biochemistry and Molecular Biology, University of Maryland School of Medicine; Nathan Smith, MD, professor of psychiatry at the University of Alabama at Birmingham; James Maddux, PhD, professor of psychology at George Mason University in Virginia; and Harold Kincaid at UAB for comments on earlier versions of this chapter. I also thank the Friends for permission to use the case in this chapter.

[2]The case of Greg Friend, as that of Robert Aller, is taken in part from public testimony before a government commission by the parents of each, testimony still available on the Web site: www.ahrp.org/testimonypresentations/NBAC1997/friend.html and www.ahrp.org/testimonypresentations/NBAC1997/aller.html

The Friend case was also described in a home-town paper of the Friends: Meredith Wadman, "Research Roulette: Are the Maryland Psychiatric Research Center's Schizophrenia Studies Harming the Patients?" (Baltimore) *City Paper,* (June 24, 1998), http://www.citypaper.com/news/story.asp?id=3709

[3]Peter Domenici, *The Hoya* (Georgetown University), February 20, 2004, http://www.thehoya.com/news/021004/news8.cfm

[4]Benedict Carey, "Most Will Be Mentally Ill At Some Point, Study Says," *The New York Times,* June 7, 2005, p. A17.

[5]Details about Mengele and Nazi physicians are from Gerald Posner and Jerome Ware, *Mengele: The Complete Story* (New York: McGraw-Hill, 1986), and Eugene Kogon, *The Theory and Practice of Hell* (New York: Farrar, Straus and Cudahy, 1950; Berkeley reprint, 1980).

[6]David Rothman, "Ethics and Human Experimentation," *New England Journal of Medicine* 317, no. 19 (November 5, 1997), p. 1198.

[7]D. Rothman, "Ethics and Human Experimentation," p. 1198.

[8]Robert Bazell, "Growth Industry," *New Republic,* March 15, 1993, p. 14.

[9]D. Rothman, "Ethics and Human Experimentation," p. 1199.

[10]Gary Matsumoto, *Vaccine A: The Covert Experiment That's Killing Our Soldiers* (New York: Basic Books, 2004), p. xiv.

[11]Henry Beecher, "The Ethics of Clinical Research," *New England Journal of Medicine* 274 (1966), pp. 1354–60.

[12]H. Pappworth, *Human Guinea Pigs* (Boston: Beacon Press, 1968).

[13]Declaration of Helsinki, item #29. See World Medical Association Web site: http://www.wma.net/e/policy/b3.htm

[14]See Gregory E. Pence, "The Tuskegee Study," *Classic Cases in Medical Ethics,* 4th ed. (New York: McGraw-Hill, 2004); James Jones, *Bad Blood* (Boston: Free Press, 1978).

[15]*Mental Disorders in America* (Bethesda, MD: National Institute of Mental Health, 2001).

[16]John W. Santrock, "Causes of Schizophrenia," *Psychology,* 7th ed. (New York: McGraw-Hill, 2004), p. 548.

[17]M.T. Tsuang, W.S. Stone, and S.V. Faraone, "Genes, Environment, and Heredity," *British Journal of Psychiatry* 40 (Supplement, 2001), pp. 18–24.

[18]R.H. Kampmeier, "The Tuskegee Study of Untreated Syphilis" (editorial), *Southern Medical Journal* 65, no. 10 (October 1972), pp. 1247–51.

[19]Franz J. Engelfinger, "Informed (but Uneducated) Consent," *New England Journal of Medicine* 287 (1972), pp. 465–66.

[20]Nell Boyce, "Informed Consent Not Always the Whole Truth," *New Scientist,* June 20, 1998.

[21]Robert Whitaker, "Lure of Riches Fuels Testing," *Boston Globe*, November 17, 1998, p. A.

[22]http://www.ahrp.org/tesitmonypresentations/NBAC1997/aller.html

[23]Sandra Boodman, "John Nash's Genius Is Extraordinary, Recovering from Schizophrenia Is Anything But," *Washington Post*, February 12, 2002.

[24]S. Boodman, "John Nash's Genius."

[25]Adil E. Shamoo and Timothy J. Keay, "Ethical Concerns about Relapse Studies," *Cambridge Quarterly of Healthcare Ethics* 5 (1996), p. 382.

[26]Gordon DuVal, "Ethics in Psychiatric Research: Study Design Issues," *Canadian Journal of Psychiatry* 49, no. 1 (January 2004), pp. 55–59.

[27]Jay Katz, "Human Experimentation and Human Rights," *Saint Louis University Law Journal* 38, no. 7 (Fall 1993).

[28]Rick Weiss, "Research Volunteers Unwittingly at Risk," *Washington Post*, August 1, 1998, p. A1. See also this article from the online journal *Target Health:* "Most IRBs, including commercial IRBs, are very demanding. Westminster IRB, a private IRB used by some clients of *Target Health*, recently required changes to informed consent three times. Unfortunately, problems can occur in clinical trials. It is, therefore, primarily up to the principal investigator, together with his or her staff, and the sponsoring company to assure patient safety and to provide adequate informed consent as to the risks and benefits of participation in a clinical trial.

"Federal investigators told a congressional panel this week that the system for policing testing of new drugs and medical devices needed changes to protect the interests of patients participating in clinical trials. In a series of reports made public at a hearing before a congressional subcommittee, the inspector general of DHHS described how excessive workloads had overwhelmed local review boards that oversee clinical trials and left them unable to insure that patients were not exposed to unsafe practices.

"The hearing before the human resources subcommittee of the House Committee on Government Reform and Oversight reflected dramatic changes in scientific research. Once the domain of federally funded university laboratories largely working alone, medical testing has expanded in amount and complexity in recent years. Today, commercial sponsors, like drug companies, finance a growing share of studies, often at multiple sites.

"A result has been more studies of greater complexity that must be approved by IRBs. These boards, required by federal regulations since 1974, were historically tied to medical schools and universities. But their number has grown and now includes independent and for-profit boards. In the reports, the inspector general recommended improving the education of clinical investigators and members of review boards; increasing the boards' accountability and ability to decide which studies merit closer scrutiny; and changing the federal oversight process so that agencies specifically examine how well the boards are protecting human test subjects.

"The reports also recommend giving the review boards greater responsibility in verifying information provided by clinical investigators. It was stressed, however, that the review and oversight system for clinical testing did not have the resources needed to strengthen protections. For example, one of the two federal groups charged with oversight of research risks in testing has one full-time investigator to review potential problems in clinical trials. Some said that more bureaucratic duties and criticism were making it increasingly difficult to find people to work on the review boards, which are voluntary." From *Target Health*, June 14, 1998; http://www.targethealth.com/

[29]Institute of Medicine, *Responsible Research: A Systems Approach to Protecting Research Participants* (Washington, D.C.: National Academy Press, 2002).

[30]For psychiatrists who abused patients in psychiatric research on schizophrenic patients, see Robert Whitaker, "Lure of Riches Fuels Testing," *Boston Globe*, November 17, 1998, p. A1; for another story about abuse of subjects and fraud in medical research, see Douglas M. Birch and Gary Cohn, "How a Cancer Drug Trial Ended in Betrayal," *Baltimore Sun*, June 24, 2001.

[31]Steve Stecklow and Laura Johannes, "Drug Makers Relied on Clinical Researchers Who Now Await Trial," *Wall Street Journal*, August 15, 1997, p. A1.

[32]R. Whitaker, "Lure of Riches Fuels Testing," p. A1.

[33]"Ketamine: A Fact Sheet," National Clearinghouse for Alcohol and Drug Information, P.O. Box 2345, Rockville, MD 20847-2345; http://www.health .org/nongovpubs/ketamine/

[34]A.C. Lahti, B. Koffel, D. LaPorte, and C.A. Tamminga, "Subanesthetic Doses of Ketamine Stimulate Psychosis in Schizophrenia," *Neuropsychopharmacology* 13 (1995), pp. 9–19; D.J. LaPorte, A.C. Lahti, B. Koffel, and C.A. Tamminga, "The Effects of Ketamine on Memory and other Cognitive Functions in Schizophrenic Patients," *Journal of Psychiatric Research* 30 (1996), pp. 321–330; A.C. Lahti, M.A. Weiler, P.K. Corey, R.A. Lahti, A. Carlsson, and C.A. Tamminga, "Antipsychotic Properties of the Partial Dopamine Agonist (-)-3PPP in Schizophrenia," *Biological Psychiatry* 43 (1998), pp. 2–11; H.H. Holcomb, A.C. Lahti, D.R. Medoff, L.W. Chen, M.A. Weiler, and C.A. Tamminga, "Serial Regional Cerebral Blood Flow Measures Demonstrate Pharmacodynamic Ketamine Effects," Submitted; G. Thaker, M. Moran, A.C. Lahti, and C.A. Tamminga, "Psychiatric Morbidity in Research Volunteers," *Archives of General Psychiatry* 47 (1990), p. 980; G. Thaker, H. Adami, M. Moran, A.C. Lahti, and S. Cassady, "Psychiatric Illnesses in Families of Subjects with Schizophrenia—Spectrum Personality Disorder: High Morbidity Risks for Unspecified Functional Psychosis and Schizophrenia," *American Journal of Psychiatry* 150 (1993), pp. 66–71; D.J. LaPorte, A.C. Lahti, P.K. Corey, and C.A. Tamminga, "Ketamine Fails to Block Memory Stage and Retrieval When Administered Following Stimulus Presentation. Submitted.

[35]M. Wadman, "Research Roulette," p. 12.

[36]Paul Appelbaum, "Drug-Free Research in Schizophrenia: An Overview of the Controversy," *Hastings Center Report* 18, no. 1, pp. 1–5.

[37]Robert Whitaker, "Drug Tested Without Disclosure," *Boston Globe*, December 31, 1998.

[38]R. Whitaker, "Drug Tested Without Disclosure."

[39]R. Whitaker, "Drug Tested Without Disclosure."

[40]P. Appelbaum, "Drug-Free Research in Schizophrenia."

[41]See Gregory E. Pence, "Animal Subjects," Chapter 10, *Classic Cases in Medical Ethics*, 4th ed. (New York: McGraw-Hill, 2004).

[42]Institute of Medicine, *Responsible Research* (Washington, D.C.: National Academy Press, 1998).

[43]*Research Involving Persons with Mental Disorders That May Affect Decision-Making Capacity* (Rockville, MD: National Bioethics Advisory Commission, 1998), http://www.georgetown.edu/research/nrcbl/nbac/capacity/TOC.htm

[44]Alliance for Protection from Research Risks, http://www.ahrp.org/

[45]S. Stecklow and L. Johannes, "Test Case."

[46]Marcia Angell, "Is Academic Medicine for Sale," *New England Journal of Medicine* 342 (May 2000), pp. 1516–18.

[47]Associated Press, "Ten Panelists in Drug Votes Had Ties to Manufacturers," *Birmingham News*, February 26, 2005, p. 4A.

[48]Gardiner Harris, "Popular Drugs for Dementia Tied to Deaths," *The New York Times*, April 12, 2005, p. A15.

[49]Vera Sharav, "Conflicts of Interest," presentation at the Clinical Investigation Symposium, U.S. Army Medical Department and Henry Jackson Foundation for the Advancement of Military Medicine, May 5–7, 2002.

[50]Thomas Laughren, "The FDA's Perspective on the Use of Placebo in Psychotropic Drug Trials," conference on Placebo in Mental Health Research: Science, Ethics and the Law, Houston, April 7 and 8, 2002. Quoted by V. Sharav, "Conflicts of Interest."

[51]*Research Involving Persons with Mental Disorders.*

[52]Jeffrey Avorn, *Powerful Medicines: The Benefits, Risks, and Costs of Prescription Drugs* (New York: Knopf, 2004); Marcia Angell, *The Truth About Drug Companies: How They Deceive Us and What to Do About It* (New York: Random House, 2004).

[53]Robert Zipursky, "Ethical Issues in Schizophrenia Research, *Current Psychiatry Reports* 1, no. 1 (October 1, 1999), pp. 13–19.

[54]M. Mello et al., "Academic Medical Centers' Standards for Clinical-Trial Agreements with Industry," *New England Journal of Medicine* 352 (May 26, 2005), pp. 2202–10.

[55]R. Whitaker, *Mad in America.*

[56]Rick Weiss, "NIH Scientists Broke Rules, Panel Says Deals with Companies Went Unreported, Probe of Potential Conflicts of Interest Finds," *Washington Post,* June 23, 2004.

[57]"Ethical Conflicts Plague NIH," *Discover* (January 2005), p. 34.

[58]Melody Petersen, "Undisclosed Ties Prompt Removal of Doctor," *The New York Times,* August 3, 2003.

[59]Richard Wysocki, "Some Scientists Say New Ethics Rules May Damage NIH," *Wall Street Journal,* March 3, 2005.

[60]J.A. Lieberman, "Effectiveness of Antipsychotic Drugs in Patients with Chronic Schizophrenia," *New England Journal of Medicine* 353 (September 22, 2005), pp. 1209–23.

Chapter 9

[1]This case is an amalgam of so many cases of Alzheimer's that it is a paradigm in the field, although it does not represent any real family or person.

[2]Associated Press, "Governor Lamm Asserts Elderly, If Very Ill, Have 'Duty to Die,'" *The New York Times,* March 29, 1984, p. 16.

[3]Richard D. Lamm, "St. Martin of Tours in a New World of Medical Ethics," *Cambridge Quarterly of Healthcare Ethics* 3 (1994), pp. 159–67.

[4]R.D. Lamm, "St. Martin."

[5]R.D. Lamm, "St. Martin."

[6]R.D. Lamm, "St. Martin."

[7]Plato, *The Trial and Death of Socrates: Four Dialogues* (New York: Dover, 1992).

[8]David Hume, "Of Suicide" (1755), in *Collected Essays of David Hume,* ed. Eugene Miller (Indianapolis, IN: Liberty Classics, 1986).

[9]Jan Narveson, "Is There a Duty to Die," in *Is There a Duty to Die?* eds. James Humber and Robert Almeder (Totawa, NJ: Humana Press, 2000).

[10]Nat Hentoff, "A Duty to Die?" *Washington Post,* May 31, 1997, p. A19; William Irvine, "The Right Not to Live," *The Freeman* 41, no. 5 (May 1991); Sidney Callahan, "A Time to Live, A Time to Die," *Sojourners Magazine* (July–August 1997); Thomas Sowell, "The Duty to Die," *Jewish World Review* (April 26, 2001); Michael Faria, "Slouching Toward a Duty to Die," *Medical Sentinel* (November–December 1999).

[11]John Hardwig, "Is There a Duty to Die?" *Hastings Center Report* 27, no. 2 (1997), pp. 34–42.

[12]See Gregory E. Pence, "Requests to Die," in *Classic Cases in Medical Ethics,* 4th ed., Chapter 3 (New York: McGraw-Hill, 2004).

[13]J. Hardwig, "Is There a Duty?"

[14]J. Hardwig, "Is There a Duty?"

[15]J. Hardwig, "Is There a Duty?"

[16]J. Hardwig, "Is There a Duty?"

[17]J. Grimley Evans et al., "Alzheimer Disease," *Oxford Textbook of Geriatric Medicine* (New York: Oxford University Press, 2000).

[18]Jennifer Dooren, "Alzheimer's Drug Shows Promise in Delaying Onset," *Wall Street Journal,* April 14, 2005, p. D5.

[19]For those who think the medical system can't be redesigned to produce more Paul Farmers, consider the University of Wisconsin at Madison, which each year for the last decade has produced more Peace Corps volunteers than any other college or university, about 130 a year, stemming from past leaders who did the same, including Governor Jim Doyle and former University of Wisconsin president Donna Shalala.

[20]Daniel Callahan, *What Kind of Life? The Limits of Medical Progress* (New York: Simon & Schuster, 1990).

[21]D. Callahan, *What Kind of Life?* p. 21.

[22]D. Callahan, *What Kind of Life?* pp. 22–23.

[23]D. Callahan, *What Kind of Life?* p. 63.

[24]D. Callahan, *What Kind of Life?* p. 286.

[25]Art Linkletter, *Parade* magazine, March 12, 2004, p. 8.

[26]Geriatric medicine professor Andrew Duxbury, MD, of the University of Alabama at Birmingham, from his lecture in the author's medical class, August 5, 2004.

[27]Charles Junkerman and David Schiedermayer, "Effects of Withdrawal of Food and Nutrition," Section II, Withdrawal of Treatment, *Practical Ethics for Students, Interns, and Residents: A Short Reference Manual,* 2nd ed. (Frederick MD: University Publishing Group, 1998), p. 11.

[28]William Cockerham, *Medical Sociology,* 9th ed. (Upper Saddle River, NJ: Pearson Publishing, 2004), p. 34.

[29]http://unstats.un.org/unsd/demographic/ww2000/table3a.htm

[30]Battin quoting John K. Inglehart, in "The American Health Care System," *New England Journal of Medicine* 340, no. 1 (January 7, 1999), pp. 70–76.

[31]Margaret Battin, "Global Life Expectancies and the Duty to Die," in J. Humber and R. Almeder, *Is There a Duty to Die?*

[32]Peter Unger, *Living High and Letting Die* (New York: Oxford University Press, 1996), pp. 4–5.

[33]I owe this point to Charles Cardwell, a reviewer of this text and philosophy professor in Tennessee. I am also indebted to him for other points he made about this chapter that improved it.

[34]Amartya Sen, *Poverty and Famines: An Essay on Entitlement and Deprivation* (New York: Oxford University Press, 1981), p. 160.

[35]Sarah-Kate Templeton, "'Better for Old to Kill Themselves than Be a Burden,' says Warnock," *Sunday-Times—Britain*, December 12, 2004.

[36]Felicia Ackerman, "'For Now I Have My Death': The Duty to Die versus the Duty to Help the Ill Stay Alive," *Midwest Studies in Philosophy* XXIV (2000).

[37]Joel Feinberg, "Duties, Rights, and Claims," *American Philosophical Quarterly* 3, no. 2 (1966), p. 139, quoted in Ackerman, above.

[38]Jan Narveson, "Is There a Duty to Die?" in *Is There a Duty to Die and Other Essays in Medical Ethics,* ed. John Hardwig (New York: Routledge, 2000).

[39]President's Council on Bioethics, *Taking Care: Ethical Caregiving in Our Aging Society,* September 2005.

[40]Stephen G. Post, *The Moral Challenge of Alzheimer Disease: Ethical Issues from Diagnosis to Dying,* 2nd ed. (Baltimore, MD: Johns Hopkins University Press, 2000), p. 115.

[41]S.G. Post, *The Moral Challenge.*

[42]Ronald Dworkin, *Life's Dominion: An Argument About Abortion and Euthanasia* (London: HarperCollins, 1993), p. 226.

[43]R. Dworkin, *Life's Dominion,* p. 226.

[44]R. Dworkin, *Life's Dominion,* p. 230.

[45]R. Dworkin, *Life's Dominion,* pp. 230–31.

[46]R. Dworkin, *Life's Dominion,* p. 232.

[47]R. Dworkin, *Life's Dominion,* p. 235.

[48]R. Dworkin, *Life's Dominion,* p. 235.

[49]SUPPORT Principal Investigators, "A Controlled Trial to Improve Care of Seriously Ill Hospitalized Patients. The Study to Understand Prognoses and Preferences for Outcomes and Risks of Treatment (SUPPORT)," *Journal of the American Medical Association* 274 (1995), pp. 1591–98.

Chapter 10

[1]Thanks to Keith Georgeson, professor of pediatric surgery at Children's Hospital in Birmingham, Alabama, for critiquing this chapter, and for Hawaii professor Ken Kipnis for originally suggesting to me that I write about this kind of case.

[2]"Jehovah" is thought by religious scholars to be an English mistranslation of the Hebrew word "Yahweh," in turn a translation of the unpronounceable "YHWH."

[3]Martin L. Smith, "Jehovah's Witnesses Refusal of Blood Products," *Encyclopedia of Bioethics* (New York: Simon & Schuster, 2004), pp. 1341–46.

[4]For salvation and early Christians, see G. Pence and G. L. Stephens, "Was Jesus a Great Teacher of Ethics?" *Seven Dilemmas in World Religions* (Paragon House Publishers, 1995). Only now on Web at: http://www.paragonhouse.com

[5]M.L. Smith, "Jehovah's Witness Refusal of Blood Products."

[6]*Holy Bible in the King James Version* (Nashville, TN: Regency Publishing House, 1976).

[7]Massachusetts Citizens for Children, *Death by Religious Exemption*, 1992; a selection reprinted in Carol Levine, ed., *Taking Sides: Clashing Views on Controversial Issues: Bioethical Issues*, 11th ed. (New York: McGraw-Hill/Duskin, 2006), p. 193.

[8]*Holy Bible in the King James Version.*

[9]Especially in translating the books of the New Testament from Greek to Latin to Old English to modern English. Also "sixteen hundred" and not "two thousand" years because what documents would be included in the New Testament did not become "canonized" or set until around A.D. 400. In the 1600s, Martin Luther questioned the legitimacy of the Book of Revelations, as did many others over the centuries. The version of the New Testament authorized by the Catholic Church contains books not recognized by many Protestant churches. For an overview of this and related issues, see "New Testament" in *Wikipedia: The Free Encyclopedia* at http://en.wikipedia.org/wiki/New_testament#The_canonization_of_the_New_Testament

[10]Kenneth Kipnis, "Pediatric Ethics and Responsibility for Children: Clearing the Ground," *Newsletter of Philosophy and Medicine* (American Philosophical Association) 2, no. 1 (Fall 2002), pp. 191–93.

[11]Alfred W. Chanda, "Human Rights and Proselytizing in Zambia," *Emory International Law Review* 14 (Summer 2000), p. 977.

[12]Plato, *Laches* in *Collected Works of Plato*, ed. E. Hamilton (Princeton, NJ: Princeton University Press, 1961).

[13]*Prince* v. *Commonwealth of Massachusetts*, 321 U.S. 1958 (1944).

[14]Angela Holder, "Adolescents," *Encyclopedia of Bioethics*, 3rd ed., vol. 1, ed. Warren Reich (New York: Simon & Schuster, 2004), p. 63.

[15]A. Holder, "Adolescents," p. 63.

[16]A. Holder, "Adolescents," p. 64.

[17]A. Holder, "Adolescents," p. 64.

[18]Carol Levine, "Do Parents Harm Their Children When They Refuse Medical Treatment on Religious Grounds?" in *Taking Sides: Clashing Views on Controversial Issues: Bioethical Issues*, 11th ed., ed. Carol Levine (New York: McGraw-Hill/Duskin, 2006), p. 207.

[19]Angela Holder, "Pediatric Adolescents," *Encyclopedia of Bioethics*, 3rd ed., vol. 4, eds. Stephen G. Post and Gale Thomson (2005), pp. 2004–12.

[20]Ann Fadiman, *The Spirit Catches You and You Fall Down: A Hmong Child, Her American Doctors, and the Collision of Two Cultures* (New York: Farrar, Straus and Giroux, 1997).

*P*hoto Credits

1: Ryan McVay/Getty Images; **21:** © Trenton Stull/Images.com/Corbis; **52:** © J.B. Forbes/St. Louis Post-Dispatch; **81:** (*left*) Copyright 2000, © Partners In Health/Moupali Das. All rights reserved.; (*right*) Copyright 2001 © Partners In Health/Mark Rosenberg. All rights reserved.; **109:** (*left*) © AP/Wide World Photos; (*middle*) © Dana Fineman/Corbis Sygma; (*right*) © Pool/Reuters/ Corbis; **137:** (*left*) The Schindler Family/The Terri Schindler-Schiavo Foundation © AP/Wide World Photos; (*right*) © David Kadlubowski/Corbis; **172:** (*left*) © Michael Stravato/The New York Times; (*right*) © Peter Thompson/ The New York Times; **203:** © Margaret Carsello/Images.com/Corbis; **233:** Life After Death by A. Manivel. Courtesy Himalayan Academy; **263:** © AP/Wide World Photos

Index

Abandoning the patients, 29
Abbott Laboratories, 221
Abnormal harm, 115–116
Abortion
  legalization of, 175–177
  moral value and, 176, 181
  parental choice and, 177, 186–188
  personhood and, 177–181
  right to choose and, 188–189,
    199–200
  Roe v. *Wade*, 175–177
  scriptural basis of prohibitions on,
    180–181
Ackerman, Felicia, 255–256
Act vs. rule utilitarianism, 65–68
Acts vs. omission doctrine, 10
Adaptation effect, 258
Addiction, 46–47
Adoption agencies, 196
Adult organ donors
  altruistic donors, 57–58, 63,
    72–73, 75
  autonomous live organ donation,
    72–73
  Kant's critique of, 55–56, 58, 64–65
  live donors and negative outcomes,
    58–61
  non-related adult donors, 62–64
  organ procurement, 57–61
  paid organ sales, 70, 73–76
  race and, 78–79
  utilitarian defense of, 61–65
Advance directives, 257–260
Adverse selection, 192
Advocacy Center for Persons with
    Disabilities, 157
AIDS (Acquired Immuno Deficiency
    Syndrome)
  challenge to ethical theories, 90–91
  cost of drugs, 104–105
  just medical care, 96–99

patient care, Kantian and utilitarian
    ideals, 91–94
  placebos/drugs in Africa, 99–103
  triage medicine, 88–90
  utilitarians v. Kantians on global
    spread of, 81–83
  virtue ethics and, 85–86, 91
Alcohol-related end-stage liver disease
    (ARESLD), 49
Alcohol sensitivity, 38
Alcoholics Anonymous (AA), 21, 35–36,
    41–44, 47
Alcoholism, 21, 34–37
  Crowfeather case, 37–38
  disease model of, 36–37, 44–46
  Fingarette's research, 42–46
  free will view, 35–36, 45
  harm reduction vs. moralism, 46–48
  liver transplants and, 17, 24, 48–50
  Native Americans and, 39, 43
  sociologist and geneticists on, 37–40
Alexander, Shana, 29, 233
Aller, Greg, 214–214, 217
Alliance for Human Research Protection
    (AHRP), 226–227
Altman, Lawrence K., 50
Altruistic donors, 57–58, 63, 72–73, 75,
    78
  virtue ethics and, 76–78
Alzheimer's disease, 245–246, 257, 259
American Civil Liberties Union, 160
American College of Obstetricians and
    Gynecologists (ACOG), 191, 193
American Lung Association, 48
American Medical Association (AMA),
    124, 229
American Society for Reproductive
    Medicine (ASRM), 130
Americans with Disabilities Act, 162
Amniocentesis, 182, 190
Andrews, Lori, 134

Angell, Marcia, 101–103, 226
Annas, George, 122
Anscombe, Elizabeth, 53–54, 65
Apologizing for mistakes, 11
Appelbaum, Paul, 223–224
Aristide, President, 106
Aristotle, 14, 126–128
Artificial insemination, 109–114
Artificial kidney machine, 22
Artificial nutrition and hydration
    (ANH), 160–161
Assemblies of God, 161
Assisted dying, 241
Assisted reproduction, 110–112
    age of parents/good of the child,
        124–126
    egg transfer, 130
    emotivism and "brainwashing"
        couples, 117–118
    multiple embryo implantation,
        119–121
    reproductive cloning, 133–133
    sex selection, 121–124
    starting vs. stopping lives, 116–117
    surrogate mothers/compensating
        donors, 128–132
Autonomy, 3–4, 14, 32–33, 56, 257
    adolescents, 273
    duty to die and, 241
    Dworkin on advance directives,
        257–260
    live organ donation, 72–73
    patient's precedent autonomy, 258
    religious beliefs, 271–272
    reproductive ethics, 118
    research subjects, 213
Awareness, 146
Ayala, Marissa and Anissa, 59, 68

Baden, Michael, 154–155
Barnard, Christiaan, 123, 143
Baseline harm, 115–116
Battin, Margaret, 251–253
Bayh-Dole Act of 1980, 220
Beckwith-Wiedemann syndrome, 112
Beecher, Henry, 208
Belmont Report, 216
Benatar, David, 116

Benjamin, Martin, 49
Bentham, Jeremy, 9, 83, 85
Bernat, James, 159
Binge drinking, 22
Bioethicist, 23
Bioethics
    acts versus omissions doctrine, 10
    genetic abortions as eugenics,
        172–173, 201
    halting AIDS, 90–91
    impartial and ethical reasoning, 30
    media and, 147–150
    public policy and healthy/unhealthy
        behavior, 17
    rule of rescue, 28–29
Bioethics committees, 23
Bioethics Council, 131
Blaming the victim, 36
Bleuler, Eugene and Manfred, 215–216
Blood transfusions, 266, 268
Bloodless surgery, 275–277
Bok, Sissela, 8
Boyd, Willie, 52, 54, 57, 61, 63–64, 67–70,
    77–79
Brain death, 140, 142–147, 233
    cognitive criteria of, 144
    Cruzan case, 146
    Harvard criteria of brain death, 144
    Quinlan case, 146
Broelsch, Christopher, 58, 63, 70
Brokaw, Tom, 257
Brown, Louise, 111, 126
Buchanan, Patrick, 85
Bull, Patricia White, 156
Bush, George W., 131, 157, 163, 165
Bush, Jeb, 157, 160, 165–167

Cadaver donors, 58, 74, 76
Callahan, Daniel, 111, 117, 248–250
Campos, Nicole Gastineau, 96
Can-you-look-him-in-the-eye? test, 14
Canterbury vs. Spence decision, 212
Carson, Rachel, 207
Castro, Fidel, 93
Categorical Imperative, 7, 53, 73
Cates, Judy, 110
Centers for Disease Control (CDC), 85,
    88, 101–103, 198, 209

Challenge studies, 217
Character, 16, 151–152
Charo, Alto, 222
Cheshire, William, 158
Children and adolescents
    emancipated minors, 274
    legal issues, 272–273
    mature minor rule, 273
    medicine and, 273–275
    parental owners vs. stewards,
        270–271
Chorionic villus sampling (CVS), 182
Christian Defense Coalition, 166
Christian News Wire, 161
Christian Scientists, 263
Circle of personhood, 139
Clinical Antipsychotic Trial of
    Intervention Effectiveness
    (CATIE) study, 231
Clinical equipoise, 100
Clinton, Bill, 222, 226, 228
Cognitive criteria of brain death, 144
Cognitive criteria of personhood, 178
Cohen, Carl, 49
Colby, William, 158
Cold-turkey view, 35
Collins, Joseph, 3
Comatose state, 142, 146, 159;
        see also Persistent vegetative
        state (PVS)
Communitarian ethics, 241
Complicity, 16
Conception; see also Assisted
    reproduction
    multiple embryo implantation,
        119–121
    paradoxes about, 114–118
    sex selection, 121–124
Consciousness, 146
    new category of, 158–160
Corn Laws (England), 84
Courage to Fail, The (Fox and Swazey), 37
Coveler, Karen, 191, 193
Cranford, Ronald, 151, 157–158
Critical interests, 258
Crowfeather, Ernie, 21–30, 33–34, 36–38,
        48, 50, 55, 95
Cruzan, Nancy, 146, 148, 151,
        157–158, 162

Cruzan decision, 160, 272
Cults, 267
Cystic fibrosis, 193

Daniels, Norman, 247–248
Darvall, Denise, 143
Darwin, Charles, 185
Death and dying, 233; see also Brain
        death; Duty to die
    biographical vs. physical life death,
        143–146
    cost of, 234
    decisions of families, 150
    Dworkin on advance directives/
        autonomy, 257–260
    end-of-life care, 250–251
    feeding tubes and starvation, 250–251
    Lamm's "duty to die" remarks,
        234–236
    upper brain death, 147
    whole-body death, 143
Deception, 16
Declaration of Helsinki, 99–100, 102,
        208, 224
Delahunty, James, 190
DeLay, Tom, 165
DeLuca, Alexander, 46–47
Dementia, 245–246
Department of Defense, 208
Department of Health and Human
        Services, 220
Dialysis, quality of life and, 33–34, 55,
        66, 73
Dickens, Charles, 84
Dickenson, Robert Latou, 110
Difference principle, 97
Disability culture, 162
Disability issues
    abortion and personhood, 180–184
    Schiavo case, 162–163
Disaster medicine, 89
Disease model, 37–37
    defense of, 44–46
    Kant's critique of, 40–42
Distributive justice, 22, 90, 230
"Do Not Resuscitate" (DNR) order, 145
Dobson, James, 161, 196
Dockery, Gary, 156

Dr. Zhivago (Pasternak), 93
Domenici, Peter, 205
Down, Langdon, 173
Down syndrome, 173–175, 183–184, 187–188, 190
Drug studies, 100–103
Dryer, Alice and John, 172–174, 176–177, 180, 184, 187–188, 200
Duty to die, 234–236
    Alzheimer's and dementia, 245–246
    Callahan's natural limits, 248–250
    as family obligation, 241
    family obligations, 257–257
    global reallocation of resources and, 251–253
    Hardwig's defense of, 240–245
    historical predecessors of, 236–237
    intergenerational justice, 235
    Lamm's remarks, 234–236
    medical professionals and medical futility, 260–261
    Rawls' theory of justice, 246–247
    right to die vs., 235, 237–239
    transfer problem, 253–255
    Warnock vs. Ackerman on, 255–256
Dworkin, Ronald, 257–260

Edmond, Jean, 59
Edwards, Robert, 111
Egg transfer, 109, 130
Emancipated minors, 274
Emotions in ethics, 126–128
    Aristotle on, 127–128
    Hume on, 126
    Kant on, 126–127
Emotivism, 109, 112–114, 130–132, 135
End-of-life cares, 233, 250–251
End-stage liver disease (ESLD), 49
End Stage Renal Disease (ESRD) Act, 30, 33, 54
Endersbe, Susan, 221
Enlightenment ethics, 3, 6, 126
Environmental issues, 92
Ethical relativism, 3–5, 53, 210–211
Ethical subjectivism, 3–5
Eugenics, 130, 175, 181–190
    grassroots eugenics, 184, 190
    parental choice and, 186–188

pre-implantation diagnosis (PID) as, 196–197
Euthanasia, 160
Experiential interests, 258
Experimental studies, 96

Factory Acts (England), 84
Falwell, Jerry, 85
Family illness, 218, 243, 256–257
Family Research Council, 161
"Famine, Affluence, and Morality" (Singer), 105
Farmer, Paul, 16, 31, 81–83, 85–87, 90–91, 93–96, 105–107, 247
    just medical care, 96–99
Federal Drug Administration (FDA), 208, 227–228, 231
Feeding tubes, 141–142, 144, 146–149, 153, 157, 160–161, 165, 169, 250–251
Feelings vs. reasoning, 4
Feinberg, Joel, 256
Felos, George, 147, 166
Fingarette, Herbert, 21, 42, 47
    Heavy Drinking research of, 42–46
Finn, Hugh, 147
Fins, Joseph, 156
Fisher, Don, 215
Fletcher, John, 177
Focus on the Family, 161, 196
Foundations of the Metaphysics of Morals (Kant), 31, 73
Fox, Rene, 37–38
Fragile X syndrome, 191, 193
Free will, 21, 26–32, 56, 189
    disease model and, 41
    drinking and, 35–36, 45
    voluntary organ donation, 62
Freedman, Benjamin, 100
Freedom of Information Act, 227
Friend, Greg and family, 204, 210–211, 215, 222, 225–227, 229
Frist, Bill, 165
Fuhrman, Mark, 169

Galton, Francis, 185
Gates Foundation, 90, 103
Gazzaniga, Michael, 179

Genetic abortions; see also Abortion
    as eugenics, 172–173, 201
Genetic criterion of personhood, 179
Genetic discrimination, 192
Genetic factors, 26
Genetic testing, 172, 181–184, 190–197
    insurance companies and, 192–193
    newborn genetic screening, 197–199
    paternalism and world views of,
        193–195
    pre-implantation diagnosis (PID),
        196–197
    screening at birth, 197
Genneralli, Thomas, 224
Genocide, 210
Giacino, Joseph, 159
Giese, Laura, 52–54, 57, 61, 63–64,
    67–72, 76–79
Gilbert, Sandra, 11
Global Fund Against AIDS, 98
God Committee, 22–31, 33, 37, 233
Golden Rule, 6, 8–9, 12, 275
Gomez-Lobo, Alfonso, 122
Gore, Al, 104
Grady, Denise, 66
Grassroots eugenics, 184, 190
Greer, George, 149, 151, 165–166, 169
GRID (Gay-Related Infectious
    Disease), 85
Gulf War Syndrome, 208
Guthrie, Robert, 198–199

Hadler, Nortin, 27
Haldane, J. B. S., 186
Hammesfahr, William, 157–158
Hard Times (Dickens), 84
Hardin, Garrett, 92
Harding, Courtenay, 216
Hardwig, John, 240–245, 248, 251–252,
    255–257
Harm
    abnormal harm, 115–116
    baseline harm, 115–116
    concept of, 115
    starting vs. stopping lives, 116–117
    total harm, 115–116
    wrongful life/birth, 115
    wronging vs. harming, 116–117

Harm Reduction Coalition (HRC), 46
Harm reduction vs. moralism, 46–48
Harvard criteria of brain death, 144
Healer/comforter role of physician, 219
Health Research Group, 101
Heavy Drinking (Fingarette), 42
Heller, Jean, 209
Hemlock Society, 239
Hemodialysis, 24–25
Hepnah, Sara, 263–264, 269, 271,
    274–276
Herrick, Richard and Ronald, 58, 68
Hiroshima and Nagasaki nuclear
    bombing, 54
Hirsch, Joy, 159
Hobbes, Thomas, 97
Holder, Angela, 273
Holocaust, 210–211
Hospital Ethics Committee, 23
Hostage-takers, 53
Hudson, Kathy, 123
Human behavior, 26–27
Human cloning, 113, 131–133
Human dignity, 33, 259
Human Fertilisation Board (England), 117
Hume, David, 126–128, 130, 136, 237
Humo immunodeficiency virus (HIV), 88
Hurewitz, Mike, 60
Hypothetical imperative, 7

Iliescu, Adriana, 109, 123–124
Ilych, Ivan, 27
Immigration Restriction Act of
    1924, 185
Impartial reasoning/reasons, 5, 28
Impartiality, 5
Implantation of embryos, 109
In the Interests of E. G., 274
In the Name of Eugenics (Kevles), 185
In vitro fertilization, 109, 111–113,
    117, 119
    pre-implantation diagnosis (PID)
        and, 196
    sex selection, 121–124
Informed consent, 61, 212–213
Ingelfinger, Franz J., 213
Institute of Medicine (IOM), 13, 221,
    226, 229

Institutional culture, 220
Institutional Review Boards (IRBs), 23,
    210, 220, 223
Insurance companies
    adverse selection, 192
    genetic testing and, 192–193
    long-term treatment, 205
Intergenerational justice, 235, 241
International Ethical Guidelines for
    Biomedical Research involving
    Human Subjects, 102
Iraqi prisoners abuse, 27

James, David, 111
Jehovah's Witnesses
    bloodless surgery, 275–277
    legal issues, 272–273, 277–278
    medical professionals and, 269
    medicine and, 263–267
    treatment refusals, 271–272
John Paul II, Pope, 136, 160–161
Johnson, Harriet McBryde, 162
Just medical care, 96–99
Justice, Rawls' theory of, 96, 246–248,
    252–253

Kampmeier, R. H., 213
Kant, Immanuel and Kantian ethics,
    21, 53, 224
    adult organ donation, 52–57, 64–65,
        67, 70
    on alcoholism as disease, 21–22, 45
    on autonomy, 3, 32–33
    Categorical Imperatives, 7, 53, 73
    central maxim of ethics, 55
    critique of disease model, 40–42
    duality of human nature, 31–32
    on emotions, 126–128
    on human dignity, 31–34
    on hypothetical and categorical
        imperatives, 7
    ideal of patient care, 224–225
    lottery method, 29
    on lying, 6–9
    Mill's critique of, 94–96
    on morality, 6, 31, 73
    patient care, 91–94, 99
    placebo drugs, 102–103

on preserving integrity of body,
    55–56, 58
Kass, Leon, 111–113, 118, 122, 131, 136,
    179, 257
Katz, Jay, 217–218
Kennedy, James, 166
Kevles, Daniel, 185
Kidder, Tracy, 106–107
Kim, Jim Yong, 86
Kindling theory of psychosis, 223
Kipnis, Kenneth, 270, 273
Kleinberg, Alvin, 270, 276
Knorr, Nathan, 265
Koontz, Dean, 136
Kravinsky, Zell, 72–73, 76
Kübler-Ross, Elisabeth, 243

Lahti, Adrienne, 222
Lamm, Richard, 92, 234–236, 240, 251
Lantos, John, 12
Last Well Person, The (Hadler), 27
Latter Day Saints, 263, 265
Laughren, Thomas, 228
Liberty principle, 97
Life Legal Defense Fund, 157
Life worth continuing, 116
Life worth starting, 116
Life's Dominion (Dworkin), 257
LifeSharers, 78
Linkletter, Art, 249
Live organ donation
    cadaver donors vs., 58, 74, 76
    utilitarian defense of, 61–65
    virtue ethics and, 76–78
Liver transplants, 58, 63, 70–71
    alcoholics and, 24, 48–50
Living High and Letting Die (Unger), 252
Living will, 146
Lurie, Peter, 101
Lying to patients
    ethical relativism and, 1–5
    ethical subjectivism and, 3–5
    impartiality and moral reasoning, 5
    Kant on lying, 6–9
    mistakes an, 11–14, 17–19
    omitting the truth vs., 10–11
    utilitarian ethics, 9–10
    virtue ethics, 14–17

McCabe, Mark, 167
McCaughney, Bobbi and Kenny, 109,
    118–121
McCullough, Gary, 161
Mad in America (Whitaker), 230
Mahoney, Patrick, 166
Malpractice, genetic testing and,
    190–197
March of Dimes Foundation, 197–198
Marseille, E., 98
Martinez, Mel, 163, 170
Maryland Psychiatric Research
    Center (MPRC), 204, 211,
    221–222, 225
Massachusetts Citizens for Children, 267
Mature minor rule, 273
Maximization principle, 87–90
Mayfield, William, 157 158
Mbeki, Thabo, 103
Medicaid, 54, 163, 239–240, 246
Medical care; see also Patient care
    handling minority views, 277–278
    insurance coverage for, 239–240
    medical professionals and medical
        futility, 260–261
    as social good, 236
    transfer problem, 253–255
Medical errors; see Mistakes
Medical ethics, 21
    autonomy and, 3–4
    ethical subjectivism and, 4–5
    harm reduction vs. moralism, 46–48
    importance of, 2
    just medical care, 96–99
    placebos and AIDS drugs, 99–103
    sanctity-of-life ethics, 89
    transplant surgeons and, 66–68
Medical experimenters, 220
Medical futility, 260–261
Medical paternalism, 3–4, 164,
    193–195, 213
Medical professionals, Jehovah's Wit-
    nesses and, 269
Medical rationing, 162
Medical research; see also Schizophrenia
    research
    American research during WWII,
        206–209
    ethical issues in, 203–204
    harm to subjects, 224–225
    informed consent, 212–213
    Nazi research, 206
    pharmaceutical companies and,
        220–221
    physician's role and, 220
    researchers defense, 222–224
    rights of patient-subjects, 208,
        226, 230
    schizophrenia and, 204–205
    social justice and, 225–226
    vulnerable subjects, 225–226
Medical saints, 85–87
Medical tools, 195–196
Medicare, 54, 163, 239–240, 246, 250
Mengele, Josef, 206
Mental illness, care for patients,
    204–205
Merit feminists, 129
MicroSort, 121–122
Mid-America Transplant Service, 56–57,
    63–64, 71
Mill, James, 9
Mill, John Stuart, 3, 9, 83, 85, 105,
    107, 118
    critique of Kantian ethics, 94–96
Minimally conscious state (MCS),
    158–159, 163, 168
Mistakes
    apologizing for, 11–14
    conceptual issues of, 17 19
    system error, 12
    taking responsibility for, 11–14
Montagnier, Luc, 88
Moral actions, feelings vs. reasoning, 4
Moral agents, 32–33
Moral Challenge of Alzheimer Disease
    (Post), 257
Moral content, 23
Moral process, 23
Moral reasoning, 5
Moral relativism, 6
Moral value, 176
Moralism, 46–48
Morality, 7, 84
    Kant on, 6, 31, 73
Mortality tables, 125
Moss, Alvin, 49
Muller, Herman J., 186

Multi-drug resistant (MDR) tuberculosis (TB), 90
Multiple embryo implantation, 119–121
Murray, Joseph, 57

Nader, Ralph, 101–102
Narveson, Jan, 238, 256
Nash, John, 215, 229
National Academy of Sciences, 13
National Alliance for the Mentally Ill, 223
National Bioethics Advisory Commission, 215, 222, 226, 228–229
National Institute of Health (NIH), 101–103, 227, 230
National Institutes of Mental Health (NIHM), 205, 211, 223, 230
Native Americans, 37, 39, 43, 50
Nattrass, Nicoli, 99
Nazi experiments, 103, 185–186, 190, 206
Nazi research, 210
Neurological criterion of personhood, 179
Newborn genetic screening, 197–199
Newcomb, Virginia, 234, 240, 245–246, 250, 257–258, 261
Newton, Isaac, 6
Nichols, Mittzi, 63
North, Oliver, 53
Nuremberg Code, 99, 102, 203, 206, 208, 216
Nussbaum, Martha, 127–128, 136

Objective standard, 212
Ofri, Danielle, 15
On Liberty (Mill), 3, 118
"On the Supposed Right to Lie from Altruistic Motives" (Kant), 8
O'Neill, Onora, 6
Operation Desert Storm, 208
Organ procurement, 57–61
    autonomous live donations, 72–73
    crossing ethical line in, 57–61
    live vs. cadaver donors, 58, 74, 76
    non-related adult donors, 62–64
    paid organ sales, 70, 73–76
    transplantation and race, 78–79
Organization of Parents through Surrogacy, 128

Origin of the Species, The (Darwin), 185
O'Rourke, Kevin, 161

Paid organ sales, 70, 73–76
Pappworth, Henry, 208
Parental authority, 270
Parental custody, 270
Parental dominion, 270
Pariente, Barbara, 165
Paris, John, 161
Partial-birth abortions, 176
Partners in Health (PIH), 86, 90, 94, 106
Pasternak, Boris, 93
Patient care
    just medical care, 96–99
    Kantian and utilitarian ideals, 91–94
Patients' rights movement, 164, 208, 213, 226, 230
Pediatric-adolescent law, 273
Peritoneal dialysis, 25
Persistent vegetative state (PVS), 140, 146, 148, 150, 155–157, 160, 163
Personal responsibility, 11–14, 16, 21, 41, 53
Personhood
    abortion and, 177–181
    cessation of, 139–140
    cognitive criterion of, 178
    criteria of, 150–154
    genetic criterion, 179
    neurological criterion of, 179
Pharmaceutical companies, 220–221, 226–227, 230
Phenylketonuria (PKU), 198–199
Physician-assisted dying, 151, 233, 255
Physician-patient relationships, 3, 8, 20
    AIDS and, 95
    communication in, 15
    genetic testing and, 193–195
    rule of rescue, 29, 95
Physician of record, 12
Placebos, 100–103, 222, 228
Plastic surgery, 56
Plato, 14, 237
Polygenic condition, 38, 45
Pontius Pilate, 10
Post, Stephen, 257

Pre-implantation diagnosis (PID), 196–197
Preimplantation genetic diagnosis
    (PGD), 59
President's Council on Bioethics,
    179, 257
Prince vs. Massachusetts, 272
Professional standard, 212
Professionalism, 269
Psychiatric research; see also
    Schizophrenia research
    NBAC's report on, 228–229
    structural critiques of, 226–228
Public Citizen, 101, 226
Public policy, healthy/unhealthy
    behavior, 17
Punishment, retributivist vs.
    utilitarians, 44

Quality of life
    dialysis and, 33–34
    Down syndrome, 174
Quill, Timothy, 151
Quinlan, Karen, 146, 148, 151, 162

Race, organ transplantation and, 78–79
Rachels, James, 53, 73, 143
Racism, 19
Randomized clinical trial (RCT),
    100–103
Rascher, Sigmund, 206
Rationality, 7, 32
Rawls, John
    on just medical care, 96–99
    theory of justice, 96, 246–248,
        252–253
Reagan, Ronald, 53, 144, 179
Reasonable standard of care, 163
Regan, Tom, 174
Religious beliefs
    handling minority views, 277–278
    legal issues, 272–273
    medicine and, 263–267
    professionalism and tolerance, 269
    treatment refusals, 271–272
Religious minorities, 267–270, 277
Reproductive cloning, 109, 132–133
Research subjects, 99

Respect for autonomy (research
    subjects), 213
Respirators, 146, 161
Responsibility, 11–14, 16, 41, 53
Rethinking Medical Ethics: A View from
    Below (Farmer and Campos), 96
Retributivists, 44
Rhoads, Cornelius, 207
Rhodes, Jackie, 139
Right not to be born, 191
Right-to-die, 147, 235, 237–239
Rifkin, Jeremy, 111
Risk Management, 11
Rodriquez, Nilda, 59
Roe v. Wade, 175–177, 181, 183
Rothman, David, 207
Rousseau, Jean Jacques, 97
Rule of fourths, 211
Rule of rescue, 28–29, 95
Rule utilitarianism, 65–66
Russell, Charles Taze, 264–265
Rutherford, Joseph, 265
Rwanda, 107

St. James, Aleta, 109–110
Sanctity-of-life ethics, 89
Sandel, Michael, 122
Satre, Jean-Peter, 15
Schiavo, Michael, 138–142, 145, 147, 149,
    152–153, 155, 160–161, 166–168
Schiavo, Terri
    autopsy results, 167–169
    background history, 137–141
    cause of problems, 154–155
    cessation of personhood, 139–140
    collapse and comatose state, 140–142
    disability issues, 162–163
    disagreements about treatment,
        157–158
    family, personhood, character issues,
        150–157, 179
    media and bioethics, 147–150
    politicization of case, 164–167
    religious issues, 160–162
Schiff, Nicholas, 159
Schindler, Robert and Michael, 138,
    141–142, 145, 147, 149–150,
    152–153, 156, 161, 165, 167, 169

Schizophrenia, 203, 211–212
    confusions and myths about,
        215–216
Schizophrenia research, 204–205
    family dilemmas, 218–219
    harm to subjects, 224–225
    informed consent and, 212–215
    kindling theory of psychosis, 223
    problems of consent in, 216–218
Scott, Sir Walter, 16
Scribner, Belding, 22–23, 25,
        28–30, 37
Second Change program, 56
Seigler, Mark, 49
Self-interest, 5, 7, 32, 97
Self-organ donation, 56
Semmelweis, Ignaz, 157
Sen, Amaryta, 253–254
Seventh-day Adventists, 263
Sewell, James and Barbara, 59
Sex selection, 121–124
Shamoo, Adil, 217
Sharav, Vera, 227
Shelton, Deborah L., 57, 67, 78
Shewmon, Alan, 159
"Should Doctors Tell the Truth?"
        (Collins), 3
Silent Spring (Carson), 207
Simeone, Jane, 120
Sims, J. Marion, 110
Singer, Peter, 105, 179
Smith, Alyssa, 58
Smith, Teri, 58, 63
Smithers Addiction Treatment and
        Research Center, 46
Snow, John, 88
Sobell, Mark and Linda, 47
Social feminists, 129
Social justice, 225–226
Social worth, 23, 29
Socrates, 14, 236–237, 243–244, 272
Sonograms, 183, 190, 195
Sorkow, Harven, 129
Soros Foundation, 90
Southern Baptist Convention, 196
Stalin, Joseph, 93
Standard of care, 18, 191
Starnes, Vaughn, 59
Starting vs. stopping lives, 116–117

Starvation, 250–251, 254
Steptoe, Patrick, 111
Stern, Bill and Elizabeth, 128–129
Stevenson, Charles, 130, 136
Stoics, 237
Structural discrimination, 163
Study in nature, 209
Suicide, 72, 241, 255
Sunderland, Trey, 223–224, 230
SUPPORT study (Study to Understand
        Prognoses and Preferences
        for Outcomes and Risks of
        Treatments), 260
Surrogacy, 109, 128–130
Swain, Rosee, 110, 118
Swazey, Judith, 37–38
System error, 12
Szasz, Thomas, 27

Taking Care: Ethical Caregiving in our
        Aging Society, 257
Tamminga, Carol, 222
Tarrant, Barbara, 60
Taub, Edward, 224
Terri's Law, 160, 164–165
Terry, Randal, 161, 166
Theistic ethics, 84
Theory of Justice, A (Rawls), 97
Thogmartin, Jon, 167
Thompson, Judith, 75
Throckmorton, Heath, 264, 268–269,
        271, 276–277
Torts (harm), 115
Total harm, 115–116
Tramont, Edmund, 103
Transfer problem, 253–255, 262
Triage medicine, 88–90
Trisomy, 173
Trolley example, 75
True moral agents, 32–33
Truman, Harry S., 54
Truthfulness, 14
Tuskegee Syphilis Study, 19, 101, 103,
        203, 208–210, 224

Unger, Peter, 252, 254
United Network for Organ Sharing
        (UNOS), 60–61, 78

United States Public Health Service
(USPHS), 209, 212
Universalizability, 6
Urban Institute, 13
Utilitarian ethics, 9–10
  history of, 83–85
  just medical care, 97–99
  patient care, 91–94
Utilitarianism, 9, 29, 44, 54, 61
  act vs. rule utilitarianism, 65–68
  assisted reproduction, 116
  defense of live organ donation,
    61–65, 68–70
  maximization principle, 87–90
  paid organ sales, 73–76
  as reform movement, 84–85
  triage medicine, 88–90
Utilitarianism (Mill), 85, 94
Utility, 9, 83, 88

Vegetative, 159
Veil of ignorance, 97, 247–248, 252–253
Veterans Administration (VA), 207
Viability, 175–176
Vichow, Rudolf, 82
Virtue ethics, 11, 14–17, 81
  AIDS and, 85–86, 91
  assisted reproduction, 116, 120
  compassion and, 164
  live organ donors and, 76–78
  moral character, 151–152
  schizophrenia research, 219–222
  wrong cause and, 272
Voluntary organ donation, 62

Wakefulness (arousal), 146
Walker, W. Campbell, 155
Wallis, Terry, 156
Wanglie, Helen, 151
Warnock, Mary and Geoffrey,
    255–256
Warren, Mary Anne, 178
Washkansky, Louis, 123, 143
Washout periods, 210–211, 214–215, 217,
    221–227, 229–230
Weijer, Charles, 100
Weldon, Dave, 165
Weller, Barbara, 166
*What Kind of Life? The Limits of Medical
  Progress* (Callahan), 248
Whistle-blowers, 16
Whitaker, Robert, 226, 229–230
Whitehead, Mary Beth, 128–129
Whittemore, James, 160
Whole-body death, 143
"Wisdom of Repugnance, The" (Kass),
    113
Wolfe, Sidney, 101
Wood, Walter, 60–61, 71
World Aids Conference, 88, 95
World Health Organization (WHO), 86,
    90, 101
Wrongful birth, 115
Wrongful birth suits, 190–191
Wrongful Death (Gilbert), 11
Wrongful life, 115
Wronging vs. harming, 116–117

Zimbardo, Philip, 27